Information Processing Speed in Clinical Populations

STUDIES ON NEUROPSYCHOLOGY, NEUROLOGY AND COGNITION

Series Editor:
Linas A. Bieliauskas, Ph.D.
VA Ann Arbor and University of Michigan, Ann Arbor, MI, USA

The series *Studies on Neuropsychology, Neurology and Cognition* provides state-of-the-art overviews of key areas of interest to a range of clinicians, professionals, researchers, instructors, and students working in clinical neuropsychology, neurology, rehabilitation, and related fields.

Topics cover a broad spectrum of core issues related to theory and practice concerning brain and behavior, and include:

- Practical and professional issues (e.g., diagnosis, treatment, rehabilitation).
- Cognitive development over the lifespan (e.g., child, geriatric).
- Domain-specific cognitive issues (e.g., sport, toxicology).
- Methodology related to brain and behavior (e.g., functional brain imaging, statistics, and research methods).
- Essential related issues (e.g., ethics, minorities and culture, forensics).

The authors, editors, and contributors to each title are internationally recognized professionals and scholars in their field. Each volume provides an essential resource for clinicians, researchers, and students wanting to update and advance their knowledge in their specific field of interest.

For continually updated information about the *Studies on Neuropsychology, Neurology and Cognition* series, please visit: **www.psypress.com/nnc/**

Other titles in this series:

Fundamentals of Functional Brain Imaging: A Guide to the Methods and their Applications to Psychology and Behavioral Neuroscience. A. C. Papanicolaou

Forensic Neuropsychology: Fundamentals and Practice. Edited by J. J. Sweet

Neuropsychological Differential Diagnosis. K. K. Zakzanis, L. Leach, & E. Kaplan

Minority and Cross-Cultural Aspects of Neuropsychological Assessment. Edited by F. R. Ferraro

Ethical Issues in Clinical Neuropsychology. Edited by S. S. Bush & M. L. Drexler

Practice of Child-Clinical Neuropsychology: An Introduction. B. P. Rourke, H. van der Vlugt, & S. B. Rourke

The Practice of Clinical Neuropsychology. A Survey of Practice and Settings. Edited by G. J. Lamberty, J. C. Courtney, & R. L. Heilbronner

Neuropsychological Rehabilitation: Theory and Practice. Edited by B. E. Wilson

Traumatic Brain Injury in Sports: An International Neuropsychological Perspective. Edited by M. R. Lovell, R. J. Echemendia, J. T. Barth, & M. W. Collins

Methodological and Biostatistical Foundations of Clinical Neuropsychology and Medical and Health Disciplines. Edited by D. V. Cicchetti & B. P. Rourke

A Casebook of Ethical Challenges in Neuropsychology. Edited by S. S. Bush

Neurobehavioral Toxicology: Neurological and Neuropsychological Perspectives. Volume I Foundations and Methods. S. Berent & J. W. Albers

Neurobehavioral Toxicology: Neurological and Neuropsychological Perspectives. Volume II Peripheral Nervous System. J. W. Albers & S. Berent

Geriatric Neuropsychology: Practice Essentials. Edited by S. S. Bush & T. A. Martin

Brain Injury Treatment: Theories and Practices. J. Leon-Carrion, K. R. H. Von Wild, & G. Zitnay

The Quantified Process Approach to Neuropsychological Assessment. Edited by A. M. Poreh

Mild Cognitive Impairment: International Perspectives. Edited by H. A. Tuokko & D. F. Hultsch

Cognitive Reserve: Theory and Applications. Edited by Y. Stern

Neuropsychology and Substance Use: State-of-the-Art and Future Directions. Edited by A. Kalechstein & W. G. van Gorp

Forthcoming titles:

Textbook of Clinical Neuropsychology. Edited by J. E. Morgan & J. H. Ricker

Executive Functions and the Frontal Lobes: A Lifespan Perspective. Edited by V. Anderson, R. Jacobs, & P. Anderson

Neurobehavioral Toxicology: Neurological and Neuropsychological Perspectives. Volume III Central Nervous System. J. W. Albers & S. Berent

Behavioural and Emotional Complications of Traumatic Brain Injury. S. F. Crowe

Geriatric Neuropsychology Casebook. J. J. Dunkin

The Neuropsychology of Epilepsy. J. I. Tracy

Fundamentals of Functional Brain Imaging, Second Edition. A. C. Papanicolaou

Information Processing Speed in Clinical Populations

Edited by
John DeLuca and Jessica H. Kalmar

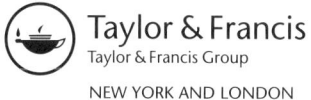
Taylor & Francis
Taylor & Francis Group
NEW YORK AND LONDON

Published 2008
by Taylor & Francis, an informa business
270 Madison Avenue
New York, NY 10016
www.taylorandfrancis.com

Published in Great Britain
by Taylor & Francis Group, an informa business
27 Church Road
Hove, East Sussex BN3 2FA

Copyright © 2008 Taylor & Francis

Typeset in Times by RefineCatch Limited, Bungay, Suffolk, UK
Printed and bound in the USA by Edwards Brothers, Inc. on acid-free paper
Cover design by Hybert Design

All rights reserved. No part of this book may be reprinted or reproduced or utilized in any form or by any electronic, mechanical, or other means, now known or hereafter invented, including photocopying and recording, or in any information storage or retrieval system, without permission in writing from the publishers.

10 9 8 7 6 5 4 3 2 1

Library of Congress Cataloging in Publication Data
Information processing speed in clinical applications / edited by John DeLuca & Jessica Kalmar.
    p. ; cm. – (Studies on neuropsychology, neurology, and cognition)
  Includes bibliographical references and index.
  ISBN 978-1-84169-476-4 (hardback : alk. paper)
  1. Human information processing. 2. Brain—Physiology. 3. Intellect—Physiological aspects. 4. Cognition—Physiological aspects. 5. Aging—Physiological aspects. I. DeLuca, John, 1956– II. Kalmar, Jessica. III. Series.
  [DNLM: 1. Mental Processes—physiology. 2. Neuropsychology—methods. 3. Aging—physiology. 4. Brain—physiology. 5. Cognition—physiology. WL 103.5 I43 2007]
QP396.I54 2007
612.8′2—dc22

2007000375

ISBN: 978-1-84169-476-4 (hbk)

To my children, Jessica, Danielle, and Robbie, who inspire me to achieve and be the best I can be.

JDL

To Wes, Rebecca, and Eliana, whose love, laughter, and support made my contribution to this book possible.

JHK

Contents

About the editors   xi
List of contributors   xiii
From the series editor   xv

1 **The history of processing speed and its relationship to intelligence**   1
AMANDA R. O'BRIEN AND DAVID S. TULSKY

2 **Assessment tools and research methods for human information processing speed**   29
THOMAS A. MARTIN AND SHANE S. BUSH

3 **Information processing speed: Measurement issues and its relationships with other neuropsychological constructs**   53
HEATH A. DEMAREE, THOMAS W. FRAZIER, AND COURTNEY E. JOHNSON

4 **The genetics of information processing speed in humans**   79
DANIELLE POSTHUMA AND ECO DE GEUS

5 **Speed of processing in childhood and adolescence: Nature, consequences, and implications for understanding atypical development**   101
ROBERT V. KAIL

6 **Processing speed and the Digit Symbol Substitution Test in schizophrenia**   125
DWIGHT DICKINSON AND JAMES M. GOLD

7	**Information processing speed in multiple sclerosis: A primary deficit?**	153
	JESSICA H. KALMAR AND NANCY D. CHIARAVALLOTI	
8	**Traumatic brain injury and processing speed**	173
	GLYNDA J. KINSELLA	
9	**Frontal-subcortical determinants of processing speed in Parkinson's disease**	195
	RODERICK K. MAHURIN	
10	**Information processing speed and aging**	221
	TIMOTHY A. SALTHOUSE AND DAVID J. MADDEN	
11	**Everyday life applications and rehabilitation of processing speed deficits: Aging as a model for clinical populations**	243
	KARLENE K. BALL AND DAVID E. VANCE	
12	**Information processing speed: How fast, how slow, and how come?**	265
	JOHN DELUCA	
	Author index	275
	Subject index	295

About the editors

John DeLuca, Ph.D., ABPP is the Director of Neuroscience Research and Vice-President for Research Training at the Kessler Medical Rehabilitation Research and Education Center (KMRREC), and Professor in the Department of Physical Medicine and Rehabilitation and the Department of Neurology and Neuroscience at the University of Medicine and Dentistry of New Jersey, USA. He studies disorders of memory and information processing in a variety of clinical populations. Dr. DeLuca has published over 300 articles, abstracts and chapters in these areas.

Jessica H. Kalmar, Ph.D. is a neuropsychologist conducting research within the Mood Disorders Research Program, Department of Psychiatry at the Yale University School of Medicine, USA. Currently, Dr. Kalmar studies neural circuitry and cognition in various adolescent psychiatric populations including: bipolar disorder, attention-deficit/hyperactivity disorder and major depressive disorder. Additionally, she has studied information processing in neurological populations, including individuals with multiple sclerosis and traumatic brain injury. Dr. Kalmar has published articles, abstracts and chapters in these areas.

List of contributors

Karlene K. Ball, Ph.D., Edward R. Roybal Center for Translational Research on Aging and Mobility, University of Alabama at Birmingham, Birmingham, AL, USA

Shane S. Bush, Ph.D., ABPP, ABPN, Independent Practice, Smithtown, New York, USA

Nancy D. Chiaravalloti, Ph.D., Kessler Medical Rehabilitation Research and Education Center, West Orange, NJ, and Department of Physical Medicine and Rehabilitation, University of Medicine and Dentistry of New Jersey, Newark, NJ, USA

Eco de Geus, Ph.D., Department of Biological Psychology, Vrije Universiteit (VU University), Amsterdam, The Netherlands

John DeLuca, Ph.D., ABPP, Kessler Medical Rehabilitation Research and Education Center, West Orange, NJ, and University of Medicine and Dentistry of New Jersey, Newark, NJ, USA

Heath A. Demaree, Ph.D., Department of Psychology, Case Western Reserve University, Cleveland, OH, USA

Dwight Dickinson, Ph.D., Department of Psychiatry, University of Maryland School of Medicine, and VISN 5 Mental Illness Research, Education and Clinical Center, Baltimore, MD, USA

Thomas W. Frazier, II, Ph.D., Psychology Department, John Carroll University, University Heights, OH, USA

James M. Gold, Ph.D., Maryland Psychiatric Research Center, and VISN 5 Mental Illness Research, Education and Clinical Center, Baltimore, MD, USA

Courtney E. Johnson, Department of Psychology, Case Western Reserve University, Cleveland, OH, USA

Robert V. Kail, Ph.D., Department of Psychological Sciences, Purdue University, West Lafayette, IN, USA

Jessica H. Kalmar, Ph.D., Department of Psychiatry, Yale University School of Medicine, New Haven, CT, USA

Glynda J. Kinsella, Ph.D., Psychological Science, La Trobe University, and Psychological Services, Caulfield General Medical Centre, Melbourne, Victoria, Australia

David J. Madden, Ph.D., Center for the Study of Aging and Human Development, and Department of Psychiatry and Behavioral Sciences, Duke University Medical Center, Durham, NC, USA

Roderick K. Mahurin, Ph.D., Department of Radiology, University of Washington Medical School, Seattle, WA, USA

Thomas A. Martin, Psy.D, ABPP, Missouri Rehabilitation Center, and Department of Health Psychology, University of Missouri-Columbia, Mt. Vernon, MO, USA

Amanda R. O'Brien, Ph.D., Kessler Medical Rehabilitation Research and Education Center, West Orange, NJ, and Department of Physical Medicine and Rehabilitation, University of Medicine and Dentistry of New Jersey, Newark, NJ, USA

Danielle Posthuma, Ph.D., Department of Biological Psychology, Vrije Universiteit (VU University), Amsterdam, The Netherlands

Timothy A. Salthouse, Ph.D., Department of Psychology, University of Virginia, Charlottesville, VA, USA

David S. Tulsky, Ph.D., Kessler Medical Rehabilitation Research and Education Center, West Orange, NJ, and Department of Physical Medicine and Rehabilitation, University of Medicine and Dentistry of New Jersey, Newark, NJ, USA

David E. Vance, Ph.D., MGS, School of Nursing, University of Alabama at Birmingham, Birmingham, AL, USA

From the series editor

Speed of information processing has been implicated as the underlying architecture for cognitive change in aging, developmental disorders, psychiatric disorders, conditions of nervous system pathology, and neurological injuries. There is no question that processing speed is related to issues of efficiency in the ability to perform critical occupational and everyday activities such as driving, operating machinery, or even simpler tasks such as sorting materials. An understanding of factors affecting processing speed is thus critical to their impact on other cognitive functions, yet it is clear that the factors are not uniform and that they are interactive.

In this volume, Drs. DeLuca and Kalmar have gathered an impressive group of authors who have focused their research on aspects of information processing speed with regard to how it is measured, how it is influenced, how it is expressed in various clinical conditions, developmental and genetic variants, and implications for everyday life. *Information Processing Speed in Clinical Populations* is a welcome addition to our series and I highly recommend it to the clinician and researcher seeking to have a concise survey of relevant research in the area and its practical application.

Linas A. Bieliauskas
Ann Arbor
January, 2007

1 The history of processing speed and its relationship to intelligence

Amanda R. O'Brien and David S. Tulsky

A review of recent theories of intelligence and research strongly supports the clinical utility of measuring processing speed (PS) in assessments of intelligence. However, the recent enthusiasm about processing speed as a significant component of intelligence is not an innovative idea in psychology. On the contrary, the use of processing speed as a major factor of intelligence and individual abilities lies at the very core of the birth of psychology as a quantitative science. During the late 1800s and early 1900s Wilhelm Wundt, Sir Francis Galton, James McKeen Cattell and other prominent psychologists strongly asserted that measures of sensory processes (e.g., processing speed) were at the heart of individuals' intellectual abilities. The field followed suit and the zeitgeist of science during the late nineteenth century and early twentieth century included the belief that anthropometric testing was the best way to measure an individual's ability, resulting in the meteoric rise of processing speed research in intelligence.

However, after the early 1900s, the notion that speed was a central component to intelligence testing had waned, only to be "rediscovered" more recently as a valuable aspect of cognitive and neuropsychological testing (e.g., Donders, Tulsky, & Zhu, 2001; Martin, Donders, & Thompson, 2000). Today, researchers assert that processing speed measures within intelligence tests are among the most sensitive indicators of "acquired cerebral dysfunction," (Hawkins, 1998). Although it is controversial, the debate over how such a "simple" factor as processing speed may contribute to higher cognitive functions has resurfaced in psychological theory. The drive to further delineate the concept of processing speed is currently a major focus of research and is discussed throughout the chapter.

The goal of this chapter is to balance the recent "rise" in the assessment of processing speed by providing the historical context of examining processing speed as a component of intelligence and cognitive ability in both clinical and research settings. Therefore, the chapter provides an historical overview of processing speed beginning with the work of Galton and ending with current research. Various methodologies used to measure and study processing speed in the experimental realm are explained. The chapter also reviews more recent history that includes the story of how processing speed was brought back into the clinical realm through the Wechsler tests (see Figure 1.1). Further analysis of what processing speed can tell us about intelligence for healthy and clinical populations is discussed. The concept of processing speed as a simple versus complex cognitive construct is evaluated, including an argument for the need for a measure of more complex processing speed. Finally, recommendations for the future directions of the study of processing speed in the field of intelligence are articulated.

The history of processing speed

The birth of psychology as a science was largely composed of research on individual differences studied by measuring reaction time. Psychology's focus on the study of individual differences in intellectual abilities occurred in the middle to late nineteenth century, partially due to the study of evolution. Darwin's theories that behavioral and mental abilities could be inherited and that variation in these abilities (and subsequent hereditary "selection" of such abilities) naturally occurred had a major impact on scientific thinking. Although psychology had grown out of the field of philosophy, Darwin's theories impacted on major thinkers in psychology and brought the study of individual differences and a more scientific approach to the field of psychology. Sir Francis Galton was a half-cousin of Darwin and was particularly influenced by his theories and his systematic approach to data collection and classification as evidenced in his 1869 book, *Hereditary Genius* (e.g., Clayes, 2001; Seligman, 2002).

Galton's "anthroprometric" lab in London and Wilhelm Wundt's first-ever psychological lab in Germany conducted the earliest research into individual differences by studying reaction time using various techniques. The initiation of research in these labs formed the foundation for formal

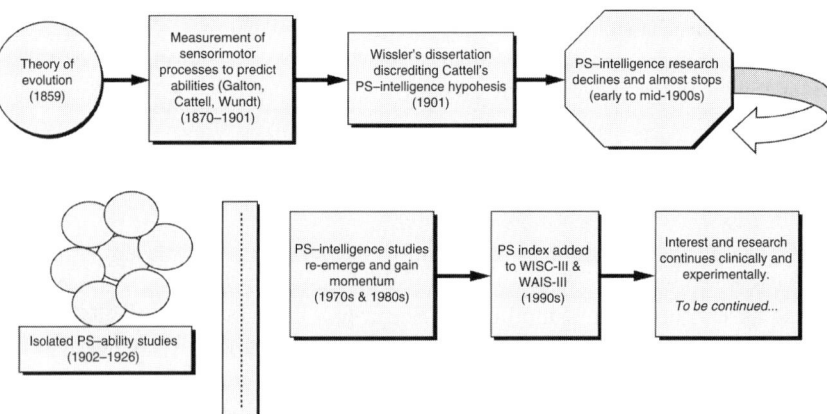

Figure 1.1 Overview timeline of the history of processing speed in the study and measurement of intelligence.

psychometric science and was the beginning of a prolific period of research in individual differences and intelligence testing. Galton is thought to be one of the first people to assert that mental processes (e.g., intelligence) could be quantitatively measured. Galton created a series of "psychometric experiments," which the general public was introduced to and could experience first hand at the International Exhibition in London in 1884. He believed that these tasks, which measured various sensory and motor processes (of which reaction time was a major focus), reflected people's intellectual strengths and weaknesses (e.g., Diamond, 1977). The popularity of Galton's work helped to generate a period referred to as the era of "brass instruments," named as such for labs with numerous apparatuses that could be adapted with various brass fittings for measuring sensory processes (e.g., speed) that he believed were at the heart of individual differences in ability. During this period, the systematic study of mostly sensorimotor abilities, including reaction time, was widely accepted as a measure of mental variables.

The instruments used in the late nineteenth century to measure individual differences are interesting contributors to the story of assessment and intelligence. As stated by Michael Sokal (Sokal, Davis, & Merzbach, 1976), "such instruments show just what was new about the 'new psychology' that led its adherents to claim it as a distinct science" (p. 59). Until Wundt began studying reaction time, the discipline of psychology had strongly asserted that the mental world could not be quantified or recorded. To attempt to do so was revolutionary, and not always well accepted by the establishment. One of the most "famous" instruments of the brass instruments era that was used to measure reaction time was the Hipp chronoscope, which essentially functioned as a very early type of stopwatch for psychological studies (see Figure 1.2). The Hipp chronoscope was quite complex, as shown by the following description:

> A chronoscope driven by Clock-work, whose movement is regulated by a vibrating tongue; it is provided with two dials of 100 divisions each, one recording seconds and 10ths, the other 100ths and 1000ths (sigma); the movement of the pointers is started and stopped by means of a clutch actuated by electromagnets, and there are connections whereby the record may either be started by making the circuit and stopped by breaking it, or vice versa.
>
> (Warren, 1934)

Although the chronoscope allowed for breakthroughs in measurements of human reaction time, the many complexities of its design led to numerous problems of calibration and inaccuracies of measurement. To correct these problems, the machine required frequent recalibration and additional pieces were often added to the machine to attempt to control for errors, making the Hipp chronometer controversial for its shortcomings and especially the variability of its measurements (http://www.chss.montclair.edu/psychology/museum/mrt.html; Sokal et al., 1976).

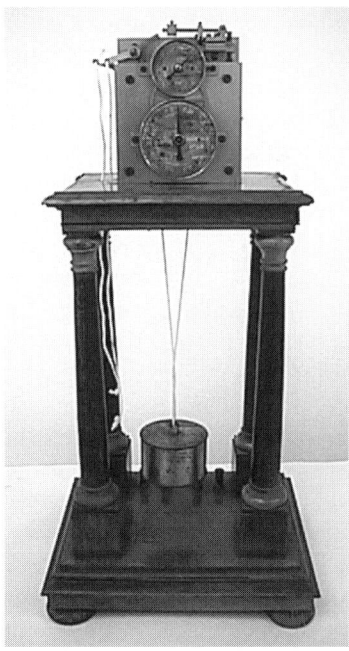

Figure 1.2 Hipp chronoscope. Photo used with permission from Dr. Thomas Perera and the Museum of the History of Reaction Time, Montclair State University, New Jersey: http://www.chss.montclair.edu/psychology/museum/mrt.html

Another primary figure in the study of processing speed and intelligence was James McKeen Cattell; one of the great proponents of measurement of individual differences and use of "brass instruments." Cattell came from a privileged background, and his scientific and professional interests, as well as a colorful and reportedly cantankerous personality, were part of a serendipitous mixture that put measuring individual differences and processing speed on the scientific map, particularly in the U.S. After graduating college in 1880, Cattell won a fellowship to Johns Hopkins University where he conducted experiments and argued about the importance of quantitative measurement of basic human abilities (e.g., reaction time) to study individual differences. However, he lost a second year of the fellowship to John Dewey, reportedly due to ongoing arguments with his supervisor, G. Stanley Hall and Johns Hopkins' administration (Ross, 1972). Cattell therefore went to Europe in 1883 and worked with Wilhelm Wundt in the world's first psychological laboratory, a decision that would have a major impact on American psychology and the field of psychological testing as a whole (Sokal, 1980). Cattell was struck by the scientific measurement and statistical analysis of human behaviors and individual differences that Wundt studied. After receiving his Ph.D. from Leipzig in 1886, Cattell continued his research under the direction of Sir Francis Galton in London, England. Galton, a pioneer in quantitative measurement of mental processes, had been measuring reaction time to study individual differences (Diamond, 1977). Cattell (1911) was heavily influenced by Galton's mentorship, theories, and research and was quoted as saying that Galton was the "greatest man [he] ever knew" (Diamond, 1977, p. 48; Sokal, 1987, p. 27).

As Cattell started his professional career at the University of Pennsylvania, he continued to be heavily influenced by Galton's work. Cattell became absorbed in the study of individual differences (see Sokal, 1987) and in 1890, he published a seminal article in *Mind* on the topic. He began the article by asserting:

> Psychology cannot attain the certainty and exactness of the physical sciences, unless it rests on a foundation of experiment and measurement. A step in this direction could be made by applying a series of mental tests and measurements to a large number of individuals.
>
> (Cattell, 1890, p. 373)

Cattell is credited with coining the term "mental tests," which were tests used to predict or measure "intelligence," although this construct was defined in various ways. Cattell's 10 "mental tasks" measured reaction time and sensory sensitivity across domains, and included tasks such as "rate of movement," "pressure causing pain," "reaction time for sound," and "number of letters remembered on once hearing," using several instruments (e.g., brass instruments) discussed earlier (Cattell, 1890). His focus on reaction time demonstrates that processing speed was a key interest for Cattell.

In the 1880s and 1890s, the cultural and scientific zeitgeist provided a very welcome reception to Cattell's mental tests and his scientific study of individual differences. New York in the 1880s was an epicenter of scientific, cultural and artistic cooperation and productivity. As a result, universities in the city were thriving as well (Sokal, 1994). This inquisitive and open environment was in place when Cattell became a professor at Columbia in 1891. Cattell was even able to negotiate the assessment of every incoming student at Columbia College and the Columbia School of Mines with his series of mental tests (Sokal, 1987).

Cattell's powerful professional positions and his work at Columbia were major factors in explaining why the study of individual differences and processing speed thrived in the late 1800s and very early 1900s. More specifically, his anthropometric laboratory was productive and highly regarded, he started the journal *Psychological Review* in 1894, took over as editor of *Science* in 1894, and helped to establish, and later became President of the American Psychological Association in 1895.

Under Cattell's presidency, the American Psychological Association (APA) created a committee on the potential collaboration between laboratories who were collecting measurements on mental and physical characteristics. The committee consisted of Cattell, Joseph Jastrow, Edmund Sanford, James

Mark Baldwin, and Lightner Witmer (a student of both Cattell and Wundt). All but one of the committee members advocated Cattell's methodology for testing individual differences and the APA recommended Cattell's anthropometric testing as the preferred methodology for studying individual differences. Only Baldwin dissented, stating that there was a need for tests that measured more complex mental processes, giving the first public criticism of the "anthropometric tests" (Sokal, 1987). Shortly thereafter, Stella Emily Sharp, a graduate student of Edward Titchener, published her dissertation in which she criticized mental testing and individual psychology. She felt that Cattell's measures of individual differences lacked any theoretical structure or useful application to functioning, which she supported with testing she had done on other graduate students (Sokal, 1987). However, these were the only two public criticisms of Cattell's methodology during a time in which he had a great deal of power in the world of psychology.

Powerful scientists' enthusiasm for measuring processing speed to determine individual differences, in the absence of clear hypothesis-driven research or sound research methodologies, continued to propel the topic, perhaps above and beyond what the evidence should have allowed. These researchers believed that the measurement of sensory processes, mainly differences in speed, would revolutionize assessment and psychology as a whole. Without any specific hypotheses about the mechanism(s) behind a relationship between speed and intelligence, these researchers still boldly asserted that their measures of processing speed could predict how successful people could be (although "success" was not specifically defined).

Research on speed and intelligence disappears

Several events in the late 1800s and very early 1900s effectively led to the significant decline of anthropometric testing and therefore to the end of the enthusiasm for measuring speed as a correlate of intellectual abilities. First, Edward Wheeler Scripture, a former student of Wundt's, had been part of the core group of psychologists using anthropometric measures in psychology. However, similar to Cattell, he reportedly had a difficult personality and was involved in many arguments and conflicts with his colleagues. As a result, he spent much of this time in the 1890s struggling to keep his job and not on testing (Sokal, 1987). At the same time, Jastrow had been struggling to publish the results of his own testing and had run into a great deal of adversity, which reportedly led to a nervous breakdown in the mid-1890s. As a result, he was no longer part of this scientific movement (Sokal, 1987). This left Witmer as one of the last "heavy hitters" in anthropometric testing, who, at the time, was switching his focus to much more specific applications of testing in clinical psychology. Additionally, as interested in individual differences as Cattell was, he openly declared that he could not say exactly what the test results would mean, but believed that it was important to gather as much empirical, scientific information as possible and discern what information it provided once it was collected. However, the true death knoll of Cattell's anthropometric testing was the 1901 dissertation of Clark Wissler, a doctoral student of Cattell's at Columbia. Cattell had collected voluminous amounts of data with regard to the testing of individual sensory differences without a hypothesis for what this information would mean or exactly how such information would be used. Wissler's dissertation examined the results of the anthropometric testing and asserted that there was virtually no relationship between Cattell's mental tests and the students' abilities, as measured by their grades, therefore indicating that such tests were not valid measures for predicting intelligence (Fancher, 1985; Plucker, 2003; Sternberg, 1990). Additionally, Wissler stated that there was very little relationship between the tasks themselves. The dissertation was widely considered definitive and is thought to be the key reason as to why Cattell gave up his line of research and assessment with his mental tests (e.g., Fancher, 1985; Plucker, 2003; Sternberg, 1990). Wissler actually left the field of psychology altogether and became a well-respected anthropologist. These events were among the most important factors that resulted in the significant decline and eventual abandonment of measuring speed as an index of more general intellectual abilities for most of the beginning and middle of the twentieth century (see Figure 1.1).

Despite Cattell's rather public failure, there were still a few researchers who continued to believe in the relationship between processing speed (i.e., reaction time) and intelligence. For example, in 1904, Charles Spearman asserted that general intelligence and sensory discrimination were almost perfectly correlated, based on his research. However, despite such positive results, Spearman did not further pursue this line of research and others could not replicate his findings (Eysenck, 1987). Cyril Burt (1909), a scientist who was largely discredited after his death, used sensory tests of touch, sound, and weight discrimination, a memory association task, and an early version of an inspection time (IT) task called the "spot pattern task" (IT is now defined as the duration of exposure to a stimulus necessary to make a simple visual discrimination with certain accuracy; e.g., 97%). He reported that the "spot pattern" test had a correlation with intelligence of .83. (Eysenck, 1987). Burt's early research on the factors comprising general intelligence made him a pioneer in educational psychology in England. However, reviews of his work completed after his death resulted in strong support for charges of falsification and fabrication of data to fit his conclusions; casting significant doubt on the veracity of his findings (e.g., Fletcher, 1991; Joynson, 1989; Kamin, 1974). A series of studies of the relationship between speed and mental tests continued experimentally in the 1910s and 1920s. However, inconsistent findings and poor methodology hampered the work and by the end of the 1920s, experimental work in speed and intelligence was slowing down as well (Fletcher, 1991; Joynson, 1989; Kamin, 1974).

More recently, some psychologists looking back on the history of this line of research assert that the dismissal of Cattell's work was based on "misunderstandings and selective reporting of historical literature" (Deary & Stough, 1996; p. 599). Jensen, in a review of the early work conducted by Galton, reports that more recent analysis of Galton's data with use of correlational techniques that did not exist in Galton's time, supports his general assertions of a relationship between elementary cognitive tasks (i.e., reaction time) and intelligence. Furthermore, Jensen asserts that in Galton's time, reaction time measures had *very* low reliability and the subjects chosen for his experiments had abilities in a very restricted range, both of which significantly limited his findings (Jensen, 1998b). Jensen's post hoc analysis of Galton's work may account for some of the shortcoming in Galton's outcomes despite a potentially groundbreaking theory. Be that as it may, this area of Galton's work was subsequently discussed as a cautionary tale of overzealous research gone wrong.

Whether justified or not, by the end of the 1920s, the study and clinical assessment of basic sensory processes to measure intelligence were essentially brought to a stop by Wissler's dissertation and other inconclusive research in this area. For approximately the next 50 years, more complex measures of intelligence, such as Binet's battery for the assessment of intelligence, were heavily favored. Prior to a resurgence of reaction time research in the 1970s, one would be hard-pressed to find any significant body of experimental or clinical studies focused on speed and mental abilities that existed after the early 1900s (Vernon, 1987). A chapter by Eysenck provides references for 14 studies that investigated mental speed in relation to mental abilities that were conducted after Wissler's dissertation between 1902 and 1926 (Eysenck, 1987). A 1928 review by MacFarland asserted that there was experimental support for a relationship between "rate" (e.g., mental speed) and mental abilities as assessed by intelligence tests. Although MacFarland added the researchers' favorite phrase "more research is needed," interest in the experimental study of intelligence significantly decreased at the end of the 1920s (Eysenck, 1987).

Research in mental speed and intelligence makes "One of the greatest comebacks in all of psychology"

Experimental research methodologies for the study of processing speed and individual abilities re-emerged beginning in the 1970s. In a 1987 book entitled, *Speed of Information Processing and Intelligence*, the editor noted that in the 10 to 15 years leading to the book, a significant re-emergence of interest and research into the connections between speed and intelligence had been undertaken, referring to the return of this research as "one of the greatest comebacks in psychology" (Vernon, 1987, p. 1). He also discussed how, despite research failures and a lack of empirical support, the idea that mental speed was related to intelligence remained. Vernon noted that there is no clear cut reason why the idea that mental speed and intelligence are integrally linked remained so robust or why it experienced a resurgence in the 1970s and

1980s. However, he speculated that scientists' increasing desire to quantify and measure individual abilities and biological systems in the most precise ways may have contributed to this phenomenon (Vernon, 1987).

To begin the volume, Vernon reviewed the work in three areas of reaction time (RT) research that were conducted in this renewal in the 1970s and 1980s. He provided significant detail of the work in each of these areas (see Vernon, 1987), but for the sake of this chapter, a brief review will suffice to summarize his major points. Vernon reviewed research that supported that RT was significantly correlated to both timed AND untimed tests of intelligence. He related these findings back to a "neural efficiency model," which stated that due to limited capacity of our cognitive systems to store and process information, faster processing is intellectually advantageous. He presented empirical support that this is true even for untimed tasks when they become more complex. More specifically, in order to take in all necessary information, retrieve information from long-term memory, and manipulate information quickly enough to solve a complicated cognitive problem/task, faster processing speed is necessary for good performance, even when there is no external time limit imposed on the task (Vernon, 1985; Vernon & Kantor, 1986). The second area of research on reaction time involved heritability and was first conducted in the mid-1980s. Research by McGue, Bouchard, Lykken, and Feuer (1984) and by Vernon and colleagues (Vernon, 1985; Vernon & Kantor, 1986) showed that reaction time and a specific type of processing speed measure demonstrated significantly higher correlations with intelligence in monozygotic versus dizygotic twins (although both groups demonstrated a significant correlation between reaction time and intelligence!) Finally, research on sex differences and mental speed was reviewed and was deemed to be inconclusive and sometimes contradictory. However, Vernon summarized that findings in this area demonstrate that gender was an important mediating factor in the relationship between level of abilities and their relationship to RT (Vernon, 1987).

Experimental research on reaction time, IT and other measures of speed in relation to intelligence has often been classified as "reductionist," meaning that researchers are searching for the most elemental components of cognition that predict higher-order cognitive processes (Deary & Stough, 1996). As much as it appears that this label is sometimes given as a criticism, it is also the eloquence of such a potential theory that drew experimental researchers back to this topic (after almost 50 years) in the same way it had earlier enticed Galton, Wundt, Cattell and others to study basic sensory processes. Arthur Jensen, a controversial yet renowned psychologist and theorist in the field of intelligence, was also drawn to this topic and its application in psychology. He has asserted that he was at least partially responsible for reviving "Galtonian" thinking in psychology after it had been abandoned by clinicians and studied purely in the experimental realm. However, Jensen's research in the late 1960s and early 1970s regarding intelligence differences between races led to huge controversy and made him a polarizing figure in intelligence research and psychology in general (e.g., Gould, 1981). Jensen argued that his work was misunderstood and taken out of context stating: "nowhere have I 'claimed' an 'innate deficiency' of intelligence in blacks ... The only genuine consensus among well-informed scientists on this topic is that the cause of the difference remains an open question" (Jensen, 1981, p. 213). Jensen was criticized, labeled by some as a racist, and for a time was ostracized by many other psychologists and researchers. It is likely that the controversy surrounding much of Jensen's work significantly hindered widespread attention to or acceptance of his research in reaction time and intelligence. In a 1998 article, Jensen reflected on the beginning of his investigations into the relationship of elementary cognitive tasks (ECT) and "g" (his hypothesized variable of general cognitive ability) and the ridicule he received from the scientific community. Jensen writes that:

> RT is obviously much too simple to reflect individual differences in anything so marvelously complex as human intelligence ... Hadn't I studied the history of psychology? ... For over half a century nearly every introductory psychology text discredited the idea that RT is related to "intelligence," while recounting the unsuccessful attempts of Galton and James McKeen Cattell.
>
> (Jensen, 1998a, p. 203)

The advent of Arthur Jensen's "Choice Reaction Time" (CRT) paradigm resulted in renewed excitement and support for a connection between speed and mental abilities in the 1980s. Jensen's CRT model breaks down the concept of reaction time into "decision time" (DT) and "movement time" (MT), which he believed better represented the fundamental reaction time component than did simple reaction time. DT is measured as the amount of time it takes for the person to react to a stimulus (e.g., to take his finger *off* of an initially depressed button). MT is defined as the period of time between when the participant releases a first button and when he or she presses a target button. CRT was shown to have a more significant relationship than simple reaction time to psychometric intelligence.

As much as CRT was an advance in studying processing speed and intelligence, it was criticized for research with small and/or restricted samples (usually students). However, a recent population-based study with 900 participants found a correlation of .5 between four CRT tasks and a measure of psychometric intelligence, which was an even stronger relationship than that reported by Jensen in a 1987 quantitative review of CRT and intelligence (Deary, Der, & Ford, 2001). Such research support in a large population-based sample has helped to assert the relevance of CRT in relation to psychometric intelligence.

Although valuable information was gained in the research on choice reaction time and psychometric intelligence, some researchers sought a more pure concept of "mental speed." As a result, the concept of IT was developed. As briefly described previously, IT is generally defined as the duration of exposure to a stimulus necessary to make a simple visual discrimination with certain accuracy (e.g., 97%). The task is so simple as to be thought of as representing basic neural speed or efficiency. The task is made more challenging by a decrease in time of exposure to the stimuli. Deary and Stough (1996) applied the theory of IT to intelligence, and outlined several advantages of IT over reaction time as an element of higher-order cognitive processes. For example, IT eliminates movement time for a more "pure" measure of processing speed or efficiency. Also, several developmental studies that have been done have prospectively demonstrated that shorter (better) IT results in higher scores on tests of psychometric intelligence, rather than IT being simply an artifact of a higher intelligence quotient (IQ) (e.g., Deary & Stough, 1996).

A review of the literature by Nettelbeck (1987) asserted that IT accounts for approximately 25% of the variance in IQ. This statistic has been replicated and even surpassed in other studies (Deary et al., 2001). However, IT consistently correlates more strongly with performance measures of intelligence than verbal measures of intelligence. (However, it is important to note that many performance measures of intelligence are timed and verbal measures are not.) A "Fluid Intelligence Hypothesis" argues that IT measures a fundamental component of cognitive ability (such as neural efficiency). Those with more efficient neural processing would be able to attend to and manipulate more information or solve novel problems due to their increased speed of processing. Although there is research support for a significant negative correlation of $-.74$ between IT and fluid intelligence (Osmon & Jackson, 2002), acceptance of IT in the framework of the Fluid Intelligence Hypothesis has not been universal by any means. Nettelbeck and colleagues (Nettelbeck, 2001; see also Burns & Nettelbeck, 2003; Burns, Nettelbeck, & Cooper, 1999) assert that IT is significantly correlated with processing speed and it is through this relationship, and not a direct relationship with fluid abilities, that IT impacts on intelligence. Although IT research supports a strong and consistent relationship between processing speed and psychometric intelligence (particularly with performance abilities), IT has remained in the experimental realm, with no tests of IT incorporated into batteries of intellectual assessment.

More recent experimental study of processing speed and intelligence focuses on the biological correlates of intelligence within the larger discussion of processing speed and intelligence. There is an extensive body of literature in this area, which is beyond the scope of this chapter (for a more extensive review see Deary & Caryl, 1997). More recent biological research into intelligence includes the study of evoked response potentials (ERPs), which represent alterations in the electrical activity in the brain in response to a sensory stimulus. ERPs have been studied in relationship to intelligence since the 1960s, and overall the research supports that individual differences in intelligence are reflected in the brain's response to elementary stimuli (Deary & Caryl, 1997). More recent research on ERPs is much more complex and investigates the different components of these potentials and the reliability of ERPs as a correlate of efficient (or inefficient) neural processes. A second area of the biological study of intelligence is the study of brain volume and its relationship to intelligence. Some researchers hypothesize that larger brains may have more neural connections and other potentially beneficial physiological features that may relate to intelligence (e.g., Walhovd et al., 2005; Wickett, Vernon, & Lee, 1994, 2000). Use of magnetic resonance imaging (MRI) has generally yielded correlations of .4 between brain volume and certain measures of psychometric intelligence (Rushton & Ankey, 1996). Measurement of glucose metabolism (with use of PET scans) has yielded mixed results. Scientists have yet to determine the direction of the relationship between intelligence and brain size or function, and exactly what aspects of brain size and function are being measured that relate to psychometric intelligence. Therefore, although some information has been gained, it appears even more questions remain (Neisser et al., 1996). Jensen continues to study biological bases of mental speed and intelligence and recently published *Clocking the Mind: Mental Chronometry and Individual Differences* (2006). He still argues for "g" (the general concept of intelligence), which he believes is influenced by neural efficiency, and states that the study of the "science of mental ability" must be based in these basic processes (see Jensen, 2006 for full review). However, biological measurements of PS have yet to be applied to the clinical assessment of intellectual functioning, although they empirically support the connection between PS and intelligence.

The return of processing speed to the clinical realm

As unlikely as it may seem given the aforementioned history and isolation of processing speed research in the experimental realm, processing speed actually did make a dramatic and unexpected return to the clinical assessment of intelligence after an absence that stretched over multiple decades.

With such a divide between experimental and clinical research, just how did processing speed re-emerge in the clinical realm? It appears that part of the credit does indeed belong to Arthur Jensen and his boldness in revisiting an area of research that was essentially discredited and considered "dead." Jensen wrote extensively about his theory of intelligence and about "g," the general cognitive ability that he believed was a part of intelligence assessments and their subtests. His research provided support for a substantial relationship between "g" and reaction time and how speed was an underlying factor that was intrinsic to "g".

During his education, Jensen was stimulated and inspired by reading the work of Galton and James McKeen Cattell. He also recognized that the study of processing speed was relegated to experimental research and very much divorced from clinical application. Despite this fact, Jensen has stated that he specifically looked for ways in which to apply his knowledge, theories, and research on reaction time and cognitive abilities in a practical and applied manner (Jensen, 1998a). His work with choice reaction time in the 1980s was the beginning of the re-emergence of processing speed research in the clinical realm. Additionally, more recent theories of intelligence have incorporated speed, in various forms, as a major component. However, as with experimental work, the clinical application of these theories in assessment has lagged behind (McGrew, 2005).

Processing speed in the assessment of intelligence

As you will recall, Galton, Cattell, and Spearman's theories that studied elementary cognitive tasks in relationship to intelligence in the late 1800s and early 1900s fell out of favor. In their place, more complex clinical measures of intellectual functioning, such as Binet's assessments of intelligence, became the norm. Even Jensen stated that Binet's test of intelligence appeared more *practically* useful. However, he argued that from a *scientific* standpoint, Galton "showed the way," and that "Galton's original intuition has now been fully confirmed" with regard to the importance of processing speed in intelligence and higher mental processing (Jensen, 1998a, p. 204).

Arguably, the most widely used and currently accepted battery to assess adult intelligence is the *Wechsler Adult Intelligence Scale Third Edition* (WAIS-III, 1997). The scale was first developed by David Wechsler in 1939. Wechsler was heavily influenced by his experiences of assessment in the military as well as becoming an employee of the Psychological Corporation (which was founded by Cattell in 1921; Tulsky, Saklofske, & Ricker, 2003a) Wechsler's battery did not necessarily generate new or unique tests of intellectual abilities, but rather synthesized tests (or modified versions of tests) that he felt best assessed various areas of intelligence. The Wechsler scales were not based on any one theory of intelligence, but rather aimed to be a comprehensive assessment instrument of intelligence that would have good *clinical* utility, but was *not* based on scientific research from the experimental realm. Although Wechsler was a student of James McKeen Cattell, he included only one measure of reaction time or processing speed (Digit Symbol subtest) in the creation of his testing battery! The first version of the Wechsler exam (in 1939) generated only a Full Scale IQ score. A second version (in 1946) added a Verbal IQ score and a Performance IQ score derived from various verbal and visual-spatial subtests. The WAIS was modified twice in Wechsler's lifetime. However, over these two revisions, only one new subtest (Vocabulary) was ever added and the scoring essentially remained the same. Until the most recent revision of the WAIS in 1997, there were no specific processing speed subtests or scoring index in the battery. However, with the WAIS-III, processing speed has been added to the testing and scoring structure of this famous intelligence test, increasing its clinical utility.

So exactly how and why was a new Processing Speed Index score added into the WAIS-III? Such a change, compared to the previous types of changes carried out in revisions of the WAIS, seems practically radical. Like many things in science, there was a bit of serendipity involved in the evolution of a Processing Speed Index score on the WAIS, which originated from changes being made to the *Wechsler Intelligence Scale for Children Third Edition* (WISC-III, 1991). During research and development for revision of the WISC, a new subtest, "Symbol Search," was added in an attempt to strengthen a factor called, "Freedom from Distractability" (Tulsky, Saklofske, & Zhu, 2003b). In the Symbol Search task, a pair of "target symbols" is positioned next to a line of five "search variables." A person is directed to mark a "yes" or "no" box to indicate if *any* of the search symbols exactly match *either* of the target symbols. There is a 2-minute time limit in which people must respond to as many of these target pairings as possible. It was expected that the new Symbol Search subtest would correlate highly with other WISC subtests including Arithmetic, Digit Span, and Coding and would therefore strengthen the "Freedom from Distractability" factor. However, the researchers conducting factor analytic studies of all the WISC subtests found an unexpected outcome—a new fourth factor, Processing Speed, emerged with Coding and Symbol Search as its subtests. The new factor reflected the measurement of speed of information processing and a Processing Speed Index was added to the structure of the WISC-III (see Prifitera, Weiss, & Saklofske, 1998). It is of note that this addition of a Processing Speed Index score to the WISC (and subsequently to the WAIS-III) was independent of the mental speed and intelligence research that had re-emerged in the 1970s; this addition was not based on a preconceived theoretical hypothesis. One can only speculate as to whether the re-emergence of processing speed in intelligence research or Jensen's work with choice reaction time allowed for greater acceptance of the WISC factor analytic studies' outcomes and the addition of processing speed to clinical intellectual assessment.

When it came time to update the WAIS-R (1981), researchers looked to the changes made to the WISC, including its new four-factor structure. The WAIS-III also delineated a set of summary scores that were organized into more specific domains of cognitive functioning, including the Verbal Comprehension Index, Perceptual Organization Index, Working Memory Index, and the new Processing Speed Index. A Symbol Search subtest was also added to the WAIS-III and it, together with Digit-Symbol Coding, were the subtests that comprised the new WAIS-III Processing Speed Index. However, in the WAIS-III, compared to the WISC-III, the Index scores (including the new Processing Speed Index) were given equal weight as the traditional IQ scores. Clinicians are actually able to decide which subtests to administer in order to generate the various Index or IQ scores, increasing the clinical utility of the battery.

Since their inception, the Index scores have increasingly been recommended over only IQ scores for their increased sensitivity and usefulness in assessing clinical populations (Tulsky et al., 2003b). In particular, the Processing Speed Index is very sensitive to neuropsychological and psychoeducational impairments in clinical populations, such as those with brain injuries (e.g., Donders et al., 2001). The development and use of the Processing Speed Index, particularly in clinical populations, is in the spirit of how Wechsler viewed intelligence tests: as clinical *tools*. As such, the clinical utility of the processing speed subtests and the Processing Speed Index score has been recognized.

It is important (and interesting) to reiterate that the addition of a Processing Speed Index to the WISC-III and therefore the WAIS-III, essentially occurred by accident. Processing speed was not added to the WISC due to one specific theoretical underpinning or agenda. It came about as the result of an exploratory factor analysis that produced something unexpected. However, with credit to the researchers, this new factor was recognized as distinct and clinically useful. This outcome, in turn, had a significant effect on the development of the WAIS-III in 1997.

Although this chapter is focused on the measurement of processing speed and intelligence in adults, it is important to note that there are other intellectual assessments (although designed for use with children) that include processing speed subtests. The Visual Matching and Cross-Out subtests of the *Woodcock–Johnson Tests of Cognitive Ability—Revised* (Woodcock & Johnson, 1989) are both tests of processing speed. The Cross-Out subtest has been subsequently moved to a diagnostic supplement in the most recent revision of the Woodcock–Johnson (W-J III). Additionally, a "Decision Speed" subtest was added to the W-J III. Incidentally, the tests included in the Woodcock–Johnson intellectual assessment are based on the Cattell–Horn–Carroll (CHC) theory of intelligence, which includes both broad and narrow ability areas. The CHC theory is discussed in more depth in the next section of this chapter. The *Differential Ability Scales* (Elliott, 1990), also an intellectual assessment designed for children, include a Speed of Information Processing test as a diagnostic subtest.

The aforementioned processing speed subtests were included in these intellectual assessment batteries in the late 1980s and early 1990s. Therefore, they were included in batteries of intellectual assessment during the time when processing speed was making its strong "comeback" in psychology. They are among the first tangible examples in which the experimental study of processing speed or theories of intelligence that included speed as a major component (i.e., the CHC theory in the case of the Woodcock–Johnson) had a tangible, clinical impact for intellectual assessment.

Recent intelligence theory as an impetus for clinical assessment of processing speed

As discussed earlier, a theoretical backing has been missing from the measurement of processing speed in intellectual assessment since the time of Galton and Wundt. This has been gradually changing, particularly over the past decade. Evidence of this is a recent review that argues that since the advent of a specific intelligence theory, the CHC theory, there has been an increase not only in theory-driven assessments, but in measures that incorporate processing speed as well (Alfonso, Flanagan, & Radwan, 2005). The CHC theory is an integration of the Cattell–Horn Gf–Gc theory and Carroll's three-stratum theory of intelligence. The Cattell–Horn Gf–Gc theory consists of eight abilities, which include speed of processing, reaction time, and decision speed, although the latter two were added in later revisions of this theory (Horn, 1991). Abilities are thought to be either "fluid" (Gf) abilities or "concrete" abilities (Gc). Carroll's three-stratum theory was composed of three "strata" of abilities that moved from the most general intellectual ability ("g"—Stratum III) to increasingly more specific abilities in Strata II and I, respectively (Carroll, 1993). Each of the more general strata subsumes the more specific ones. Speed is in the second stratum of Carroll's theory, recognizing it as an important intellectual factor. According to Alfonso et al. (2005), the CHC theory is the most comprehensive and empirically supported psychometric theory of the structure of cognitive and academic abilities to date. The integration of these two theories kept the three-stratum model, with 10 broad abilities (of which processing speed and decision speed/reaction time are two), and 70 narrow abilities. The CHC emphasizes the importance of multiple abilities and, therefore, when used as a guide for assessment, multiple abilities should be assessed.

Alfonso et al. (2005) argue that the CHC influenced many intelligence test revisions after the late 1990s. Subtests for speed (or additional subtests to assess processing speed) were added to the WISC-IV, WAIS-III, Wechsler Preschool and Primary Scale of Intelligence™—Third Edition (WPPSI-III), and the Woodcock–Johnson-III/Diagnostic Supplement. Although the developers of the WAIS-III did not specifically assert any one theory as a guide, Alfonso et al. (2005) argue that acknowledgement of the research of Cattell, Horn, and Carroll by the authors of these scales (Psychological Corporation, 2002) supports the argument that, at the very least, the CHC theory was used as a guide during the development and revision processes. However, scientists who worked on the revision of the WAIS-III have noted that Wechsler did not use any modern intelligence theory in the development of his scales. However, they also note that whether deliberate or not, the Wechsler intelligence scales mirror concepts included in modern intelligence theory, including the CHC theory (Zhu & Weiss, 2005). For example Tulsky and Price (2003) demonstrated a six-factor model for the WAIS-III scores (Verbal Comprehension, Perceptual Organization, Processing Speed, Working Memory, Visual Memory, and Auditory Memory). These domains are very similar to the concepts espoused in the CHC theory. Regardless of the direct impact on the development of the most recent Wechsler scales, the CHC theory provides a model of a sound, empirically supported theoretical underpinning to guide future revisions and interpretations of intellectual assessments, with speed as a prominent and important component. It also demonstrates that theory-driven assessment has high clinical utility that can be empirically supported, increasing its value.

Cautions about processing speed and intellectual assessment

Given all the recent enthusiasm about the concept and measurement of processing speed in relationship to intellectual faculties, it is important to reflect on the aforementioned history of this topic. As reviewed earlier, the single-minded enthusiasm for measuring processing speed during the time of Galton and Cattell, without hypothesis-driven research or appropriate methodological rigor and peer review, led to the swift downfall of processing speed in clinical research. So the way we can be sure that this newest wave of excitement for processing speed research in intelligence doesn't meet the same fate is by paying attention to the history, relying more heavily on research-supported theories of intelligence, and avoiding dichotomous thinking that processing speed either does or does not fully explain intellectual abilities.

Researchers and clinicians alike need to recognize the limitations and the need for additional research in this area. For example, it is of note that depending on the measure of "processing speed" the correlation between PS and intelligence ranges from about .4 to an impressive .7. This would mean that processing speed accounts for anywhere from 16% to 49% of psychometric intelligence. That leaves another 51% to 84% of the variance in psychometric intelligence unaccounted for. Recognition of the importance and sensitivity of processing speed, balanced with the knowledge that there is still *much* to be discovered and learned about intelligence is a primary need.

Additionally, clinicians and researchers alike also need to carefully consider their interpretations of tests of "processing speed." A recent study attempted to clarify the interpretation of five frequently used measures of processing speed in intellectual tests, including the Coding and Symbol Search subtests of the WISC-III, the Visual Matching and Cross-Out Subtest of the Woodcock–Johnson Tests of Cognitive Ability—Revised (Woodcock & Johnson, 1989), and the Speed of Information Processing test from the Differential Ability Scales (Elliott, 1990). The researchers hypothesized that there may be factors other than pure mental speed that affect performance on these tests, including motor speed and "number facility" ("the ability to perform basic arithmetic operations with speed and accuracy," Ekstrom, French, Harman, & Dirmen, 1976, p. 115). They did find that there was a significant motor speed component to all the subtests they measured. Additionally, there was a numeric component to visual matching, Speed of Information Processing on the DAS, and, oddly, Symbol Search. The authors argue that there are other variables or cognitive abilities at play in the performance of these "processing speed" measures (Feldmann, Kelly, & Diehl, 2004).

However, rather than simply criticize these tests, researchers and clinicians need to ask themselves how to place assessments of processing speed, reaction time, inspection time, and so on, into distinct, more informative categories within intellectual batteries. The very basis for including processing speed measures in intellectual assessment stems from a history in which tests of sensorimotor abilities (e.g., reaction time) were thought to provide valuable information in intellectual assessment. Although motor-free assessments of processing speed have value (particularly for clinical samples who may have impaired or no motor function), tests of processing speed that include motor speed may also have unique and valuable information to share. Additionally, there are so many conceptualizations of mental speed and of intelligence (and how to measure these concepts), that much work needs to be done before enough empirical evidence will have been compiled to support any of these views. Just one example of this is R. B. Cattell's multidimensional view of mental speed. In this theory Cattell provides research evidence for *seven* types of mental speed (Cattell, 1971), and he is able to define and discuss the relevance of each of them. However, the best way to measure any one of these seven types of mental speed, or what performance in any of them means for intelligence, remains unclear. Quite simply, despite over 100 years of interest and research, there is not enough research on individual processing speed tests to make a determination as to an absolutely "right" administration methodology for processing speed tests, or which types of test will best predict various intellectual outcomes definitively.

Finally, the authors of the aforementioned study note that these supposedly simple tests of processing speed may also require other cognitive skills such as working memory, attention, or visual memory for successful completion (Feldmann et al., 2004). It is very difficult to assess or discuss any one cognitive skill in isolation from all others. Therefore, although these commonly used tests of processing speed appear to be impacted by motor speed and task content (Feldmann et al., 2004), they also appear to provide valuable information on the assessment of processing speed and intellectual abilities.

Simple or complex processing speed?

Processing speed is a complex construct that is defined and measured in many ways and cannot be fully understood in isolation from other cognitive abilities. Therefore, to simply state that slowed processing speed results in decreased intelligence is an inaccurate and gross oversimplification. There is a large body of evidence that demonstrates the interaction of information processing speed with other cognitive domains. It is well documented that slowed processing speed can negatively impact other cognitive skills such as verbal abilities (Sherman, Strauss, & Spellacy, 1997), long-term memory (e.g., DeLuca, Barbieri-Berger, & Johnson, 1994; DeLuca, Gaudino, Diamond, Christodoulou, & Engel, 1998; Gaudino, Chiaravalloti, DeLuca, & Diamond, 2001), and working memory (Chiaravalloti, Christodoulou, Demaree, & DeLuca, 2003; Demaree, DeLuca, Gaudino, & Diamond, 1999, see chapter 3 in this volume for further details). It is entirely possible that someone with impaired processing speed will, as a result, also be impaired in other cognitive domains, which may be reflected in certain assessments of intelligence (Chiaravalloti et al., 2003). However, this is not necessarily always the case and cognitively compromised is not equivalent to "less intelligent."

The need for defining and measuring complex PS

As processing speed has been studied in the experimental domain (i.e., RT, CRT), it has largely been thought of as a unitary construct, and that construct is "simple" processing speed (Chiaravalloti et al., 2003). Even inspection time may be considered a measure of simple processing speed, not requiring any manipulation of information. This is not to suggest that complex processing speed entails the manipulation of information; that description would belong to working memory, which is discussed at length in a later chapter in this volume (see chapter 3). There is a qualitative difference between the need to respond to a stimulus as quickly as possible (as in simple or choice RT tasks) and the need to efficiently or quickly process information in order to come to some correct conclusion while holding information in one's mind. If one's complex processing speed were impaired, it may take too long to process the information, and the information would be lost from working memory before one was able to process it. This type of processing speed is qualitatively different from simple processing speed and therefore must be measured differently as well.

Salthouse (1996) very eloquently describes how processing speed is a complex cognitive ability and how it may impact other cognitive abilities through either a *limited time mechanism* or a *simultaneity mechanism*. The limited time mechanism hypothesis asserts that the time spent on more basic cognitive functions will impact on the ability to complete more complex cognitive functions that are needed later in a cognitive sequence when a time limit is imposed. The simultaneity mechanism hypothesis asserts that cognitive actions performed early in a complex task will be "lost" by the time more complex cognitive tasks are (or should be) taking place, whether or not a time limit is imposed. In other words, cognitive tasks that would be conducted later in the sequence of a complex cognitive task may never occur because information from earlier tasks in the sequence is forgotten or cannot be completed in a given amount of time and is essentially lost. Salthouse's model (1996) provides a theoretical framework for understanding how impairment in processing speed can have a significantly negative impact on other cognitive skills, and ultimately on global cognitive functioning in complex situations. His theory also illustrates how processing speed can be viewed as simple, or can be involved and confounded with much more complex cognitive abilities.

If, as suggested, processing speed can be viewed as either simple or complex, there is a need to measure this more complex processing speed as well. Several suggestions for measuring complex processing speed have been made, including use of the Paced Auditory Serial Addition Test (PASAT, Gronwall

& Wrightson, 1981), Digit Symbol Subtest of the WAIS-III, the Symbol Digit Modality Test, and the Trail Making Test, although no consensus exists on how to measure complex information processing speed. However, if we accept that the PASAT is indeed measuring complex processing speed (as shown by Chiaravalloti et al., 2003 using factor analysis), and that complex processing speed is related to several other cognitive skills, then the PASAT should also be related to measures of psychometric intelligence. Indeed, a brief review of the literature verifies that this is indeed the case (Crawford, Obsonsawin, & Allan, 1998; Deary, Langan, Hepburn, & Frier, 1991; Egan, 1988; Wills & Leathem, 2004). In fact, several of these studies describe the PASAT's relationship with general intellectual abilities as "substantial," with a loading of .72 with general intelligence in one study (Crawford et al., 1998), while another study found the PASAT scores significantly correlated with *all* WAIS-R subtests (Deary et al., 1991). It may be that for the construct of processing speed to remain clinically useful, a more complex processing speed domain must be specifically defined and measured. More research on existing neuropsychological measures, as well as the development of new measures to validly and reliably measure complex processing speed in relationship to intelligence, is necessary to further explore this possibility.

Processing speed and clinical populations: Considerations for clinicians

In everyday life, there is clearly a cost for slowed processing speed, such as safety concerns or occupational problems due to real-world demands. Additionally, there is research that supports that impairment in information processing speed is significantly correlated to decrements in quality of life in clinical populations such as persons with multiple sclerosis (Barker-Collo, 2006), and to the ability to perform tasks of daily living (Kalmar, Gaudino, Moore, Halper, & DeLuca, submitted). Problems in everyday living or decreased quality of life are distinct issues from the fact that slowed processing speed does not necessarily equate with decrements in certain types (i.e., "crystalized") of psychometric intelligence. Verbal abilities such as vocabulary and knowledge are often robust skills that do not decline with age or many types of illnesses or injuries. Intact verbal abilities are helpful in compensating for processing speed deficits. Therefore, although one may experience declines in psychometric measures of fluid abilities when processing speed time increases, "crystalized" abilities are likely to remain the same. This demonstrates the complexity of discussing psychometric intelligence and articulating what the exact impact of processing speed impairments is on such measures.

Several clinical populations frequently demonstrate impairments in processing speed, including multiple sclerosis (MS), chronic fatigue syndrome (CFS), and traumatic brain injury (TBI) (see also chapters 7 and 8 of this volume). Assessments of processing speed (compared to assessment of other cognitive domains) have consistently been found to be most sensitive and able to differentiate between clinical groups and healthy control groups (e.g., Demaree et al., 1999; Donders et al., 2001; Martin et al., 2000). As measures of psychometric intelligence (with processing speed subtests) may predict future functioning in daily life, such measures are frequently included in assessments in several clinical populations (e.g., Kalmar et al., submitted; Leahy & Lam, 1998).

Slowed processing speed is one of the most commonly reported and significant cognitive impairments in persons with TBI (Madigan, DeLuca, Diamond, Tramontano, & Averill, 2000; Mathias et al., 2004; Ponsford & Kinsella, 1992; Stuss, Stethem, Hugenholtz, Picton, Pivik, & Richard, 1989; see chapter 8 in this volume for more detailed discussion). Research using persons with TBI has shown significant support for the sensitivity of processing speed measures to differentiate between severity of TBI and between healthy controls and those with a TBI (Donders et al., 2001; Hawkins, 1998; Martin et al., 2000). Particularly, the Processing Speed Index of the WAIS-III, consisting of Digit Symbol Coding and Symbol Search, has demonstrated sensitivity consistently in this clinical group (Donders et al., 2001; Hawkins, 1998; Martin et al., 2000). However, researchers caution that, as sensitive as these measures are, additional assessments should be utilized in a complete neuropsychological assessment of persons with TBI.

In numerous studies of persons with multiple sclerosis, information processing speed is asserted as one of the primary cognitive deficits seen in various subtypes of MS, independent of physical slowing (e.g., DeSousa, Albert, & Kalman, 2002; Rao, 1991). Several studies have utilized the PASAT and other measures to demonstrate that measures of information processing speed are sensitive to cognitive impairments, even mild impairments, particularly in this clinical group (Achiron et al., 2005; Demaree et al., 1999; Kail, 1998; Kalmar, Bryant, Tulsky, & DeLuca, 2004; Snyder, Cappelleri, Archibald, & Fisk, 2001). Please see chapter 7 of this volume for a comprehensive discussion of MS and processing speed.

Research in TBI and MS provides strong support for the clinical utility of measures of processing speed when used with these groups. However, the real challenge for clinicians and researchers alike is how to integrate the information gathered from these and other clinical groups. What does the robust finding of decreased processing speed mean for overall intellectual functioning and daily functioning? Outcomes from tests of processing speed in these clinical populations should not be interpreted in isolation. Rather (like any other individual neuropsychological assessment), measurement of processing speed must be incorporated and interpreted as only part of a comprehensive battery of neuropsychological assessments to maximize the utility of what we can learn from the assessment of processing speed in clinical groups. Slowed processing speed does not mean that persons with TBI or MS are incapable of accurately completing other cognitively demanding tasks. In fact, there is research support that, although processing speed is significantly impacted in these clinical groups, given more time, they can often perform similarly to healthy adults (e.g., speed–accuracy trade off) (Lengenfelder, Bryant, Diamond, Kalmar, Moore, & DeLuca, 2006; Madigan et al., 2000; Ponsford & Kinsella, 1992).

Individuals with TBI and MS are often frustrated by the increased amount of time it may take them to complete a daily task or to solve a problem. People in these clinical groups will sometimes describe themselves as less intelligent, or as feeling "stupid," due to the increased time it takes them to complete certain tasks. These sentiments reflect the frustration of not being able to complete cognitive tasks or solve complex problems in the same manner (i.e., as quickly) as prior to their diagnosis. However, asking if a person is more or less "intelligent" is the wrong question and is largely dependent on how one defines the concept of intelligence (a topic that is much beyond the scope of this chapter). Asking in what way one is intelligent is a more accurate query. The latter question would acknowledge that intelligence is a complex and multifaceted construct, of which processing speed is only one, albeit salient, dimension that will impact daily functioning. This is not to minimize the personal experience of persons with TBI and MS who have to cope with impaired processing speed, and the impact that such an impairment has on daily functioning and quality of life. Rather, it is simply to note that even if one requires more time to complete a task, he or she may do equally as good a job as someone who requires less time. A greater focus on existing abilities, rather than on how quickly one can complete a task, may often be a clinically salient point in the discussion of processing speed and intelligence in clinical populations.

Conclusions and future directions

At the present time, it seems that the story of processing speed has come full circle, having received a great deal of attention in the time of Galton and Cattell, being subsequently discredited and, in recent decades, regaining prominence in both experimental and clinical psychology, particularly in its relationship to intellectual abilities. The sensitivity of measures of processing speed to detect impairment and differentiate between clinical and healthy groups has been strongly supported across several research studies and across several clinical populations. Such sensitivity may allow for early detection of cognitive problems in aging, multiple sclerosis, and other potentially vulnerable groups who would benefit from such diagnosis and early intervention. The addition of the Symbol Search and Digit Symbol Coding to the third edition of the WAIS and the genesis of a Processing Speed Index score have greatly increased awareness of the value of processing speed in relation to psychometric intelligence. The significant impact that impaired processing speed can have on other cognitive skills is also well documented. All of these valuable findings taken together rightfully generate a lot of excitement about processing speed research and the application of this work.

However, it is important to learn from the complex early history of the study of processing speed. For example, it is necessary to temper excitement with critical analysis of the research, thoughtful deliberations about the applications of such research, and the vision to see what remains to be investigated. At this point in the history of processing speed research, there are several areas left to be explored or clarified. First, as discussed earlier, processing speed must be studied as a multidimensional variable. It is yet to be determined how to best define and measure "complex" processing speed. Second, additional longitudinal research is needed in clinical groups, aging, and healthy adults to better understand how early detection of processing speed impairments relates to type and severity of later cognitive impairments, to daily functioning, quality of life and overall intellectual functioning. Third, attempts to figure out how to best compensate for or remediate processing speed impairment have yet to be fully explored. Neuroimaging studies of both clinical and healthy groups may help to answer questions about how people do compensate for such impairments and how this differs between groups. More specifically, research should determine whether or not neural reorganization occurs to compensate for processing speed impairments and how this process may be facilitated.

The study of processing speed to determine individual differences is one of the oldest areas of research in psychology. Although quickly abandoned in the early twentieth century, this area has re-emerged as a valuable and complex domain that deserves the attention of clinical researchers. Whatever direction the future of this field takes, a solid foundation has been laid by the earliest researchers as well as more contemporary scientists such as Jensen, Carroll, and many others. With hypothesis-driven, peer-reviewed, thoughtful work, much can still be learned about the complex relationship between processing speed and intelligence.

Acknowledgements

This work was supported by the Henry H. Kessler Foundation. We also thank John DeLuca and Jessica Kalmar for their helpful comments on a draft of this manuscript.

References

Achiron, A., Polliack, M., Rao, S. M., Barak, Y., Lavie, M., Appelboim, N., et al. (2005). Cognitive patterns and progression in multiple sclerosis: Construction and validation of percentile curves. *Journal of Neurology, Neurosurgery, and Psychiatry*, 76, 744–749.

Alfonso, V. C., Flanagan, D. P., & Radwan, S. (2005). The impact of the Cattell–Horn–Carroll theory on test development and interpretation of cognitive and academic abilities. In D. P. Flanagan & P. L. Harrison (Eds.), *Contemporary intellectual assessment: Theories, tests, and issues* (pp. 185–202). New York: Guilford Press.

Barker-Collo, S. L. (2006). Quality of life in multiple sclerosis: Does information processing speed have an independent effect? *Archives of Clinical Neuropsychology*, *21*, 167–174.

Burns, N. R., & Nettelbeck, T. (2003). Inspection item in the structure of cognitive abilities: Where does IT fit? *Intelligence*, *31*, 237–255.

Burns, N. R., Nettelbeck, T., & Cooper, C. J. (1999). Inspection time correlates with general speed of processing but not with fluid ability, *Intelligence*, *27*, 37–44.

Burt, C. (1909). Experimental tests of general intelligence. *British Journal of Psychology*, *3*, 94–177.

Carroll, J. B. (1993). *Human cognitive abilities: MDBO MDNMA survey of factor-analytic studies*. New York: Cambridge University Press.

Cattell, J. McK. (1890). Mental tests and measurements. *Mind*, *15*, 373–381.

Cattell, J. McK. (1911). Francis Galton. *Popular Science Monthly*, *78*, 309–311.

Cattell, R. B. (1971). *Abilities: Their structure, growth, and action*. Boston: Houghton-Mifflin.

Chiaravalloti, N. D., Christodoulou, C., Demaree, H. A., & DeLuca, J. (2003). Differentiating simpler versus complex processing speed: Influence on new learning and memory performance. *Journal of Clinical and Experimental Neuropsychology*, *25*, 489–501.

Clayes, G. (2001). Introducing Francis Galton, "Kantsaywhere" and "The Donoghues of Dunno Weir." *Utopian Studies*, *12* (2), 188–190.

Crawford, J. R., Obonsawin, M. C., & Allan, K. M. (1998). PASAT and components of WAIS-R performance: Convergent and discriminant validity. *Neuropsychological Rehabilitation*, *8* (3), 255–272.

Deary, I. J., & Caryl, P. G. (1997). Neurosciences and human intelligence differences. *Trends in Neuroscience*, *20*, 365–371.

Deary, I. J., Der, G., & Ford, G. (2001). Reaction times and intelligence differences: A population-based cohort study. *Intelligence*, *29*, 389–399.

Deary, I. J., Langan, S. J., Hepburn, D. A., & Frier, B. M. (1991). Which abilities does the PASAT test? *Personality and Individual Differences*, *10*, 983–987.

Deary, I. J., & Stough, C. (1996). Intelligence and inspection time: Achievements, prospects, and problems. *American Psychologist*, *6*, 599–608.

DeLuca, J., Barbieri-Berger, S., & Johnson, S. K. (1994). The nature of memory impairments in multiple sclerosis: Acquisition versus retrieval. *Journal of Clinical and Experimental Neuropsychology*, *16* (2), 183–189.

DeLuca, J., Gaudino, E. A., Diamond, B. J., Christodoulou, C., & Engel, R. A. (1998). Acquisition and storage deficits in multiple sclerosis. *Journal of Clinical and Experimental Neuropsychology*, *20* (3), 376–390.

Demaree, H. A., DeLuca, J., Gaudino, E. A., & Diamond, B. J. (1999). Speed of information processing as a key deficit in multiple sclerosis: Implications for rehabilitation. *Journal of Neurology, Neurosurgery, and Psychiatry*, *67*, 661–663.

DeSousa, E. A., Albert, R. H., & Kalman, B. (2002). Cognitive impairment in multiple sclerosis: A review. *American Journal of Alzheimer's Disease and Other Dementias*, *17*, 23–29.

Diamond, S. (1977). Francis Galton and American psychology. *Annals of the New York Academy of Sciences*, *291*, 47–55.

Donders, J., Tulsky, D. S., & Zhu, J. (2001). Criterion validity of the new WAIS-III subtest scores after traumatic brain injury. *Journal of the International Neuropsychological Society*, *7*, 892–898.

Egan, V. (1988). PASAT: Observed correlations with IQ. *Personality and Individual Differences, 9,* 179–180.

Ekstrom, R. B., French, J. W., Harman, H. H., & Dirmen, D. (1976). *Manual for kit of factor-referenced cognitive tests* (3rd ed.). Princeton, NJ: Educational Testing Service.

Elliott, C. D. (1990). *Differential Ability Scales.* San Antonio, TX: Psychological Corporation.

Eysenck, H. J. (1987). Speed of information processing, reaction time, and the theory of intelligence. In P. A. Vernon (Ed.), *Speed of information processing and intelligence* (pp. 21–68). Norwood, NJ: Ablex Publishing Corp.

Fancher, R.E. (1985). *The intelligence men: Makers of the IQ controversy.* New York: W. W. Norton.

Feldman, G. M., Kelly, R. M., & Diehl, V. A. (2004). An interpretative analysis of five commonly used processing speed measures. *Journal of Psychoeducational Assessment, 22,* 151–163.

Flanagan, D. P., & Harrison, P. L. (Eds.). (2005). *Contemporary intellectual assessment: Theories, tests, and issues.* New York: Guilford Press.

Fletcher, R. (1991). *Science, ideology, and the media.* New Brunswick, NJ: Transaction.

Gaudino, E. A., Chiaravalloti, N. D., DeLuca, J., & Diamond, B. J. (2001). A comparison of memory performance in relapsing-remitting, primary progressive and secondary progressive, multiple sclerosis. *Neuropsychiatry, Neuropsychology and Behavioral Neurology, 14* (1), 32–44.

Gould, S. J. (1981). *The mismeasure of man.* W. W. Norton.

Gronwall, D., & Wrightson, P. (1981). Memory and information processing capacity after closed head injury. *Journal of Neurology, Neurosurgery, and Psychiatry, 44,* 889–895.

Hawkins, K. A. (1998). Indicators of brain dysfunction derived from graphic representations of the WAIS-III/WMS-III technical manual clinical samples data: A preliminary approach to clinical utility. *Clinical Neuropsychologist, 12,* 535–551.

Horn, J. L. (1991). Measurement of intellectual capabilities: A review of theory. In K. S. McGrew, J. K. Werder, & R. W. Woodcock, *WJ-R technical manual* (pp. 197–232). Chicago: Riverside.

Jensen, A. R. (1981). *Straight talk about mental tests.* New York: Free Press.

Jensen, A. R. (1998a). Jensen on "Jensenism." *Intelligence, 26,* 181–208.

Jensen, A. R. (1998b). Information processing and g. In A. R. Jensen, *The g factor: The science of mental ability* (pp. 203–269). Westport, CT: Praeger.

Jensen, A. R. (2006). *Clocking the mind: Mental chronometry and individual differences.* Oxford, UK: Elsevier Science.

Joynson, R. B. (1989). *The Burt affair.* New York: Routledge.

Kail, R. (1998). Speed of information processing in patients with multiple sclerosis. *Journal of Clinical and Experimental Neuropsychology, 20,* 98–106.

Kalmar, J. H., Bryant, D., Tulsky, D., & DeLuca, J. (2004). Information processing deficits in multiple sclerosis: Does choice of screening instrument make a difference? *Rehabilitation Psychology, 49,* 213–218.

Kalmar, J. H., Gaudino, E. A., Moore, N. B., Halper, J., & DeLuca, J. (submitted). The relationship between cognitive deficits and everyday functional activities in multiple sclerosis.

Kamin, L. J. (1974). *The science and politics of IQ.* Potomac, MD: Lawrence Erlbaum Associates, Inc.

Leahy, B. J., & Lam, C. S. (1998). Neuropsychological testing and functional outcome for individuals with traumatic brain injury. *Brain Injury, 12,* 1025–1035.

Lengenfelder, J., Bryant, D., Diamond, B. J., Kalmar, J. H., Moore, N. B., & DeLuca, J. (2006). Processing speed interacts with working memory efficiency in multiple sclerosis. *Archives of Clinical Neuropsychology, 21,* 229–238.

Madigan, N. K., DeLuca, J., Diamond, B., Tramontano, G., & Averill, A. (2000). Speed of information processing in traumatic brain injury: A modality specific impairment? *Journal of Head Trauma Rehabilitation, 15,* 943–956.

Martin, T. A., Donders, J., & Thompson, E. (2000). Potential of and problems with new measures of psychometric intelligence after traumatic brain injury. *Rehabilitation Psychology, 45,* 402–408.

Mathias, J. L., Bigler, E. D., Jones, N. R., Bowden, S. C., Barrett-Woodbridge, M., Brown, G. C., et al. (2004). Neuropsychological and information processing performance and its relationship to white matter changes following moderate and severe traumatic brain injury: A preliminary study. *Applied Neuropsychology, 11,* 134–152.

McGrew, K. S. (2005). The Cattell-Horn-Carroll theory of cognitive abilities: Past, present and future. In D. P. Flanagan & P. L. Harrison (Eds), *Contemporary intellectual assessment* (pp. 185–202). New York: Guilford Press.

McGue, M., Bouchard, T. J., Lykken, D. T., & Feuer, D. (1984). Information processing abilities in twins reared apart. *Intelligence, 8,* 239–258.

Neisser, U., Boodoo, G., Bouchard, T. J., Boykin, A. W., Brody, N. Ceci, S. J., et al. (1996). Intelligence: Knowns and unknowns. *American Psychologist, 51,* 77–101.

Nettelbeck, T. (1987). Inspection time and intelligence. In P. A. Vernon (Ed.), *Speed of information processing and intelligence* (pp. 295–346). Norwood, NJ: Ablex Publishing Corp.

Nettelbeck, T. (2001). Correlation between inspection time and psychometric abilities. A personal interpretation. *Intelligence, 29,* 459–474.

Osmon, D. C., & Jackson, R. (2002). Inspection time and IQ fluid or perceptual aspects of intelligence? *Intelligence, 30,* 119–127.

Plucker, J. (2003). Available at http://www.indiana.edu/~intell/wisslers.shtml.

Ponsford, J., & Kinsella, G. (1992). Attentional deficits following closed head injury. *Journal of Clinical and Experimental Neuropsychology, 14,* 822–838.

Prifitera, A., Weiss, L. G., & Saklofske, D. H. (1998). The WISC-III in context. In A. Prifitera & D. H. Saklofske (Eds.), *WISC-III: Clinical use and interpretation.* San Diego, CA: Academic Press.

Psychological Corporation (2002). *WAIS-III and WMS-III technical manual.* San Antonio, TX: Psychological Corporation.

Rao, S. (1991). Cognitive function in patients with multiple sclerosis: Impairment and treatment. *International Journal of MS Care, 1,* 9–22.

Ross, D. (1972). *Stanley Hall: The psychologist as prophet.* Chicago: Chicago University Press.

Rushton, J. P., & Ankey, C. D. (1996). Brain size. *Psychnomic Bulletin and Review, 3* (1), 21–36.

Salthouse, T. A. (1996). The processing speed of theory of adult age differences in cognition. *Psychological Review, 103,* 403–428.

Seligman, D. (2002). Good breeding. *National Review, 54* (1), 53–54.

Sherman, E. M. S., Strauss, E., & Spellacy, F. (1997). Validity of the Paced Auditory Serial Addition Test (PASAT) in adults referred for neuropsychological assessment after head injury. *Clinical Neuropsychologist, 11,* 34–45.

Snyder, P. J., Cappelleri, J. C., Archibald, C. J., & Fisk, J. D. (2001). Improved detection of differential information processing speed deficits between two disease-course types of multiple sclerosis. *Neuropsychology, 15*, 617–625.

Sokal, M. M. (1980). Science and James McKeen Cattell, 1894–1945. *Science, 209*, 43–52.

Sokal, M. M. (1987). James McKeen Cattell and mental anthropometry: Nineteenth-century science and reform and the origins of psychological testing. In M. M. Sokal (Ed.), *Psychological testing and American society 1890–1930* (pp. 21–45). New Brunswick, NJ: Rutgers University Press.

Sokal, M. M. (1994). James McKeen Cattell, the New York Academy of Sciences and the American Psychological Association, 1891–1902. *Annals of the New York Academy of Sciences, 727*, 13–35.

Sokal, M. M., Davis, A. B., & Merzbach, U. C. (1976). Laboratory instruments in the history of psychology. *Journal of the History of the Behavioral Sciences, 12*, 59–64.

Spearman, C. (1904). "General intelligence": Objectively determined and measured. *American Journal of Psychology, 15*, 201–292.

Sternberg, R. J. (1990). *Metaphors of mind: Conceptions of the nature of intelligence*. Cambridge: Cambridge University Press.

Stuss, D. T., Stethem L. L., Hugenholtz, H., Picton T., Pivik J., & Richard M. T. (1989). Reaction time after head injury: Fatigue, divided and focused attention, and consistency of performance. *Journal of Neurology, Neurosurgery, and Psychiatry, 52*, 742–748.

Tulsky, D. S., & Price, L. R. (2003). The joint WAIS-III and WMS-III factor structure: Development and cross-validation of a six-factor model of cognitive functioning. *Psychological Assessment, 15* (2), 149–162.

Tulsky, D. S., Saklofske, D. H., & Ricker, J. (2003a). Historical overview of intelligence and memory: Factors influencing the Wechsler Scales. In D. S. Tulsky, D. H. Saklofske, G. J. Chelune, R. K. Heaton, R. J. Ivnik, R. Bornstein, et al., *Clinical interpretation of the WAIS-III and WMS-III*. San Diego, CA: Academic Press.

Tulsky, D. S., Saklofske, D. H., & Zhu, J. (2003b). Revising a standard: An evaluation of the origin and development of the WAIS-III. In D. S. Tulsky, D. H. Saklofske, G. J. Chelune, R. K. Heaton, R. J. Ivnik, R. Bornstein, et al., *Clinical interpretation of the WAIS-III and WMS-III* (pp. 43–93). San Diego, CA: Academic Press.

Vernon, P. A. (1985). Individual differences in general cognitive ability. In L. C. Hartlage & C. F. Telzrow (Eds.), *The neuropsychology of individual differences: A developmental perspective*. New York: Plenum.

Vernon, P. A. (Ed.). (1987). *Speed of information processing and intelligence*. Norwood, NJ: Ablex Publishing Corp.

Vernon. P. A., & Kantor, L. (1986). Reaction time correlations with intelligence test scores obtained under either timed or untimed conditions. *Intelligence, 10*, 315–330.

Walhovd, K. B., Fjell, A. M., Reinvang, I., Lundervold, A., Fischl, B., Salat, D., et al. (2005). Cortical volume and speed-of-processing are complementary in prediction of performance intelligence. *Neuropsychologia, 43*, 704–713.

Warren, H. C. (1934). *Dictionary of psychology*. Boston: Houghton-Mifflin.

Wechsler, D. (1939). *Wechsler-Bellevue Intelligence Scale*. New York: Psychological Corporation.

Wechsler, D. (1946). *Wechsler-Bellevue Intelligence Scale—Form II*. New York: Psychological Corporation.

Wechsler, D. (1955). *Wechsler Adult Intelligence Scale*. New York: Psychological Corporation.

Wechsler, D. (1981). *Wechsler Adult Intelligence Scale—Revised*. New York: Psychological Corporation.

Wechsler, D. (1991). *Wechsler Intelligence Scale for Children—Third Edition*. San Antonio, TX: Psychological Corporation.

Wechsler, D. (1997). *Wechsler Adult Intelligence Scale—Third Edition*. San Antonio, TX: Psychological Corporation.

Wickett, J. C., Vernon, P. A., & Lee, D. H. (1994). In vivo brain size, head perimeter, and intelligence in a sample of healthy adult females. *Personality and Individual Difference, 16*, 831–838.

Wickett, J. C., Vernon, P. A., & Lee, D. H. (2000). Relationships between factors of intelligence and brain volume. *Personality and Individual Differences, 29*, 1095–1122.

Wills, S., & Leathem, J. (2004). The effects of test anxiety, age, intelligence level, and arithmetic ability on Paced Auditory Serial Addition Test performance. *Applied Neuropsychology, 11*, 178–185.

Woodcock, R. W., & Johnson, M. B. (1989). *Woodcock–Johnson Psycho-Educational Battery—Revised*. Allen, TX: DLM.

Zhu, J., & Weiss, L. (2005). The Wechsler scales. In D. P. Flanagan & P. L. Harrison (Eds.), *Contemporary intellectual assessment* (pp. 297–324). New York: Guilford Press.

2 Assessment tools and research methods for human information processing speed

Thomas A. Martin and Shane S. Bush

An interest in measuring processing speed (PS) has been prevalent since the early days of psychology. For example, while investigating individual differences in mental ability, British scientist Sir Frances Galton, theorized that higher intelligence is a result of faster "mental speed" (Galton, 1883). Although his attempts to demonstrate an association between reaction time (RT) and IQ were unsuccessful, subsequent research suggests that differences in psychometric intelligence may be largely dependent on mental speed (Eysenck, 1986; Jensen, 1982; Vernon, 1987; see Deary & Stough, 1996 for a review). As psychology's appreciation of the relationship between PS and intelligence has evolved, efforts to refine PS as a construct and to identify the variables that contribute to individual differences in PS have been undertaken. This line of research suggests that PS is related to a number of factors, including age, education, gender, and intelligence (Barrett, Eysenck, & Lucking, 1986; Brittain, La Marche, Reeder, Roth, & Boll, 1991; Stuss, Stethem, & Pelchat, 1988; Wiens, Fuller, & Crossen, 1997). The reader is referred to chapter 1 in this book for a review of PS and intelligence.

The field of psychology has investigated the vulnerability of PS to aging and various neurological disorders. For example, diminished speed of processing has been found to be associated with normal aging, with this decrease in PS noted to be a significant contributor to age-related decline of other cognitive domains (Salthouse & Coon, 1993; Sliwinski & Bushke, 1997). PS has also been found to be compromised by a number of neurocognitive disorders, including chronic fatigue syndrome, dementia, traumatic brain injury, symptomatic HIV, Parkinson's disease and multiple sclerosis (Chiaravalloti, Christodoulou, Demaree, & DeLuca, 2003; DeLuca, Christodoulou, Diamond, Rosenstein, Kramer, & Natelson, 2004; Demaree, DeLuca, Guadino, & Diamond, 1999; Lezak, 1995; Llorente et al., 1998; Madigan, DeLuca, Diamond, Tramontano, & Averill, 2000; Martin, Donders, & Thompson, 2000; Sawamoto, Honda, Hanakawa, Fukuyama, & Shibasaki, 2002; Tiersky, Johnson, Lange, Natelson, & DeLuca, 1997).

Growing awareness of the vulnerability of PS to aging and neurological insult has fueled efforts to identify the impact that declining speed of processing has on cognitive functioning. This research has found that impaired PS contributes to deficits in a number of cognitive domains, including information processing, working memory, long-term episodic memory, verbal abilities, and visuospatial skills (DeLuca, Barbieri-Berger, & Johnson, 1994; DeLuca, Gaudino, Diamond, Christodoulou, & Engel, 1998; Demaree et al., 1999; Sherman, Strauss, & Spellacy, 1997).

Given the deleterious influence impaired PS has on multiple cognitive domains, it is not surprising that decreased speed of processing has been found to contribute to compromised functional status. For instance, deficits in information processing and memory functioning have been found to adversely affect the functional status of persons with multiple sclerosis, independent of demographic or physical disability variables (Kessler, Cohen, Lauer, & Kausch, 1992; Shawaryn, Schultheis, Garay, & DeLuca, 2002).

Over the years, psychology's efforts to interpret and measure PS have yielded exciting findings that have shaped our understanding of intelligence. Given the importance of PS with regard to cognitive functioning and quality of life, and the known vulnerability of PS to aging and neurological insult, the field of psychology is likely to continue in its investigation and assessment of this construct. An appropriate appreciation of psychology's current understanding of PS, and the research methods and clinical tools that have been used to assess PS, will facilitate this endeavor. Accordingly, this chapter provides an overview of the current conceptualization of PS, followed by a review of the strengths and weaknesses of the research methods and assessment tools that have been used to measure PS. Ensuing discussion examines how research methods and clinical tools can be used to facilitate the rehabilitation of PS deficits, and identifies challenges for the future.

Conceptualization of processing speed

A rich history of experimental and clinical research has led to the current conceptualization of PS. Along the way, these efforts have also contributed to some confusion regarding the meaning of this construct and how it is affected by neurological insult. For example, varied terminology, including complex attention, mental speed, reaction time, inspection time, and information processing have all been used to define how fast information is processed cognitively. Similarly, the labeling of clinical tools that assess multiple cognitive domains as measures of PS has led to inconsistent findings regarding the vulnerability of PS to disease (e.g., DeLuca, Chelune, Tulsky, Legenfelder, & Chiaravalloti, 2004).

Although the term "information processing" has been used to refer to PS, this construct can be viewed as a broader concept that incorporates both working memory (WM) and PS (Archibald & Fisk, 2000). While WM refers to a limited capacity memory system that provides temporary storage to manipulate information for complex cognitive tasks (Baddeley, 1986: Baddeley & Hitch, 1994), PS refers to either the time required to execute a cognitive task or the amount or work that can be completed within a finite period of time (J. DeLuca, personal communication, July 14, 2005). While most processing of information is probably a reflection of both WM and PS, it is clear that WM and PS are not identical constructs, and that not all tasks that are dependent on PS involve WM. The individuality of these constructs is supported by developmental research that has found that these abilities develop largely independently of one another and mature at different points during adolescence (Luna, Garver, Urban, Lazar, & Sweeney, 2004). However, this research also suggests that these abilities are related, as the development of WM is modestly influenced by PS, with faster processing of information thought to contribute to more efficient encoding in WM. These findings lend support for the theory that compromised PS associated with aging and neurological insult is a primary contributor to deficits in WM and other cognitive abilities (DeLuca et al., 2004; Salthouse, 1996).

Psychology's understanding of PS has also been complicated by the tendency of clinical tools to assess multiple cognitive domains simultaneously. While it could be argued that any task with a speeded component places some demand on PS, the clinical tools typically employed to assess PS also tap other cognitive domains, including attention, WM, and motor and sensory functioning. While the simultaneous assessment of multiple cognitive domains is largely unavoidable given the integrative nature of the human central nervous system, it becomes the task of the clinician to identify the multiple domains being assessed and appreciate how these various influences have contributed to the findings. For example, DeLuca and colleagues (DeLuca, Chelune, et al., 2004) noted that virtually all of the research studies examining the PS ability of individuals with multiple sclerosis have employed clinical methodology that included a significant WM component. This methodology complicates the interpretation of findings and can have treatment implications, as the rehabilitation of WM and PS requires different treatment interventions.

The construct PS may itself be a source of confusion for understanding the ability it is supposed to represent. For example, Salthouse (1993) made a distinction between motor speed, which often requires minimal cognitive demands, and cognitive processing speed, which demands more cognitive energy. Similarly, recent research has identified two distinct forms of PS, "simple" and "complex" PS, with "complex" information PS being largely distinct from tests of simple and complex reaction time (Chiaravalloti et al., 2003). The authors concluded that PS is not a unitary construct and that the distinct forms of PS should be assessed with different neuropsychological measures.

While PS can be defined as the execution time needed to complete a cognitive task, or the amount of work that can be completed within a finite period of time, a working conceptualization of this construct demands an appreciation of how PS operates and interacts with other cognitive abilities. Salthouse (1996) postulated that the speed with which an individual performs a cognitive activity is a reflection of their ability to carry out many different types of processing operations. He offers two distinct mechanisms for understanding how diminished speed of processing can compromise intellectual functioning, the *limited time mechanism* and the *simultaneity mechanism*. The *limited time mechanism* indicates that slower speed of executing many processing operations means that less processing can be completed in a given amount of time. The *simultaneity mechanism* refers to the notion that products from early processing may no longer be available by the time later processing is completed. Through these two mechanisms, it is hypothesized that slowed PS diminishes the encoding strength of information, resulting in a cascade of inadequate learning that contributes to poor recall and recognition (Kail, 1997, 1998; Kail & Salthouse, 1994). This explanation of how slow PS impacts other cognitive domains provides a framework for conceptualizing PS and its relationship with other cognitive abilities.

Research methods used to assess speed of information processing

According to Salthouse (2000) a number of different experimental methods have been employed to assess PS, with these procedures varying according to the research tradition. For instance, psychometric researchers have tended to rely on measures of perceptual and decision speed. *Perceptual speed* refers to the speed of responding to simple test content in which errorless performance would be expected if there were no time limit (e.g., elementary comparison and search and substitution operations). Comparatively *decision speed* refers to the time utilized to respond in cognitive tests with moderately complex content. Given the cognitive demands of the task, response errors would be expected even in the absence of time restrictions. Both psychometric and experimental researches have frequently utilized relatively simple tasks (e.g., reaction time tasks), such as repetitive finger tapping, to assess *psychomotor speed*. *Psychophysical speed* has also been examined by looking at decision accuracy following briefly presented auditory or visual stimuli (e.g., inspection time tasks). Lastly, psychophysiological researchers have utilized methods thought to reflect the *time course of internal responses*, such as measuring the latency of particular aspects of event-related potentials (Salthouse, 2000).

Letter and pattern comparison are two frequently used experimental measures of perceptual speed that were developed by Salthouse and Babcock (1991). Since their inception these tests have been used by a number of experimental researchers (e.g., Hedden, Lautenschlager, & Park, 2005), with subtle differences in administration sometimes noted between studies (Salthouse, 1993). Assessing PS via elementary comparison, letter and pattern comparisons are paper and pencil tests that are very similar in design and administration. Within each test, there are three separately timed sections (30-second time limit for each section), with each successive section offering letter or pattern strings of increased length. For example, in the letter comparison test, an examinee is presented with pairs of letter strings consisting of three, six, or nine letters each. The examinee is required to quickly determine if the two letter strings are the same or different, and to respond by writing an S or a D on the answer sheet. Pattern comparison is identical to letter comparison except that the examinee is presented with pairs of line drawings consisting of three, six, or nine line segments. The total score for both measures reflects the number of correct responses that are provided within the time limit for all three trials. Consistent with typical measures of perceptual speed, letter and pattern comparisons employ a relatively simple task that must be completed in a limited amount of time. Despite the simplicity of their respective tasks, letter and pattern comparisons tap a number of cognitive domains in addition to PS, including visual and motor functioning and WM.

As noted previously, reaction and inspection time studies are two research paradigms that have frequently been used to assess speed of processing. Reaction time (RT) can be broadly defined as the amount of time between a stimulus and a response. Psychologists have utilized three basic types of reaction time experiments (Luce, 1986; Welford, 1980). In *simple* reaction time experiments, there is a single stimulus and single response (e.g., press a button in response to a light). In *recognition* reaction time experiments, there are certain stimuli that should be responded to, while other stimuli should be ignored (e.g., symbol recognition tasks). In *choice* reaction time experiments, the examinee must give a response that corresponds to an identified stimulus; such as pressing a specific key in response to the display of a corresponding letter on a computer screen (Kosinski, 2005).

Dutch physiologist, Francisco Donders (1868), was one of the first scientists to systematically assess RT. He reasoned that the time required for a mental process could be identified by subtracting the RT of a simple task from the time needed to complete a more complex task that incorporated the easier task as part of the activity. Donders believed that the time difference indicated how much time was needed for the added element of complexity. It was later argued that the subtraction method was problematic for a number of reasons, including its assumption that the sum of a task is equal to the individual parts of the activity (Boring, 1952). In fact, adding another task to an activity may substantially increase the difficulty level of the activity, thereby altering the entire process. These issues of subtraction (or relative deviation scores) to assess "pure" processing speed continue today (Heaton, Nelson, Thompson, Burks, & Franklin, 1985; Lamberty, Putnam, Chatel, Bieliauskas, & Adams, 1994). Nonetheless, Donders was a pioneer in the study of RT and was able to demonstrate that simple reaction time is shorter than a recognition reaction time, and that choice reaction time is the longest of all (Kosinski, 2005).

Subsequent research has confirmed that reaction to sound is faster than reaction to light (Brebner & Welford, 1980; Welford, 1980; Woodworth & Schlosberg, 1954). This speed difference is probably related to the fact that an auditory stimulus takes 8–10 milliseconds to reach the brain (Kemp, 1973), while a visual stimulus can take 20–40 milliseconds (Marshall, Talbot, &

Ades 1943). These differences in RT between stimuli are noted to persist whether the examinee is asked to make a simple or a complex response (Kosinski, 2005; Sanders, 1998).

RT variables also have a long history of use in studies of human cognitive aging, and in research on the information processing foundations of psychometric intelligence (e.g., Deary & Der, 2005). This area of investigation has frequently utilized the Ravens Progressive Matrices (Raven, Court, & Raven, 1982) as a measure of psychometric intelligence. Not surprisingly, RT has demonstrated a moderate but consistent negative correlation with psychometric intelligence. That is, higher psychometric intelligence is associated with lower (i.e., quicker) reaction times (Neubauer, 1997; Neubauer, Spinath, Riemann, Angleitner, & Borkenau, 2000).

While the long history of experimental designs using RT methods to assess PS suggests that these research paradigms will continue to be used in the future, it is important to note that RT is affected by a number of variables. In addition to the sensory modality utilized for stimulus processing (e.g., auditory vs. visual), RT has been found to be influenced by stimulus intensity, the use of direct versus peripheral vision, and individual variables such as arousal level, age, gender, fatigue, breathing cycle, personality, brain injury and psychiatric illness (Brebner, 1980; Brebner & Welford, 1980; Buchsbaum & Callaway, 1965; Collins et al., 2003; Deary & Der, 2005; Kosinski, 2005; Lenzenweger, 2001; Luce, 1986; Welford, 1980). Additionally, the nature of RT tasks (e.g., requiring an examinee response) makes them inherently vulnerable to confounds associated with carrying out the response activity (e.g., motor speed). Thus the interpretation of RT as a measure of PS must be done with caution.

Inspection time (IT) studies are another popular paradigm that has been used to investigate PS. In contrast to RT paradigms, IT is not based on response latencies but rather on accuracy rate as a function of the length of time a stimulus is presented (Chaiken & Young, 1993). More simply, IT is the briefest target stimulus duration needed to achieve a specified accuracy rate, which is often set at 97.5% (Nettelbeck, 1982). The typical IT procedure includes the presentation of a target stimulus (e.g., two vertical lines of different length), with the examinee instructed to indicate which line is longer. The offset of the stimulus is immediately followed by the onset of an overlapping backward-masking figure that closely resembles the target. Stimulus exposure typically occurs for a fixed number of trials that occur for durations of time that are varied randomly from trial to trial. Stimulus exposure typically ranges between 20 and 180 milliseconds. The examinee's percentage of correct responses is plotted against stimulus exposure duration, with IT identified as the briefest duration of time needed to achieve the predetermined level of response accuracy (Vickers & Smith, 1986).

Because IT paradigms ignore the examinee's speed of responding to a stimulus, IT is believed to offer a purer measure of PS as compared to RT measures, which are confounded by motor speed and executive processes (e.g., decision-making time) (Osmon & Jackson, 2002). Accordingly, IT paradigms have been conceptualized as research strategies designed to isolate a general dimension of information processing that is thought to be free from the influence of higher order cognitive activities (Brand & Deary, 1982; Deary & Stough, 1996). Similar to RT, IT has been found to correlate strongly with psychometric intelligence (Bates & Rock, 2004; Deary & Stough, 1996; Stough, Brebner, Nettelbeck, Cooper, Bates, & Mangan, 1996). However, despite the elimination of motor speed as a confounding factor, IT has been found to be related predominantly to the performance intelligence quotient (PIQ) of the Wechsler Adult Intelligence Scales (Psychological Corporation, 1997), with little relationship to the verbal intelligence quotient (VIQ) (e.g., Deary, 1993, Nettelbeck, 1987). This strong correlation with PIQ has led some authors (e.g., Deary & Stough, 1996; Nettelbeck & Rabbitt, 1992) to suggest that IT is a measure of the fluid aspects of intelligent behavior (Horn & Cattell, 1967). However, the fact that PIQ subtests, and other measures (e.g., Raven's Progressive Matrices) that are frequently compared to IT, also tap into visual processing raises the question that IT may be related to visual aspects of intelligence. Support for this theory was provided by a confirmatory factor analytic study (Crawford, Deary, Allan, & Gustafsson, 1998). These investigators found that visual IT could be better explained by a model that incorporated both general intelligence and an orthogonal visual processes aspect of intelligence.

Osmon and Jackson (2002) examined whether IT was related more to visual perceptual abilities or to basic neuronal efficiency processing that is represented in fluid intelligence. Their findings suggested that IT is related to fluid intelligence, with the relationship between IT and visual processing eliminated when the common variance between visual processes and fluid intelligence is controlled. They concluded that the relationship between IT and fluid intelligence reflects some fundamental underlying aspect of intelligence, such as neural processing efficiency. However, not all authors agree that IT is a measure of fluid intelligence. For instance, IT has been conceptualized as representing a class of visual tasks sharing the characteristic that they require identification of a highly distinctive target under time constraints (Burns, Nettelbeck, & Cooper, 1999; Burns, Nettelbeck, & White, 1998; Burns, Nettelbeck, White, & Wilson, 1999). This conceptualization suggests that IT will share variance with tests that define a broad general speediness factor (Burns, 1998; Burns, Nettelbeck, & Cooper, 1999; Nettelbeck, 1994). Working to alleviate design weaknesses that had been identified in prior research studies used to investigate the relationship between IT and intelligence, Burns and Nettelbeck (2003) once again examined the relationship between IT and fluid intelligence. Their results were consistent with their previous findings that suggested IT is not a measure of fluid intelligence, but rather a measure of a broad general speediness factor.

Just as there are questions about what IT represents, there is dispute about what factors contribute to the differences in IT between individuals. For example, there is debate as to whether individual differences in IT are related to high-level cognitive strategies, learning, motivation, or the result of low-level "basic" information processing limitations (Deary, Simonotto, et al., 2001). In an attempt to shed light on this topic and further extend the biological study of IT, Deary and colleagues (Deary, Simonotto, et al., 2001) conducted a pilot study in which they had seven healthy adult participants (with high levels of education) undergo functional magnetic resonance imaging (fMRI) of the brain while they were performing an IT task. They theorized that given the association between IT and intelligence, performance of an inspection task would result in activation of brain areas that have been found to be active when individuals are completing common psychometric measures. For example, the cingulate gyrus, lateral areas of the frontal lobes, and areas related to the executive control of working memory have been found to be activated by psychometric tests, such as the Paced Auditory Serial Addition Task and the Raven's Progressive Matrices (Deary et al., 1994; Duncan et al., 2000; Prabhakaran, Smith, Desmond, Glover, & Gabrieli, 1997). Consistent with their expectations, the authors found that their IT task resulted in a widespread pattern of significant brain activation that included those areas of the brain that are involved in higher level cognitive processing.

Overall, it is clear that the investigation of IT has enriched our understanding of intelligence and information processing. It is hopeful that ongoing research will further clarify what IT represents and identify the factors that account for the variability of IT between individuals. While IT paradigms, compared to RT paradigms, may offer a purer measure of PS, it is important to note that confounding variables may also influence IT. For instance, there is evidence that central cholinergic pathways influence IT (Deary, Hunter, Langan, & Goodwin, 1991). Consistent with this assertion, patients with Alzheimer's disease (and diminished cholinergic function) have been found to have significantly reduced IT (Deary et al., 1991), while pharmacologically increased cholinergic transmission has been found to improve IT (Hutchison, Nathan, Mrazek, & Stough, 2001). Additionally, glucose levels can affect PS, with moderate levels of hypoglycemia known to adversely impact both IT and RT (Ewing, Deary, McCrimmon, Strachan, & Frier, 1998; McCrimmon, Deary, Huntly, MacLeod, & Frier, 1996).

Investigation of the underlying neurophysiology of PS has been initiated, with the latencies of event related electrophysiological potentials (ERPs) identified as a means to carry out this line of research (Deary, Der, & Ford, 2001). While studies have identified a moderate relationship between intelligence and the ERP component P300 (Bazana & Stelmack, 2002), disagreement exists regarding the exact cognitive significance of the P300. Nonetheless, it has been argued that P300 latency represents the timing of a cognitive process and can be regarded as a measure of PS (Walhovd et al., 2005). While studies investigating speed of processing defined by an ERP component have been conducted (Walhovd et al., 2005), and may prove useful in identifying the neurophysiological basis of PS, this line of research is yet in its infancy.

Clinical tools used to assess speed of information processing

While there is a long history of experimental research on PS, its application clinically is relatively recent. Neuropsychological measures that have been utilized to assess PS include the Paced Auditory Serial Addition Test (PASAT) (Kalmar, Bryant, Tulsky, & DeLuca, 2004), the Digit Symbol-Coding subtest from the Wechsler Adult Intelligence Scale (Krupp, Sliwinski, Masur, Friedberg, & Coyle, 1994), the Trail Making Test (Azouvi, Jokic, Van der Linden, Marlier, & Bussel, 1996), and various RT measures (Collins & Long, 1996). While sharing a common goal, measures used in the assessment of PS employ a number of different task demands and thus also measure cognitive constructs other than PS. For example, the PASAT requires the ongoing manipulation of information, while simple RT measures require persistent attention to a single stimulus (Chiaravalloti et al., 2003).

Because clinical tools typically assess multiple cognitive domains simultaneously, when assessing PS, clinicians should consider the assessment goals and select measures accordingly. That is, choose tests that target "primarily" PS or WM, or both WM and PS (Kalmar et al., 2004), as appropriate, to meet the needs of each evaluation. Additionally, it is important to be aware of test characteristics that may influence findings. For example, many of the clinical tools that have been developed to assess PS require intact motor and visual functioning, and place demands on executive processes (e.g., decision-making). The following clinical tools are reviewed because they have been identified as measures of PS and are used with relative frequency in clinical practice.

The Adult Memory and Information Processing Battery (AMIPB) includes a test of information PS that consists of 105 rows of five numbers. The examinee is instructed to cross out the second highest number in each row. The total score is the number of correct answers completed within a 4-minute time limit. The task is considered to be minimally stressful and relatively easy to perform. Investigation of a modified version of this measure (e.g., enlarged print size, reduced number of stimuli, acceptance of a verbal response) provided preliminary support for this test as a reliable and feasible assessment of speed of information processing in individuals with multiple sclerosis. However, it is important to note that the demands associated with this test require a motor or verbal response and also tap WM functioning. The authors conclude that the utility of the AMIPB as a simple measure of one aspect of cognitive functioning has yet to be established (Vlaar & Wade, 2003).

The PASAT (Gronwall, 1977) has been used in clinical and experimental settings as a measure of speed of information processing, attention, and concentration (O'Donnell, MacGregor, Dabrowski, Oestreicher, & Romero, 1994). Traditional administration includes presentation of four audiotaped recorded series of 61 single-digit numbers. The examinee is required to add each digit to the digit immediately preceding it, and to announce the total after each of the 60 pairs. Each series is presented at a fixed rate, with the speed of presentation increasing for each successive series. Performance on each of the four trials is scored as the total number of correct responses. Performance on the PASAT is dependent on a number of cognitive processes, including WM to maintain and manipulate the numbers, and speed of processing because examinees are provided limited time to process the information and respond. Accordingly, impaired performance on the PASAT can result from deficits in WM, slow speed of information processing, or both (Bryant, Diamond, & DeLuca, 2003; Kalmar et al., 2004).

The PASAT has been found to be sensitive to changes in PS associated with neurological insult (e.g., DeLuca, Chelune et al., 2004), and it has been noted to load on the same factor as the Symbol Digit Modalities Test (see below) in a sample of individuals with severe head injury (Haslam, Batchelor, Fearnside, Haslam, & Hawkins, 1995). While the PASAT it is not confounded by visuomotor factors, it is dependent on auditory functioning. Additionally, it demands a fast speech response, which may prevent its use with individuals who have speech impairment or dysarthria. Also, the PASAT may be inappropriate for persons with low cognitive functioning or who have mathematical deficits (Sherman et al., 1997). Lastly, some examinees may become anxious during the task and experience the test as stressful, although recent data suggest that such anxiety has little impact on performance (Wills & Leathem, 2004). It has also been suggested that the PASAT may be particularly challenging and frustrating for older individuals who are cognitively impaired (Woodard & Axelrod, 2005).

Successive subtraction of 7 starting from 100 (Serial 7s) and reciting the alphabet backwards (Alphabet Backwards) have been included in neuropsychological test batteries as measures of complex attention and speed of information processing (LaMarche, Alexander, Stanford, Beth, Dolske, & Morthland, 1994; Shum, McFarland, & Bain, 1990). Their brief administration time and the lack of special equipment needed contribute to the utility of these measures, particularly in settings where extensive evaluation is not practical (Williams, LaMarche, Alexander, Stanford, Fielstein, & Boll, 1996). Factor analysis of the Serial 7s and Alphabet Backwards tests, along with other commonly used speeded performance measures (e.g., Symbol Digit Modalities Test and Trail Making Test) identified a factor structure consisting of two factors, visual-motor scanning speed and information PS. It was concluded that the Serial 7s and Alphabet Backwards tests could be seen as time efficient and technically simple measures of PS. However, the authors cautioned that practice and education effects might impact test performance (Williams et al., 1996). Additionally, the task demands associated with Serial 7s and Alphabet Backwards suggest that WM is also probably involved in this processing.

The Stroop Test measures the relative speed of reading names of colors, naming colors, and naming colors used to print an incongruous color name (e.g., the color *green* is used to print the word "blue") (Mitrushina, Boone, & D'Elia, 1999). Many different versions of the Stroop Test exist, with the common versions incorporating a timed performance component. Historically, the Stroop Test has been seen as a measure of executive functioning involving cognitive inhibition (Boone, Miller, Lesser, Hill, & D'Elia, 1990). Factor analysis of sets of executive measures suggested the Stroop Test has more in common with timed executive measures (e.g., verbal fluency) and measures of information PS and WM (e.g., WAIS Digit Symbol-Coding) than executive tests that involve set shifting (e.g., Wisconsin Card Sorting Test) (Boone, 1999; Mitrushina et al., 1999). While the timed performance component of the Stroop Test undoubtedly places demands on PS, it is obvious that it taps multiple cognitive abilities. Accordingly, impaired performance on the Stroop Test cannot be assumed to be an indication of compromised PS.

The Symbol Digit Modalities Test (SDMT; Smith, 1991) is a speeded task that has been used extensively with diverse clinical groups. It requires an examinee to look at a series of nine geometric figures that have each been paired with a number. Test items present the geometric figure only and the examinee must quickly write in the target number that goes with each figure. The score is the number of correct substitutions completed within 90 seconds. The test also allows for an oral administration in which the examinee simply reads off the correct number to the examiner, who records the answers. Unlike the PASAT, the SDMT does not involve the manipulation of information held in short-term memory, and thus has only minimal WM (i.e., phonological loop) involvement. Accordingly, it may be a "purer" measure of PS. The oral administration of the test also provides an assessment of PS that is unaffected by the motor activity associated with writing out the answers, although the verbal output may be influenced by motor-speech factors such as dysarthria.

The Trail Making Test (TMT; Army Individual Test Battery, 1944) is a commonly used neuropsychological assessment instrument (Arbuthnott & Frank, 2000; Reitan & Wolfson, 1993) that consists of two subtests. TMT-A involves drawing a line that connects consecutive numbers from 1 to 25, while TMT-B involves drawing a line connecting alternating numbers and letters in sequence (i.e., 1–A–2–B, etc.). Traditional scoring is the time in seconds required to complete each part of the test. The TMT provides information regarding attention, visual scanning, speed of eye–hand coordination, and information processing (Mitrushina et al., 1999). Parts A and B correlate only .49 with each other (Heilbronner, Henry, Buck, Adams, & Fogle, 1991), with Part B a more demanding task that also assesses the ability to alternate between sets of stimuli. Accordingly, while PS influences performance on both Parts A and B, a number of other factors also impact test performance. An oral version of the TMT is also available in which the examinee simply counts from 1 to 25 (Part A) and then alternates between numbers and letters up to 13 (Part B). The oral and written versions of the TMT have been found to be strongly correlated (Ricker, Axelrod, & Houtler, 1996), with the oral version probably tapping the same multiple cognitive domains as the written test, with the exception of motor speed, but with the added demands associated with producing a verbal response.

The most recent revision of the Wechsler Adult Intelligence Scale (WAIS-III; Psychological Corporation, 1997) includes two subtests that assess the ability to process visual information quickly. The first subtest, Digit Symbol-Coding, is very similar to the SDMT, and consists of a series of numbers each of which is paired with a corresponding symbol. Using this key, the examinee must copy down the symbol that goes with the given number. Total score is the number of correctly identified symbols that are provided within the 120-second time limit. This subtest has been available in former versions of the WAIS, and although it is clearly influenced by motor and WM functions, it is known to be a measure of mental speed (Matarazzo, 1972). Symbol Search is a new subtest introduced with the WAIS-III that requires the examinee to scan two groups of symbols: a target group (composed of two symbols), and a search group (composed of five symbols), and then indicate whether either of the target symbols matches any of the symbols in the search group. The total score is the number of correct responses within the 120-second time limit. In addition to assessing PS, Symbol Search also places demands on motor (minimal) and WM functions. As noted above, each of these tests takes only 2 minutes to administer, and when both tests are completed a Processing Speed Index (PSI) score can be calculated.

As would be expected, the PSI has been found to be sensitive to the effects of normal aging and a variety of neurological conditions (Donders, Tulsky, & Zhu, 2001; Hawkins, 1998; Psychological Corporation, 1997). The WAIS-III is able to provide four index scores and comparison of the PSI to the Perceptual Organization Index is thought to reveal differences between individuals' visual-spatial and fluid reasoning skills and their ability to process information quickly (Psychological Corporation, 1997). A study comparing the PSI to the Working Memory Index (WMI) following traumatic brain injury highlights the uniqueness of these two constructs, as the PSI was found to be sensitive to injury severity, while the WMI was not (Martin et al., 2000). While the PSI is proving to be an efficient and reliable measure of PS, it is important to remember that the tests required to calculate this index score are dependent on visual processing, WM, and motor speed.

Computerized measures of processing speed

The ability of computerized measures to provide highly accurate measurement of simple and complex RT has been viewed as a significant advancement in the field of neuropsychological research (Bleiberg, Kane, Reeves, Garmoe, & Halpern, 2000). Initial investigation of the relationship between select computerized neuropsychological measures and traditional neuropsychological tests found a strong concordance between the measures (Bleiberg et al., 2000). While computerized assessment measures may have advantages over traditional neuropsychological tests used to assess PS (e.g., more exact timing), it is important to note that computerized RT measures, like most traditional RT measures, are dependent on an examinee's visual or sensory functioning and motor speed. Computerized RT measures are also probably influenced by the same confounds noted in the experimental RT literature (e.g., stimulus intensity, the use of direct versus peripheral vision). The following computerized assessment tools have been identified as measures of PS.

ImPACT (Immediate Post-Concussion Assessment and Cognitive Testing; Maroon, Lovell, Norwig, Podell, Powell, & Hartl, 2000) is a computerized neuropsychological test battery that has been used to assess the cognitive functioning of athletes with concussion. Version 2.0 of ImPACT consists of six individual test modules that measure different aspects of cognitive functioning, including RT and PS. The test battery was designed to provide multiple types of information, with each test module contributing to multiple composite scores. The RT composite score represents the average response time on a go/no-go task, a choice reaction time task, and a symbol–number matching task. The PS composite represents the weighted average of three tasks that serve as interference measures for the memory paradigms (e.g., selecting numbered buttons in backward order as quickly as possible) (Iverson, Lovell, & Collins, 2005). In addition to assessing RT and PS, the tasks used to calculate the RT and PS composite scores also place demands on visual and motor functions, and WM. Recent research examining the construct validity of ImPACT with a sample of concussed amateur athletes found a significant correlation between the PS and RT composites and the SDMT, suggesting that all three measures were assessing a similar underlying construct (Iverson et al., 2005).

MicroCog (Powell, Kaplan, Whitla, Weintraub, Catlin, & Funkenstein, 1993) was designed to measure adult cognitive functioning through unsupervised computer administration. The test offers a standard form that consists of 18 subtests or a shortened version consisting of 12 subtests. The standard form yields the following five ability-based domain scores; attention/mental control, memory, reasoning/calculation, spatial processing, and RT. Tasks involve alphabet recitation, abstract reasoning, object matching, story recall, and assessment of RT. The demands associated with these tasks tap multiple domains, including motor and visual functioning and WM. Independent analysis of the factor structure of MicroCog with a clinical sample was consistent with the initial validity examination of a nonclinical sample, supporting a two-factor structure that includes information processing speed and information processing accuracy (Lopez, Summerall, & Ryan, 2002). However, the authors cautioned that much of the variance was left unaccounted for by these two factors and that MicroCog is best viewed as a screening program that does not replace a comprehensive neuropsychological examination.

The Useful Field of Vision test (UFOV; Visual Awareness, Inc., Chicago, IL) is a standardized and commercially available test that quantifies the visual field area (useful field of view) over which the examinee can process rapidly presented information (Ball & Roenker, 1998). The test consists of three subtests: visual information processing, divided attention, and selective attention, which are used to generate an overall composite index. Each subtest consists of visually presented graphics that the examinee must correctly identify after a brief exposure. Tasks become increasingly difficult as distracting visual stimuli are added and exposure time is decreased. Test administration has evolved from the standard version, which was administered via touch screen with the Visual Attention Analyzer, to two newer versions that can be administered with a personal computer (PC) in 15 minutes or less (Edwards, Vance, Wadley, Cissell, Roenker, & Ball, 2005). The PC versions of the test utilize either a touch screen or a mouse response to document an examinee's response. Performance scores calculated in milliseconds for each subtest indicate the length of exposure time required by the individual to process the information accurately. The UFOV test has been found to be predictive of driving competency in older adults and related to their everyday functioning abilities (Edwards et al., 2005; Owsley, McGwin, & Ball, 1998; Sekuler, Bennett, & Mamelak, 2000). While the UFOV test is similar to an IT task in that it assesses the length of exposure time required to accurately assess visually presented stimuli, test performance is dependent on a motor response.

The Visual Threshold Serial Addition Test (VT-SAT; Demaree et al., 1999) sequentially presents a series of 50 single digits on a computer monitor. Administration procedures are similar to the standardized protocol of the PASAT, with the examinee instructed to add each visually presented number to the immediately preceding number and to report the sum aloud. The VT-SAT uses a method-of-limits procedure to determine the rate of stimulus presentation for each participant to achieve a 50% success rate. This rate of presentation, referred to as threshold speed, represents an index of PS while controlling for accuracy of performance. By holding accuracy (i.e., working memory) constant, the VT-SAT may allow for a more direct measure of PS than is provided via traditional administration of the PASAT. Nonetheless, like the PASAT, the VT-SAT is a measure of both PS and WM, and requires a fast speech response. However, while VT-SAT administration is not dependent on hearing ability, it does place demands on the visual system.

Research methods and clinical tools used to facilitate the treatment of processing speed deficits

Research has established the important contribution of PS to cognitive functioning, functional status, and quality of life. For example, compromised PS is believed to contribute to deficits in a number of cognitive domains, including working memory, long-term episodic memory, verbal abilities, and visuospatial skills (DeLuca et al., 1994; DeLuca et al., 1998; Demaree et al., 1999; Sherman et al., 1997). Deficits in PS have also been found to significantly affect the functional status of persons with multiple sclerosis (Kessler et al., 1992), including driving ability (Schultheis, Garay, & DeLuca, 2001; Shawaryn et al., 2002). Additionally, PS deficits are noted to significantly compromise the driving ability of older adults (Edwards et al., 2005).

Given the above findings, it has been suggested that efforts designed to enhance PS in clinical populations may lead to improved functional status and sense of autonomy (Shawaryn et al., 2002). This line of reasoning is gaining support in the literature. For example, UFOV test performance has been found to be enhanced by speed of processing training (Ball, Beard, Roenker, Miller, & Ball, 1988; Ball & Owsley, 2000; Edwards, Wadley, Myers, Roenker, Cissell, & Ball, 2002; Roenker, Cissell, Ball, Wadley, & Edwards, 2003). PS training also led to improved performance on laboratory measures of timed independent activities of daily living and on-the-road driving performance (Ball & Owsley, 2000, Ball, Berch, Helmers, Jobe, Leveck, & Marsiske, 2002; Edwards et al., 2002; Roenker et al., 2003). These findings are encouraging and argue for a broader utilization of cognitive rehabilitation interventions specifically designed to promote PS. Continued research assessing the efficacy of these interventions and the impact of improved PS on quality of life is also needed.

Challenges for the future

Research efforts and psychology's understanding of PS have evolved considerably since the pioneering work of Sir Francis Galton and Francisco Donders. Numerous research paradigms and clinical tools have been developed to assess PS, and there is growing evidence of the important contribution of PS to cognitive functioning and activities of daily living. However, a number of barriers hindering the investigation and conceptualization of PS can be identified and addressed. For instance, clarification of the multiple constructs that have been used to define PS (e.g., IT, RT, and information processing) would alleviate confusion stemming from the use of similar, but distinct, terms to define how fast information is processed cognitively. Additionally, the identification of at least two distinct forms of PS (Chiaravalloti et al., 2003) suggests that the clinical utility of the term "PS" itself should be investigated. Using more descriptive terminology, such as simple PS and complex PS, may promote our conceptualization of PS and lead to refined assessment tools and treatment interventions. Developing assessment tools that target PS, while minimizing the influence of confounding variables (e.g., motor speed) and clarifying the constructs that are assessed by our current measures of PS, will also advance our assessment of PS. Lastly, efforts to facilitate the exchange and application of information between laboratory and clinical settings would promote the development of "real world" assessment measures and treatment interventions.

References

Arbuthnott, K., & Frank, J. (2000). Trail Making Test, part B as a measure of executive control: Validation using a set-switching paradigm. *Journal of Clinical and Experimental Neuropsychology, 22*, 518–522.

Archibald, C. J., & Fisk, J. D. (2000). Information processing efficiency in patients with multiple sclerosis. *Journal of Clinical and Experimental Neuropsychology, 22* (5), 686–701.

Army Individual Test Battery. (1944). *Manual of directions and scoring*. Washington, DC: War Department, Adjutant General's Office.

Azouvi, P., Jokic, C., Van der Linden, M., Marlier, N., & Bussel, B. (1996). Working memory and supervisory control after severe closed-head injury. A study of dual task performance and random generation. *Journal of Clinical and Experimental Neuropsychology, 18*, 317–337.

Baddeley, A. D. (1986). *Working memory*. Oxford, UK: Clarendon Press.

Baddeley, A. D., & Hitch, G. J. (1994). Developments in the concept of working memory. *Neuropsychology, 8*, 485–493.

Ball, K., Beard, B., Roenker, D., Miller, R., & Ball, D. (1988). Visual search: Age and practice. *Investigative Ophthalmology and Visual Science, 29*, 448.

Ball, K., Berch, D. B., Helmers, K. F., Jobe, J. B., Leveck, M. D., & Marsiske, M. (2002). Effects of cognitive retraining interventions with older adults. A randomized controlled trial. *Journal of American Medical Association, 288*, 2271–2281.

Ball, K., & Owsley, C. (2000). Increasing mobility and reducing accidents in older drivers. In K.W. Schaie & M. Pietrucha (Eds.), *Mobility and transportation in the elderly* (pp. 213–251). New York: Springer Publishing Company, Inc.

Ball, K. K., & Roenker, D. L. (1998). *Useful field of view*. San Antonio, TX: The Psychological Corporation; Harcourt Brace & Company.

Barrett, P., Eysenck, H. J., & Lucking, S. (1986). Reaction time and intelligence: A replicated study. *Intelligence, 10*, 9–40.

Bates, T. C., & Rock, A. (2004). Personality and information processing speed: Independent influences on intelligent performance. *Intelligence, 32*, 33–46.

Bazana, P. G., & Stelmack, R. M. (2002). Intelligence and information processing during an auditory discrimination task with backward masking: An event-related potential analysis. *Journal of Personality and Social Psychology, 84*, 998–1008.

Bleiberg, J., Kane, R. L., Reeves, D. L., Garmoe, W. S., & Halpern, E. (2000). Factor analysis of computerized and traditional tests used in mild brain injury research. *The Clinical Neuropsychologist, 14* (3), 287–294.

Boone, K. B. (1999). Neuropsychological assessment of executive functions: Impact of age, education, gender, intellectual level, and vascular status on executive test scores. In B. L. Miller & J. Cummings (Eds.), *The frontal lobes* (pp. 247–260). New York: Guilford Press.

Boone, K. B., Miller, B. L., Lesser, I. M., Hill, E., & D'Elia, L. (1990). Performance on frontal lobe tests in healthy, older individuals. *Developmental Neuropsychology, 6* (3), 215–223.

Boring, E. G. (1952). *A history of experimental psychology* (2nd ed.). New York: Appleton-Century-Crofts.

Brand, C. R. & Deary, I. J. (1982). Intelligence and "inspection time." In H. J. Eysenck (Ed.), *A model for intelligence* (pp. 133–148). New York: Springer-Verlag.

Brebner, J. T. (1980). Reaction time in personality theory. In A. T. Welford (Ed.), *Reaction times* (pp. 309–320). New York: Academic Press.

Brebner, J. T. & Welford, A. T. (1980). Introduction: An historical background sketch. In A. T. Welford (Ed.), *Reaction times* (pp. 1–23). New York: Academic Press.

Brittain, J. L., La Marche, J. A., Reeder, K. P., Roth, D. L., & Boll, T. J. (1991). Effects of age and IQ on Paced Auditory Serial Addition Task (PASAT) performance. *The Clinical Neuropsychologist, 5*, 163–175.

Bryant, D. S., Diamond, B., & DeLuca, J. (2003). Processing speed interacts with working memory efficiency in multiple sclerosis. *Journal of the International Neuropsychological Society, 9*, 229.

Buchsbaum, M., & Callaway, E. (1965). Influence of respiratory cycle on simple RT. *Perceptual and Motor Skills, 20*, 961–966.

Burns, N. R. (1998). *Inspection time and cognitive abilities: An event-related potential study*. Unpublished PhD thesis, University of Adelaide, South Australia.

Burns, N. R., & Nettelbeck, T. (2003). Inspection time in the structure of cognitive abilities: Where does IT fit? *Intelligence, 31*, 237–255.

Burns, N. R., Nettelbeck, T., & Cooper, C. J. (1999). Inspection time correlates with general speed of processing but not fluid ability. *Intelligence, 27*, 37–44.

Burns, N. R., Nettelbeck, T., & White, M. (1998). Testing the interpretation of inspection time as a measure of speed of sensory processing. *Personality and Individual Differences, 24*, 25–39.

Burns, N. R., Nettelbeck, T., White, M., & Willson, J. (1999). The effects of car window tinting on visual performance: A comparison of elderly and young drivers. *Ergonomics, 42*, 428–443.

Chaiken, S. R., & Young, R. K. (1993). Inspection time and intelligence: Attempts to eliminate the apparent movement strategy. *American Journal of Psychology, 106*, 191–210.

Chiaravalloti, N. D., Christodoulou, C., Demaree, H. A., & DeLuca, J. (2003). Differentiating simple versus complex processing speed: Influence on new learning and memory performance. *Journal of Clinical and Experimental Neuropsychology, 25* (4), 489–501.

Collins, L. F., & Long, C. J. (1996). Visual reaction time and its relationship to neuropsychological test performance. *Archives of Clinical Neuropsychology, 11*, 613–623.

Collins, M. W., Field, M., Lovell, M. R., Iverson, G., Johnston, K. M., Maroon, J., & Fu, F. H. (2003). Relationships between postconcussion headache and neuropsychological test performance in high school athletes. *The American Journal of Sports Medicine, 31* (2), 168–174.

Crawford, J. R., Deary, I. J., Allan, K. M., & Gustafsson, J. E. (1998). Evaluating competing models of the relationship between inspection time and psychometric intelligence. *Intelligence, 26*, 27–42.

Deary, I. J. (1993). Inspection time and WAIS-R-IQ subtypes: A confirmatory factor analysis study. *Intelligence, 17*, 223–236.

Deary, I. J., & Der, G. (2005). Reaction time, age, and cognitive ability: Longitudinal findings from age 16 to 63 years in representative population samples. *Aging, Neuropsychology, and Cognition (Neuropsychology, Development and Cognition: Section B), 12* (2), 187–215.

Deary, I. J., Der, G., & Ford, G. (2001). Reaction times and intelligence differences: A population-based cohort study. *Intelligence, 29*, 389–399.

Deary, I. J., Ebmeier, K. P., MacLeod, K. M., Dougall, N., Hepburn, D. A., Frier, B. M., et al. (1994). PASAT performance and the pattern of uptake of 99mTc-exametazime in brain estimated with single photon emission tomography. *Biological Psychology*, *38*, 1–18.

Deary, I. J., Hunter, H., Langan, S. J., & Goodwin, G. M. (1991). Inspection time, psychometric intelligence and clinical estimates of cognitive ability in pre-senile Alzheimer's disease and Korsakoff's patients. *Brain*, *114*, 2543–2554.

Deary, I. J., Simonotto, E., Meyer, M., Marshall, A., Marshall, I., Goddard, N., et al. (2001). The functional anatomy of inspection time: A pilot fMRI study. *Intelligence*, *29*, 497–510.

Deary, I. J., & Stough, C. (1996). Intelligence and inspection time: Achievements, prospects and problems. *American Psychologist*, *51*, 599–608.

DeLuca, J., Barbieri-Berger, S., & Johnson, S. K. (1994). The nature of memory impairments in multiple sclerosis: Acquisition versus retrieval. *Journal of Clinical and Experimental Neuropsychology*, *16*, 183–189.

DeLuca, J., Chelune, G. J., Tulsky, D. S., Lengenfelder, J., & Chiaravalloti, N. D. (2004). Is speed of processing or working memory the primary information processing deficit in multiple sclerosis? *Journal of Clinical and Experimental Neuropsychology*, *26* (4), 550–562.

DeLuca, J., Christodoulou, C., Diamond, B. J., Rosenstein, E. D., Kramer, N., & Natelson, B. H. (2004). Working memory deficits in chronic fatigue syndrome: Differentiating between speed and accuracy of information processing. *Journal of the International Neuropsychological Society*, *10*, 101–109.

DeLuca, J., Gaudino, E. A., Diamond, B. J., Christodoulou, C., & Engel, R. A. (1998). Acquisition and storage in multiple sclerosis. *Journal of Clinical and Experimental Neuropsychology*, *20*, 376–390.

Demaree, H. A., DeLuca, J., Guadino, E. A., & Diamond, B. J. (1999). Speed of information processing as a key deficit in multiple sclerosis: Implications for rehabilitation. *Journal of Neurology, Neurosurgery, and Psychiatry*, *67*, 661–663.

Donders, F. C. (1868). On the speed of mental processes (trans. W. G. Koster, 1969). *Acta Psychologica*, *30*, 412–431.

Donders, J., Tulsky, D. S., & Zhu, J. (2001). Criterion validity of new WAIS-III subtest scores after traumatic brain injury. *Journal of the International Neuropsychological Society*, *7*, 892–898.

Duncan, J., Seitz, J., Kolodny, J., Bor, D., Herzog, H., Ahmed, A., et al. (2000). A neural basis for general intelligence. *Science*, *289*, 457–460.

Edwards, J. D., Vance, D. E., Wadley, V. G., Cissell, G. M., Roenker, D. L., & Ball, K. K. (2005). Reliability and validity of Useful Field of View test scores as administered by personal computer. *Journal of Clinical and Experimental Neuropsychology*, *27*, 529–543.

Edwards, J. D., Wadley, V. G., Myers, R. S., Roenker, D. L., Cissell, G. M., & Ball, K. K. (2002). Transfer of a speed of processing intervention to near and far cognitive functions. *Gerontology*, *48*, 329–340.

Ewing, F. M. E., Deary, I. J., McCrimmon, R. J., Strachan, M. W. J., & Frier, B. M. (1998). Effect of acute hypoglycemia on visual information processing in adults with Type 1 diabetes mellitus. *Physiology and Behavior*, *64*, 653–660.

Eysenck, H. J. (1986). Inspection time and intelligence: A historical introduction. *Personality and Individual Differences*, *7*, 603–607.

Galton, F. (1883). *Inquiries into human faculty and its development*. London: Macmillan.

Gronwall, D. M. A. (1977). Paced auditory serial-addition task: A measure of recovery from concussion. *Perceptual Motor Skills, 44*, 367–373.

Haslam, C., Batchelor, J., Fearnside, M. R., Haslam, A. S., & Hawkins, S. (1995). Further examination of post-traumatic amnesia and post-coma disturbance as non-linear predictors of outcome after head injury. *Neuropsychology, 9*, 599–605.

Hawkins, K. A. (1998). Indicators of brain dysfunction derived from graphic representations of the WAIS-III/WMS-III technical manual samples: A preliminary approach to clinical utility. *The Clinical Neuropsychologist, 12*, 535–551.

Heaton, R. K., Nelson, L. M., Thompson, D. S., Burks, J. S. & Franklin, G. M. (1985). Neuropsychological findings in relapsing–remitting and chronic-progressive multiple sclerosis. *Journal of Consulting and Clinical Psychology, 53*, 103–110.

Hedden, T., Lautenschlager, G., & Park, D. C. (2005). Contributions of processing ability and knowledge to verbal memory tasks across the adult life span. *The Quarterly Journal of Experimental Psychology, 58A* (1), 169–190.

Heilbronner, R. L., Henry, G. K., Buck, P., Adams, R. L., & Fogle, T. (1991). Lateralized brain damage and performance on Trail Making A and B, Digit Span Forward and Backward, and TPT memory and location. *Archives of Clinical Neuropsychology, 6*, 251–258.

Horn, J. L., & Cattell, R. B. (1967). Age differences in fluid and crystallized intelligence. *Acta Psychologica, 26*, 107–129.

Hutchison, C. W., Nathan, P. J., Mrazek, L. & Stough, C. (2001). Cholinergic modulation of speed of early information processing: The effect of Donepezil on inspection time. *Psychopharmacology, 155*, 440–442.

Iverson, G. L., Lovell, M. R., & Collins, M. W. (2005). Validity of ImPACT for measuring processing speed following sports-related concussion. *Journal of Clinical and Experimental Neuropsychology, 27*, 683–689.

Jensen, A. R. (1982). Reaction time and psychometric g. In H. J. Eysenck (Ed.), *A model for intelligence*. Heidelberg, Germany: Springer.

Kail, R. (1997). The neural noise hypothesis: Evidence from processing speed in adults with multiple sclerosis. *Aging, Neuropsychology, and Cognition, 4*, 157–165.

Kail, R. (1998). Speed of information processing in patients with multiple sclerosis. *Journal of Clinical and Experimental Neuropsychology, 20*, 98–106.

Kail, R., & Salthouse, T. A. (1994). Processing speed as a mental capacity. *Acta Psychologica, 86*, 199–225.

Kalmar, J. H., Bryant, D., Tulsky, D., & Deluca, J. (2004). Information processing deficits in multiple sclerosis. Does choice of screening instrument make a difference? *Rehabilitation Psychology, 49* (3), 213–218.

Kemp, B. J. (1973). Reaction time of young and elderly subjects in relation to perceptual deprivation and signal-on versus signal-off condition. *Developmental Psychology, 8*, 268–272.

Kessler, H. R., Cohen, R. A., Lauer, K., & Kausch, D. F. (1992). The relationship between disability and memory dysfunction in multiple sclerosis. *International Journal of Neuroscience, 62*, 17–34.

Kosinski, R. J. (2005). A literature review on reaction time. Retrieved June 28, 2005 from http://biowww.clemson.edu/bpc/bp/Lab/110/reaction.htm.

Krupp, L. B., Sliwinski, M., Masur, D. M., Friedberg, F., & Coyle, P. K. (1994). Cognitive functioning and depression in patients with chronic fatigue syndrome and multiple sclerosis. *Archives of Neurology, 51*, 705–710.

LaMarche, J. A., Alexander, R. W., Stanford, L. D., Beth, R. E., Dolske, M. C., & Morthland, M. (1994). A descriptive study of cognitive efficiency: Verbal and numerical cognitive fluency. *Archives of Clinical Neuropsychology*, 9, 152.

Lamberty, G. J., Putnam, S. H., Chatel, D. M., Bieliauskas, L. A. & Adams, K. M. (1994). Derived trail making test indices. *Neuropsychiatry, Neuropsychology, and Behavioral Neurology*, 7, 230–234.

Lenzenweger, M. F. (2001). Reaction time slowing during high-load, sustained-attention task performance in relation to psychometrically identified schizotypy. *Journal of Abnormal Psychology*, 110, 290–296.

Lezak, M. D. (1995). *Neuropsychological assessment* (3rd ed). New York: Oxford University Press.

Llorente, A. M., Miller, E. N., D'Elia, L. F., Selnes, O. A., Wesch, J., Becker, J. T., et al. (1998). Slowed information processing in HIV-1 disease: The multicenter AIDS cohort study (MACS). *Journal of Clinical and Experimental Neuropsychology*, 20, 60–72.

Lopez, S. L., Summerall, S. W., & Ryan, J. J. (2002). Factor structure of MicroCog in a clinical sample. *Applied Neuropsychology*, 9 (3), 183–186.

Luce, R. D. (1986). *Response times: Their role in inferring elementary mental organization*. New York: Oxford University Press.

Luna, B., Garver, K. E., Urban, T. A., Lazar, N. A., & Sweeney, J. A. (2004). Maturation of cognitive processes from late childhood to adulthood. *Child Development*, 75 (5), 1357–1372.

Madigan, N. K., DeLuca, J., Diamond, B., Tramontano, G., & Averill, A. (2000). Speed of information processing in traumatic brain injury: A modality specific impairment? *Journal of Head Trauma Rehabilitation*, 15, 943–956.

Martin, T. A., Donders, J., & Thompson, E. (2000). Potential of and problems with new measures of psychometric intelligence after traumatic brain injury. *Rehabilitation Psychology*, 45 (4), 402–408.

Maroon, J. C., Lovell, M. R., Norwig, J., Podell, K., Powell, J. W., & Hartl, R. (2000). Cerebral concussion in athletes: Evaluation and neuropsychological testing. *Neurosurgery*, 47, 659–672.

Marshall, W. H., Talbot, S. A., & Ades, H. W. (1943). Cortical response of the anaesthetized cat to gross photic and electrical afferent stimulation. *Journal of Neurophysiology*, 6, 1–15.

Matarazzo, J. D. (1972). *Wechsler's measurement and appraisal of adult intelligence* (5th ed). Baltimore: Williams & Wilkins.

McCrimmon, R. J., Deary, I. J., Huntly, B. J. P., MacLeod, K. J., & Frier, B. M. (1996). Visual information processing during controlled hypoglycemia in humans. *Brain*, 119, 1277–1287.

Mitrushina, M. N., Boone, K. B., & D'Elia, L. F. (1999). *Handbook of normative data for neuropsychological assessment*. New York: Oxford University Press.

Nettelbeck, T. (1982). Inspection time: An index for intelligence? *Quarterly Journal of Experimental Psychology*, 34, 299–312.

Nettelbeck, T. (1987). Inspection time and intelligence. In P. A. Vernon (Ed.), *Speed of information processing and intelligence*. Norwood, NJ: Ablex.

Nettelbeck, T. (1994). Speediness. In R. J. Sternberg (Ed.), *Speed of information processing and intelligence* (pp. 295–346). Norwood, NJ: Ablex.

Nettelbeck, T., & Rabbitt, P. M. A. (1992). Aging, cognitive performance, and mental speed. *Intelligence*, 16, 189–205.

Neubauer, A. C. (1997). The mental speed approach to the assessment of intelligence. In J. Kingma & W. Tomic (Eds.), *Advances in cognition and education: Reflections on the concept of intelligence*. Greenwich, CT: JAI Press.

Neubauer, A. C., Spinath, F. M., Riemann, R., Angleitner, A., & Borkenau, P. (2000). Genetic and environmental influences on measures of speed of information processing and their relation to psychometric intelligence: Evidence from the German observational study of adult twins. *Intelligence, 28* (4), 267–289.

O'Donnell, J. P., MacGregor, L. A., Dabrowski, J. J., Oestreicher, J. M., & Romero, J. J. (1994). Construct validity of neuropsychological tests of conceptual and attentional abilities. *Journal of Clinical Psychology, 50* (4), 596–600.

Osmon, D. C., & Jackson, R. (2002). Inspection time and IQ: Fluid or perceptual aspects of intelligence? *Intelligence, 30*, 119–127.

Owsley, C., McGwin, G., Jr., & Ball, K. (1998). Vision impairment, eye disease, and injurious motor vehicle crashes in the elderly. *Ophthalmic Epidemiology, 5* (2), 101–113.

Powell, D. H., Kaplan, E. F., Whitla, D., Weintraub, S., Catlin, R., & Funkenstein, H. H. (1993). *MicroCog: Assessment of cognitive functioning: Manual*. San Antonio, TX: The Psychological Corporation.

Prabhakaran, V., Smith, J. A. L., Desmond, J. E., Glover, G. H., & Gabrieli, J. D. E. (1997). Neural substrates of fluid reasoning: An fMRI study of neurocortical activation during performance of the Raven's Progressive Matrices Test. *Cognitive Psychology, 33*, 43–63.

Psychological Corporation (1997). *WAIS-III WMS-III technical manual*. San Antonio, TX: Author.

Raven, J. C., Court, J. H., & Raven, J. (1982). *Manual for the Raven's Progressive Matrices and Vocabulary Scales*. London: H. K. Lewis and Co.

Reitan, R. M., & Wolfson, D. (1993). *The Halstead-Reitan neuropsychological test battery* (2nd ed.). Tucson, AZ: Neuropsychology Press.

Ricker, J. H., Axelrod, B. N., & Houtler, B. D. (1996). Clinical validation of the Oral Trail Making Test. *Neuropsychiatry, Neuropsychology, and Behavioral Neurology, 9*, 50–53.

Roenker, D. L., Cissell, G. M., Ball, K. K., Wadley, V. G., & Edwards, J. D. (2003). Speed-of-processing and driving simulator training result in improved driving performance. *Human Factors, 45* (2), 218–233.

Salthouse, T. A. (1993). Speed mediation of adult age differences in cognition. *Developmental Psychology, 29*, 722–738.

Salthouse, T. A. (1996). The processing-speed theory of adult age differences in cognition. *Psychological Review, 103*, 403–428.

Salthouse, T. A. (2000). Aging and measures of processing speed. *Biological Psychology, 54*, 35–54.

Salthouse, T. A., & Babcock, R. L. (1991). Decomposing adult age differences in working memory. *Developmental Psychology, 27*, 763–776.

Salthouse, T. A., & Coon, V. E. (1993). Influence of task specific processing speed on age differences in memory. *Journal of Gerontology, 48*, P245–P255.

Sanders, A. F. (1998). *Elements of human performance: Reaction processes and attention in human skill*. Mahwah, NJ: Lawerence Erlbaum Associates, Inc.

Sawamoto, N., Honda, M., Hanakawa, T., Fukuyama, H., & Shibasaki, H. (2002). Cognitive slowing in Parkinson's disease: A behavioral evaluation independent of motor slowing. *The Journal of Neuroscience, 22* (12), 5198–5203.

Schultheis, M. T., Garay, E., & DeLuca, J. (2001). The influence of cognitive impairment on driving performance in multiple sclerosis. *American Academy of Neurology, 56* (8), 1089–1094.

Sekuler, A. B., Bennett, P. J., & Mamelak, M. (2000). Effects of aging on the useful field of view. *Experimental Aging Research, 26*, 103–120.

Shawaryn, M. A., Schultheis, M. T., Garay, E., & DeLuca, J. (2002). *Archives of Physical Medicine and Rehabilitation, 83*, 1123–1129.

Sherman, E. S. E., Strauss, E., & Spellacy, F. (1997). Validity of the Paced Auditory Serial Addition Test (PASAT) in adults referred for neuropsychological assessment after head injury. *The Clinical Neuropsychologist, 11*, 34–45.

Shum, D. H. K., McFarland, K. A., & Bain, J. D. (1990). Construct validity of eight tests of attention: Comparison of normal and closed head injury samples. *The Clinical Neuropsychologist, 4*, 151–162.

Sliwinski, M., & Bushke, H. (1997). Processing speed and memory in aging and dementia. *Journal of Gerontology, 52B*, 308–318.

Smith, A. (1991). *Symbol Digit Modalities Test*. Los Angeles: Western Psychological Services.

Stough, C., Brebner, J., Nettelbeck, T., Cooper, C. J., Bates, T. C., & Mangan, G. L. (1996). The relationship between intelligence, personality, and inspection time. *British Journal of Psychology, 87*, 255–268.

Stuss, D. T., Stethem, L. L., & Pelchat, G. (1988). Three tests of attention and rapid information processing: An extension. *The Clinical Neuropsychologist, 2*, 246–250.

Tiersky, L. A., Johnson, S. K., Lange, G., Natelson, B. H., & DeLuca, J. (1997). Neuropsychology of chronic fatigue syndrome: A critical review. *Journal of Clinical and Experimental Neuropsychology, 19*, 560–586.

Vernon, P. A. (1987). Speed of information-processing and intelligence. In P. A. Vernon (Ed.), *Biological approaches to the study of human intelligence*. Norwood, NJ: Ablex.

Vickers, D., & Smith, P. L. (1986). The rationale for the inspection time index. *Personality and Individual Differences, 7*, 609–623.

Vlaar, A. M. M., & Wade, D. T. (2003). The Adult Memory and Information Processing Battery (AMIPB) test of information-processing speed: A study of its reliability and feasibility in patients with multiple sclerosis. *Clinical Rehabilitation, 17*, 386–393.

Walhovd, K. B., Fjell, A. M., Reinvang, I., Lundervold, A., Fischl, B., Salat, D., et al. (2005). Cortical volume and speed-of-processing are complementary in prediction of performance intelligence. *Neuropsychologia, 43* (5), 704–713.

Welford, A. T. (1980). Choice reaction time: Basic concepts. In A. T. Welford (Ed.), *Reaction times* (pp. 73–128). New York: Academic Press.

Wiens, A. N., Fuller, K. H., & Crossen, J. R. (1997). Paced Auditory Serial Attention Test: Adult norms and moderator variables. *Journal of Clinical and Experimental Neuropsychology, 19*, 473–483.

Williams, M. A., LaMarche, J. A., Alexander, R. W., Stanford, L. D., Fielstein, E. M., & Boll, T. J. (1996). Serial 7s and Alphabet Backwards as brief measures of information processing speed. *Archives of Clinical Neuropsychology, 11* (8), 651–659.

Wills, S. & Leathem, J. (2004). The effects of test anxiety, age, intelligence level, and arithmetic ability on Paced Auditory Serial Addition Test performance. *Applied Neuropsychology, 11*, 180–187.

Woodard, J. L., & Axelrod, B. N. (2005). Neuropsychological batteries for older adults. In S. S. Bush and T. A. Martin (Eds.), *Geriatric neuropsychology: Practice essentials* (pp. 41–84). New York: Psychology Press.

Woodworth, R. S. & Schlosberg, H. (1954). *Experimental psychology*. New York: Henry Holt.

3 Information processing speed: Measurement issues and its relationships with other neuropsychological constructs

Heath A. Demaree, Thomas W. Frazier, and Courtney E. Johnson

Information processing speed is a frequently used term in the field of neuropsychology and, when used in the literature, there is little debate about its meaning. However, operationalization of the construct is extremely varied across studies. In general, the operationalization of processing speed involves one or more of the following functions: the amount of time required to perceive information, process that information, and/or formulate/enact a response.

The primary purpose of this chapter is to identify neuropsychological constructs that are related to information processing speed. To accomplish this goal, an extremely brief review of clinical research is first presented (see chapters 1–2 for more detailed discussion), with particular attention paid to the most frequently used information processing paradigms. Second, comprising the bulk of the chapter, theoretical and empirical work supporting the relationship between information processing speed, working memory, information acquisition/recall, and executive abilities is presented (processing speed is also related to intellectual functioning, see chapter 1). Next, it is proposed that many processing speed tasks possess relatively poor discriminant validities (i.e., they measure other neuropsychological domains as well), and this fact may lead to the false conclusion that processing speed is associated with other cognitive constructs when, in fact, they may result from simple operational confounds. Examples of these relationships are cited and data from research designed to better discriminate between neuropsychological constructs are presented. We conclude with ideas for future research that may improve the specificity and accuracy with which processing speed and related constructs are evaluated in both healthy and clinical populations.

A brief review of processing speed research within clinical populations

Clinicians and researchers alike have suggested that neurological dysfunction—stemming from multiple sclerosis (MS), traumatic brain injury (TBI), chronic fatigue syndrome (CFS), and systemic lupus erythematosus (SLE), to name a few—is associated with slowed information processing speed. Findings appear to be relatively robust, with researchers noting impairment on many commonly used processing speed measures. For example, it has been reported that persons with MS show significant impairment on the Processing Speed Index (PSI) of the Wechsler Adult Intelligence Scale—3rd edition (WAIS-III; Wechsler, 1997a), which is a composite of the Symbol Search and Digit-Symbol Coding subtests (Chelune, 2002; DeLuca, Chelune, Tulsky, Lengenfelder, & Chiaravalloti, 2004). In addition, Denney, Lynch, Parmenter, and Horne (2004) found that persons with MS evidenced significant impairment on a factor-analyzed set of "processing speed" tasks—initial planning time on the Tower of London (Krikorian, Bartok, & Gay, 1994) and the word reading, color naming, and color–word times on the Stroop Color–Word Task (Stroop, 1935). Persons diagnosed with MS also have impaired performance on the classic Paced Auditory Serial Addition Test (PASAT; Gronwall, 1977), a task that requires participants to add the last two numbers of a series presented at a constant interstimulus interval, ranging from long (2.4 s/digit) to short (1.2 s/digit) (e.g., DeLuca, Johnson, & Natelson, 1993; Diamond, DeLuca, Kim, & Kelley, 1997; Hillary et al., 2003). Similar results have been found for the Paced Visual Serial Addition Test (PVSAT), which is identical to the PASAT with the exception that stimuli are visually presented (Diamond et al., 1997). Relative to healthy controls, persons experiencing TBI, CFS, or SLE, also evidence impaired PASAT performance (Cicerone, 1997; DeLuca, Johnson, Beldowicz, & Natelson, 1995; DeLuca et al., 1993; Shucard, Parrish, Shucard, McCabe, Benedict, & Ambrus, 2004). Other measures used to evaluate information processing speed in clinical populations include visual/auditory simple/choice reaction time tasks (e.g., Chiaravalloti, Christodoulou, Demaree, & DeLuca, 2003) and the slope comparing number set size to response time on the Sternberg Memory Scanning Test (SMST; Sternberg, 1966) (e.g., Archibald et al., 2004; Hillary et al., 2003).

Constructs related to processing speed

Evidence has accumulated that processing speed may be related to working memory, and episodic memory, as well as some executive abilities. A review of these literatures follows.

Working memory

Working memory is the cognitive system that temporarily stores, processes, and manipulates information. Baddeley developed the "multiple component" model of working memory, which has received significant empirical support over the years. According to this model, working memory consists of a central executive system that works in conjunction with two slave subsystems. The central executive serves as an attentional control system that oversees working memory operations. By manipulating attentional resources, the central executive controls the two slave subsystems (Baddeley, 1992, 1997; Baddeley, 1986; Baddeley & Hitch, 1974). Each slave system processes different types of information. The first slave system (the *phonological loop*) is involved in processing verbal information, while the second (the *visuospatial sketchpad*) processes visuospatial information. The phonological loop can be conceptualized as a phonological store similar to an audiotape that stores verbally encoded (speech-based) information. According to Baddeley's theory, this verbal information will be lost within a few seconds to decay/interference if it is not rehearsed or transferred to long-term memory. The visuospatial sketchpad is similar to the phonological loop except that it handles nonverbal information such as the visual appearance and location of an object. Much like the verbal information, nonverbal information that is not rehearsed or transferred to long-term memory will be lost in a matter of seconds. The two slave systems operate independently from each other as evidenced by the observations that a visuospatial stimulus, such as a moving point of light, will not interfere with rehearsal or performance within the phonological loop and vice versa. Interference of attentional control within the central executive (induced by counting backwards, for example) will, however, disrupt rehearsal and performance within both slave subsystems (Baddeley, 1998).

Importantly, according to Baddeley (1981, 1986), processing speed may predict working memory capacity because faster rehearsal helps with the creation/maintenance of working memory stores. That is, faster processing speeds should be associated with better working memory ability (although other factors, such as stimulus familiarity, may also affect working memory). Unfortunately, most studies of working memory do not assess processing speed, or attempt to evaluate its influence. Of studies that have examined working memory and processing speed, the majority find a positive relationship where deficits in working memory are related to slower processing speed (Kennedy, Clement, & Curtiss, 2003; Lengenfelder, Bryant, Diamond, Kalmar, Moore, & DeLuca, 2006; Madigan, DeLuca, Diamond, Tramontano, & Averill, 2000; Nebes et al., 2000; Shucard et al., 2004). These studies are discussed in more detail throughout the chapter. It should be noted, however, that a smaller portion of research investigating working memory and processing speed does not find a relationship (Keri, Szendi, Kelemen, Benedek, & Janka, 2001; Perlstein, Cole, Demery, Seignourel, Dixit, & Larson, 2004; Salmond, Chatfield, Menon, Pickard, & Sahakian, 2005). For example, Keri and colleagues (2001) found working memory and processing speed were unrelated in a small group of individuals with remitted schizophrenia. Results from this study should be considered with caution because the sample size was very small ($N = 14$) and the lack of correlation may be attributable to other factors (e.g., poor attention/concentration).

Early development of information processing and working memory in healthy individuals

A recent review by Fry and Hale (2000) summarized the cognitive development of children/adolescents, with emphasis placed on processing speed, working memory, and intelligence. According to their review, processing speed and working memory show similar rates of improvement with age. With regard to processing speed, Hale (1990) administered four processing speed tasks to children aged 10 to 19 and determined that age improves processing speed at a *global* level (i.e., independent of task type). To further test this global development hypothesis, Kail (1991) performed a meta-analysis using data from 72 studies incorporating various reaction time measures. He supported Hale's (1990) assertion that processing speed improvement acted as a function of age (through young adulthood) and was global. The mathematical function that best described the age–speed relationship was exponential in nature, in which the greatest processing speed improvements were observed relatively early and then became more gradual during childhood/adolescence (Fry & Hale, 2000; Kail, 1991).

With regard to working memory, Dempster (1981) noted in his meta-analysis that working memory span increased most dramatically during the early school years, with further improvement slowing thereafter. The non-linear, exponential relationships between age–processing speed and age–working memory are parallel, and it has been widely accepted that working memory improvements during development are largely accounted for by the faster processing speeds (Dempster, 1981, 1985, 1992; Gathercole & Baddeley, 1993). Empirically, short-term verbal memory span may be predicted by processing speed as well as articulation rate, which purportedly reflects covert rehearsal rate. This has been well demonstrated by Kail (1992) (see chapter 5 of this book for a more complete review of processing speed in children and adolescents).

Other studies have demonstrated the predictive ability of processing speed on working memory. In four experiments incorporating over 2000 young adults, Kyllonen and Christal (1990) found that processing speed measures correlated moderately ($r = .35-.38$) with their working memory composite score. Using a similar methodology but incorporating 9-year-olds, a considerably higher correlation ($r = .60$) was found between speed and working memory composites (de Jong & Das-Smaal, 1995). Moreover, among 109 4- to 7-year-olds, a path coefficient of $-.70$ was revealed between reaction time and working memory (Miller & Vernon, 1996), suggesting that quicker processing speed predicted better working memory performance. Finally, Fry and Hale (1996) administered four information processing speed and four working memory tasks to 219 children and young adults (aged 7 through 19). Again revealing the importance of processing speed underlying working memory, a path coefficient of $-.51$ was revealed (collapsing across age groups).

Healthy adults

Performance on both information processing speed and working memory tasks has been found to deteriorate after young adulthood (Cerella & Hale,

1994; Chaytor & Schmitter-Edgecombe, 2004). However, similar to what is observed among individuals with MS (Demaree, DeLuca, Gaudino, & Diamond, 1999), it appears that working memory decline during normal aging is at least partially attributable to slowed processing speed (for a more detailed discussion on processing speed and aging see chapter 10 in this book). For example, Diamond and colleagues (2000) administered the Auditory and Visual Threshold Serial Addition Tests (AT-SAT and VT-SAT) to 12 younger (mean age = 27) and 12 older (mean age = 77) participants. Unlike the PASAT, which uses fixed inter-stimulus intervals (ISIs) for number presentation (e.g., 1.2, 1.6, 2.0, 2.4 s), the AT-SAT and VT-SAT were designed to alter ISI during the task to ensure that each participant achieves a 50% accuracy rate. Thus working memory accuracy is controlled in order to attain a purer measure of processing speed. Older participants processed visual and auditory information more slowly as compared to their younger counterparts, but the older individuals were able to maintain comparable working memory accuracy levels when provided with additional time. This suggests that better working memory performance is intimately related to faster processing speed. In Salthouse's (1994a) review of research on aging and working memory, he highlighted the importance of speed in age-related working memory decline. For example, Salthouse (1994a) has demonstrated that when age is entered into a regression equation after controlling for information processing speed, age-related effects on working memory are significantly attenuated. More recently, using an abstract design version of the Self-Ordered Pointing Task to measure working memory ability, Chaytor and Schmitter-Edgecombe (2004) found that processing speed performance significantly explained working memory decline during aging.

Overall, results from these studies suggest that information processing speed may be a core determinant of working memory ability (during both developmental gains and age-related declines).

Acquisition/recall

Numerous studies have documented the relationship between measures of information processing speed and long-term memory across the adult lifespan (for examples see Bryan & Lusczcz, 1996; Salthouse, 1994b; for a meta-analytic review see Verhaeghen & Salthouse, 1997). Much of this work has supported the notion that age-related decreases in information processing speed mediate declines in memory (Kail & Salthouse, 1994; Salthouse, 1996a, 1996b) (see also chapter 10 of this text). Furthermore, Salthouse and Coon (1993) identified that general, and not task-specific, information processing speed capacity mediates the relationship between age and declarative/episodic memory (see also Bryan & Luszcz, 1996). Thus task- and modality-specific processing speed measures do not appear to contribute significant incremental variance over and above general processing speed to the mediation of episodic memory abilities in normal aging. Rather, declines in general information processing speed with age appear to drive age-related decreases in episodic memory.

In addition to information processing speed, working memory capacity has also been found to mediate age-related declines in episodic memory (Verhaeghen & Salthouse, 1997). Some research has suggested that declines in working memory capacity mediate declines in processing speed, which then mediate age-related declines in episodic memory (Kirasic, Allen, Dobson, & Binder, 1996). However, it remains unclear if both information processing speed and working memory mediate declines in episodic memory independently of one another or in conjunction. Previous conflicting findings, the potential confound of working memory capacity, and other methodological problems have led some researchers to question the hypothesis that age-related declines in information processing speed mediate declines in episodic memory function (Sliwinski & Buschke, 1997). However, in spite of the existing confusion, this literature remains at a advanced stage, where models are tested and mediational hypotheses are pitted against one another (Baron & Kenny, 1986).

Many studies have examined processing speed and episodic memory deficits in clinical populations, as the chapters in this book will attest. Additionally, multiple studies have reported a significant positive relationship between measures of processing speed and measures of episodic memory (for two examples, see Gladsjo, McAdams, Palmer, Moore, Jeste, & Heaton, 2004; Joy, Kaplan, & Fein, 2003), suggesting that processing speed is a potential moderator of episodic memory deficits. However, while almost all measures of cognitive abilities show positive relationships (Carroll, 1993; Salthouse, 2005), finding a significant positive relationship is only one step in determining moderation or mediation. Researchers must also show that the relationship between the independent variable (i.e., disease status, present versus absent), and the dependent variable (i.e., episodic memory) decreases significantly or becomes non-significant after controlling for individual differences in the mediator, processing speed. Unfortunately, few studies using clinical populations have actually examined whether processing speed mediates the relationship between disease presence and episodic memory deficits. Thus the generalizability of studies demonstrating processing speed as a mediator of episodic memory decline in normal aging to psychiatric or neurological conditions remains unclear. The following text reviews studies in schizophrenia, geriatric depression, bipolar disorder, elevated thyroid stimulating hormone, dementia, TBI, and multiple sclerosis, with an emphasis on studies directly examining processing speed as a moderator or mediator of episodic memory deficits.

Schizophrenia

Multiple studies have noted both information processing speed and episodic memory deficits in schizophrenia (for a review, see Cirillo & Seidman, 2003;

see also chapter 6 of this text). This work has indicated that most of the deficits in episodic memory observed in schizophrenia are as a result of problems with encoding. However, only a few studies have examined the role of processing speed as a mediator of episodic memory deficits. Holthausen, Wiersma, Sitskoom, Dingemans, Schene, and van den Bosch (2003) directly examined processing speed as a mediator of verbal learning, verbal retrieval, visual memory, and semantic memory in a sample of 118 patients with schizophrenia and 45 control participants. Processing speed was measured by combining the results from a modified Trail Making Test (Vink & Jolles, 1985) and the word and color reading trials from the Stroop task (Stroop, 1935). Verbal learning and retrieval were assessed using the total score for the five learning trials and the difference between long delay recall and recognition, respectively, on the California Verbal Learning Test (Delis, Kramer, Kaplan, & Ober, 1987). Visual learning was assessed using the immediate and delayed recall trials of a complex figure test (Duley, Wilkins, Hamby, Hopkins, Burwell, & Barry 1993), and semantic memory was assessed using a single 1-minute trial of a category fluency task (Lezak, 1995). Hierarchical regression analyses were performed in the total sample to examine whether processing speed and other cognitive constructs reduced the variance explained in memory scores by schizophrenia status, following the method outlined by Salthouse (1996b). This analytic procedure is common in these studies and, as stated above, is intended to assess whether changes in processing speed moderate or mediate the changes in memory associated with the disease. Results indicated that processing speed partially mediated disease-related memory decrements for all memory measures. However, results of analyses performed separately within the patient and control groups indicated that other cognitive constructs, particularly executive functions, contributed unique variance to the prediction of memory variables. These results suggest that processing speed deficits may account for some of the decrements in episodic memory functions observed in schizophrenia. A study by Brebion, David, Pilowsky, and Jones (2004) supported this conclusion and suggested that, in individuals with schizophrenia, processing speed is related to memory efficiency, defined by measures of recall, recognition, and organization, but not to memory errors, defined by measures of intrusions and source memory errors.

Taken together, these two studies strongly suggest that processing speed at least partially mediates decline in episodic memory in schizophrenia. The fact that they employed different measures of processing speed and episodic memory suggests that task- and modality-specific factors are not artificially driving the observed mediation.

Geriatric depression

Several studies have examined the bivariate relationships between measures of depression, episodic memory, and processing speed. However, only one study directly examined whether processing speed mediates depression-related declines in episodic memory in depressed and non-depressed older adults. Specifically, Nebes and colleagues (2000) examined the relationship between processing speed, working memory, and episodic memory in healthy older adults ($N = 19$) and older adults with depression ($N = 39$). These authors operationalized processing speed as the difference between the copy trial and the coding trial of the digit symbol subtest of the Wechsler Adult Intelligence Scale—Revised (Wechsler, 1981). This procedure was used to remove the effects of motor functioning from the processing speed measure. Working memory was measured using a version of the N-back test (Dobbs & Rule, 1989) and episodic memory was assessed using the logical memory subtest of the Wechsler Memory Scale—3rd edition (WMS-III; Wechsler, 1997b), the total recall from trials 1–5 of the CVLT, and immediate recall of a complex figure. Thus the study evaluated the effects of processing speed and working memory on structured and unstructured verbal and visual memory. A similar hierarchical regression procedure was used to the one described above. They found that processing speed and working memory mediated depression-related decline in measures of structured (story memory) and unstructured (list learning) verbal and visual (complex figure) memory. They also reported analyses indicating that working memory accounted for additional variance in depression-related decline in memory when processing speed was entered into the equation first. They interpreted these findings to imply that both processing speed and working memory mediated depression-related memory decline, but that working memory accounts for additional unique variance after controlling for processing speed.

Elevated thyroid stimulating hormone

One study has examined processing speed as a mediator of verbal episodic memory deficits in patients with and without elevated thyroid stimulating hormone (TSH; Cook et al., 2002). This study found that processing speed deficits did *not* mediate declines in measures of episodic memory due to elevated TSH. The design employed two measures of processing speed; however, both measures (digit symbol-coding and a digit comparison task) involved the visual modality, suggesting that this finding may be restricted to instances where processing speed is operationalized in this fashion.

Dementia

Numerous studies have examined cognitive deficits in various forms of dementia (for a brief review, see Fields, 1998). These studies have generally found both processing speed and episodic memory deficits in dementia, with episodic memory deficits being most prominent in dementia of the Alzheimer's type, but processing deficits being more prominent in cerebrovascular dementia. Unfortunately, only one study has directly examined whether processing speed deficits observed in dementia (defined generally without reference to a specific type) mediate episodic memory deficits (Sliwinski & Buschke, 1997). Specifically, this study examined a large sample of individuals with normal aging ($N = 140$) and a smaller sample of individuals diagnosed with DSM-IV dementia ($N = 29$). They examined cued recall from two variants of an associative memory task (Buschke, Sliwinski, Kuslansky, & Lipton, 1997) and free recall using the logical memory subtest of the WMS-III (Wechsler, 1997b). Processing speed was operationalized by combining the digit symbol task of the WAIS-R and response time during a computerized number copy task. Results indicated that processing speed mediated the relationship between aging and memory, but not dementia and memory. These results suggest that processing speed is an important component, and possibly sole determinant, of age-related memory decline, but that the memory deficit in dementia is primary and not a result of impaired processing speed. The latter conclusion should be tempered by the fact that both processing speed measures used in this study involved visual stimuli and thus generalizability may be limited. Alternatively, the combination of two measures decreases the possibility that findings are due to task-specific factors.

Bipolar disorder

One study has examined the mediational hypothesis in bipolar disorder (Kieseppa et al., 2005). This study operationalized processing speed using digit symbol-coding from the WAIS-III (Wechsler, 1997a) and reaction time to correct responses from a continuous performance test. Verbal and nonverbal episodic memory were measured using multiple tasks. Results indicated that both measures of processing speed did *not* mediate deficits in episodic memory in bipolar disorder. This suggests that the episodic memory problems observed in bipolar disorder are independent of the relatively mild processing speed deficits.

Traumatic brain injury (TBI)

Several studies present data regarding processing speed and episodic memory deficits in traumatic brain injury (Madigan et al., 2000; Sherman, Strauss, & Spellacy, 1997; Tiersky, Cicerone, Natelson, & DeLuca, 1998; see also chapter 8 of this volume). These studies have found significant decrements in both processing speed and episodic memory measures. While no studies could be found directly examining the mediational hypothesis, two studies provide conflicting data regarding the mediation of episodic memory deficits by processing speed. Sherman and colleagues (1997) examined the relationship between processing speed, indexed by the PASAT, and verbal and visual memory function in a sample of 441 individuals referred for possible closed head injury. They found moderate associations between PASAT scores and various verbal and visual memory scores. This study did not directly test the mediational hypothesis, presumably due to the fact that PASAT scores were not significantly related to head injury severity, precluding the possibility of significant mediation. Thus the results of this study imply that the memory deficits in head injury are not mediated by processing speed deficits, at least as indexed by the PASAT. However, Hillary and colleagues (2003) present data indicating that spacing of repetitions of verbal information improves episodic memory in TBI. These data may indicate that when information is presented in such a fashion as to allow more thorough processing (thereby accounting for problems with processing speed), individuals with TBI are able to show greatly improved episodic memory. However, these data could also be interpreted as indicating that the spacing improves episodic memory through enhanced consolidation and not processing speed per se. Future work is needed to directly examine whether processing speed deficits completely or partially mediate episodic memory deficits in TBI. This work should also carefully attend to the level of TBI severity, as this may influence the mediational findings.

Chronic fatigue syndrome

In a review of cognitive deficits in CFS, Michiels and Cluydts (2001) indicate that processing speed, working memory, and verbal learning are all impaired in CFS. Other studies have supported this contention for processing speed (Marshall, Forstot, Callies, Peterson, & Schenck, 1997; van der Werf, de Vree, van der Meer, & Bleijenberg, 2002), but results for working memory and episodic memory are less clear, with some studies finding deficits and others not (DeLuca, Christodoulou, Diamond, Rosenstein, Kramer, & Natelson, 2004; DeLuca et al., 1995; Tiersky et al., 1998). To attempt to better characterize the relationship between processing speed and episodic memory in CFS, Michiels and Cluydts (2001) administered a battery of cognitive measures to 29 patients with CFS and 22 controls matched on demographic factors and IQ. Results indicated deficits in both processing speed and episodic memory for verbal information. Additionally, the deficit in episodic memory was due to poor initial encoding and storage of information. This pattern may suggest that difficulties with processing speed resulted in problems with encoding. Unfortunately, however, this possibility was not directly examined. Chiaravalloti, Christodoulou, and colleagues (2003) examined verbal learning and memory using a modified selective reminding procedure (Buschke & Fuld, 1974) in a mixed medical sample that included patients with CFS and patients with rheumatoid arthritis. Their results indicated a significant correlation between a factor score representing processing speed and measures of working memory. Episodic memory was not examined in this study. This finding further suggests that information processing speed may play a role in the acquisition of new information, however the hypothesis concerning whether processing speed mediates deficits in episodic memory was again not tested directly.

Multiple sclerosis

Several studies have examined information processing speed and long-term memory function concurrently in patients with MS. These studies have indicated significant processing speed and learning and episodic memory deficits in MS subtypes (for examples see Archibald & Fisk, 2000; Gaudino, Chiaravalloti, DeLuca, & Diamond, 2001) that are consistent across the visual and auditory domains (Diamond et al., 1997). Also, episodic memory deficits in multiple sclerosis seem to be greatest for the acquisition of verbal and visual information, with no differences between modalities. Individuals with primary and secondary progressive multiple sclerosis also appear to show additional deficits in recall, even after equating individuals with multiple sclerosis and controls on acquisition (Gaudino et al., 2001).

Multiple studies have found significant positive relationships between measures of processing speed and episodic memory, particularly for measures of acquisition of unstructured verbal information (DeLuca, Barbieri-Berger, & Johnson, 1994; DeLuca, Gaudino, Diamond, Christodoulou, & Engel, 1998; Demaree, Gaudino, DeLuca, & Ricker, 2000). Arnett (2004) showed that speed of presentation influences episodic memory, as indexed by immediate recall of a short story in patients with MS and college students. This further supports the notion that processing speed influences the acquisition of information in episodic memory. However, simple bivariate correlations and manipulations such as that reported above are not sufficient to establish mediation. Unfortunately, only one study has provided results directly examining whether information processing speed mediates MS-related declines in episodic memory. Chiaravalloti, Demaree, and Gaudino (2003) directly examined processing speed as a mediator of verbal learning and memory in MS patients. Processing speed was indexed using a composite score derived from the average of performances on digit span, PASAT total score, AT-SAT percent correct, and VT-SAT total score. They found that individuals with MS, who required a larger number of trials to learn words, had poorer recall and shallower depth of encoding. However, when information processing speed was entered as a covariate in ANCOVA, individuals requiring a higher number of learning trials no longer differed significantly from individuals requiring a lower number of learning trials. This finding may suggest that information processing speed mediates the deficits observed on an episodic memory test (selective reminding) in patients with MS.

We are unaware of any studies directly examining whether working memory contributes incrementally to the mediation of episodic memory deficits in MS (but see Kalmar & Chiaravalloti, chapter 7 in this volume). Results from DeLuca, Christodoulou, and colleagues (2004) suggest that information processing speed deficits are more common and prominent than working memory deficits in individuals with MS. However, these involved simple comparisons between average levels and individual scores. Studies directly examining this issue are necessary for more accurately characterizing the cause of memory problems in multiple sclerosis.

Executive functioning

Although infrequent, a few individual studies designed to investigate the influence of processing speed on various aspects of executive functioning have been performed. These studies are described below.

Subjective time estimation (STE)

It is well known that individuals report the duration of a task—known as subjective time estimation (STE)—to be shorter when that task requires higher levels of their cognitive resources (Hicks, Miller, & Kinsbourne, 1976; McClain, 1983; Zakay, Nitzan, & Glicksohn, 1983). For example, Hicks and colleagues (1976) found that individuals judged the duration of a card sorting task to be shorter when the information requiring processing on each card was increased. In terms of individual difference research, Fink and Neubauer (2001) found that individuals with higher levels of intelligence, as measured by the Raven's Advance Progressive Matrices test (Raven, 1958), rated the duration of two processing speed tasks they performed to be longer (and more realistic) than individuals with lower intelligence. The reason for this, the authors surmised, is that individuals with higher intelligence have faster information processing speeds (e.g., Neubauer & Bucik, 1996; Neubauer & Knorr, 1998), and thus would use less of their cognitive resources to perform the tasks.

To directly test the impact of processing speed on STE, Fink and Neubauer (2005) asked 96 undergraduate students to perform one working memory and one processing speed task, providing an STE for each. The working memory task was a Computation Span (CS) task in which participants were asked to perform 28 mathematical calculations by adding and/or subtracting 10 numbers presented to them on a computer screen for 12 seconds. Participants were asked to make the calculation, report their result verbally, and use any remainder of their 12 seconds to memorize the answer (the working memory component of the task). Following the task, resulting in their working memory score, participants were asked to correctly report their results in the order attained. They were then asked to judge the amount of time needed to perform this working memory task (i.e., the STE). The processing speed and working memory tasks were identical, except that the speeded task included no memory component (i.e., participants were not asked to remember their calculations). Again, participants were asked to provide STEs for the processing speed task. As a control, participants provided STEs during a "cognitive rest" condition in which a fixation cross was presented for the same duration as the mathematical stimuli (i.e., 12 seconds). Finally, participants also performed the Raven's Advance Progressive Matrices test. Results showed that, collapsed across all participants, STEs were significantly shorter for the cognitively demanding tasks (i.e., working memory, processing speed) than those requiring no processing (i.e., the rest condition). Linear regression analyses revealed that persons with higher intelligence scored significantly higher on both working memory and processing speed tasks, and that the high-IQ STEs for the cognitively demanding tasks were significantly longer than for those with lower intelligence. Most importantly, processing speed was significantly correlated with STE on both the processing speed ($r = .39$, $p < .01$) and working memory tasks ($r = .30$, $p < .01$), with faster processing speed strongly predicting more accurate (i.e., longer) time of duration. Thus it appears that processing speed may be an important factor influencing accuracy of time estimation. That said, some of the relationship between processing speed and STE accuracy in this study may be explained by the significant overlap between working memory and processing speed tasks (e.g., visual processing, mathematical ability, etc.). Future research may benefit from using more disparate measures.

An index of executive abilities as a function of age

It has been well documented that executive abilities decline as a function of age (Brennan, Welsh, & Fisher, 1997; Corey-Bloom, Wiederholt, Edelstein, Salmon, Cahn, & Barrett-Connor, 1996; Fisk & Warr, 1996), and some have postulated that such deterioration results from slowed processing speed (for a review, see Salthouse, 1996b). To directly test the influence of age-related processing speed decline on executive functioning, Keys and White (2000) administered a series of executive tasks to 46 healthy young adults (age range 17–23) and 40 healthy older adults (age range 56–82). Within their battery, there were three tasks that are commonly administered within the neuropsychological community (i.e., they were experimental tasks being evaluated within the study). These three tasks were the Controlled Oral Word Association Test (COWAT; Benton, Hamsher, & Sivan, 1994), Part I of the RUFF Figural Fluency Test (RUFF; Ruff, 1988), and Trails B (U.S. Army, 1944). To subsequently partial out the influence of psychomotor speed on executive task performance, the authors administered psychomotor speed tasks that were similar to the COWAT, RUFF, and Trails B, repsectively (the psychomotor tasks were subsequently used as covariates in analyses). For example, Trails A was the psychomotor speed task for Trails B. For the other tasks, the researchers needed to become more creative: For example, the psychomotor speed task for the COWAT was the time it took participants to repeat 10 times a series of one-, two-, and three-syllable words beginning with "F" (e.g., fire, flower, family), "A," and "S." In their sample, age was found to significantly predict RUFF and Trails B (but not COWAT) performance. The shared variance between RUFF performance and age was .18 but, after controlling for psychomotor speed, this relationship declined to .07. Likewise, controlling for psychomotor speed (in this case, Trails A) reduced the shared variance between age and Trails B from .41 to .03. Although Keys and White's (2000) main point was that age adversely influences executive functioning *even after controlling for age-related psychomotor speed slowing*, their data are even more robust in demonstrating that psychomotor speed accounts for the vast majority of executive performance decline associated with the normal aging process.

Tower of London in MS

Arnett, Higginson, and Randolph (2001) performed research designed to disentangle the relative contributions of depression and psychomotor speed among MS patients on the performance of a task requiring planning ability, the Tower of London (TOL; Davis, Bajszar, & Squire, 1994). The need to disentangle this relationship was for two reasons: (1) both MS patients and persons with depression tend to show impairment on processing speed tasks (Demaree et al., 1999; Tsourtos, Thompson, & Stough, 2002) and cognitively demanding tasks (like the TOL) (Arnett et al., 1997; Foong, Rozewicz, Davie, Thompson, Miller, & Ron, 1999; Hartlage, Alloy, Vazquez, & Dykman, 1993), and (2) the comorbidity between MS and depression is significant (e.g., Minden & Schiffer, 1990). In addition to the TOL, these authors also administered three information processing speed tasks—the PASAT, the Symbol-Digit Modalities Test (Smith, 1982), and total time per switch on the Visual Elevator subtest from the Test of Everyday Attention (Robertson, Ward, Ridgeway, & Nimmo-Smith, 1994). Arnett and colleagues (2001) found that (a) the time per trial (TOL time/trial) index score on the TOL, and (b) the three information processing speed measures both accounted for 25% of the variance in depression. Remarkably, the variance accounted for by these measures overlapped 100%! Thus, it appears that one commonly used measure of planning ability (TOL time/trial) is significantly affected by impairments in processing speed. Of note, the authors found that the TOLs moves per trial score accounted for an additional (non-overlapping) 8% of the variance in depression score, suggesting that this purely non-time-dependent measure may be a useful proxy for pure executive planning ability.

Operational confounds

No neuropsychological processing speed measure is entirely pure; that is, they all tap other constructs as well. Given its frequent use, let us analyze the PASAT further and discuss research designed to parse apart the myriad constructs it additionally measures. Figure 3.1 illustrates three potential confounds of the PASAT (Figure 3.1(a)–(c)) and one potential relationship between processing speed and information acquisition/recall (Figure 3.1(d)). Researchers have deconstructed these relationships using different strategies, and these are presented as good examples of methods designed to differentiate between the constructs underlying PASAT performance.

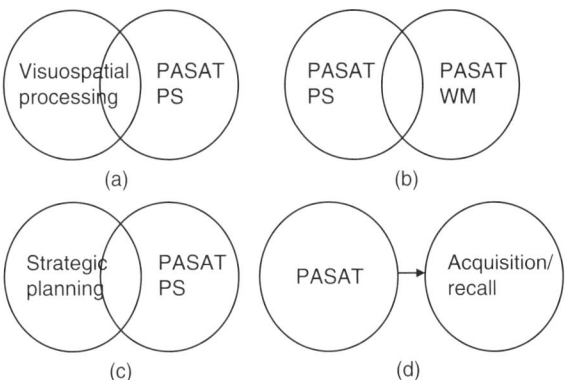

Figure 3.1 Potential PASAT confounds, (a), (b), and (c), and relationships, (d). PS = processing speed; WM = working memory.

Using a concrete example (Figure 3.1(a)), given the propensity for MS to affect myelin sheaths within the optic nerve (Sharpe & Sanders, 1975), one may logically suspect that persons with MS might have impaired performance on processing speed tasks requiring visual perception because of the poor quality and hence integration of visual input. In this example, Diamond and colleagues (1997) determined that impaired visual processing among MS patients does not selectively affect PASAT performance by demonstrating that persons with MS were similarly impaired on both the PASAT and PVSAT. Another way that the visual acuity–processing speed confound has been controlled is by ensuring that MS and control groups are equated on visuospatial perception ability, as inferred by performance on such tasks as the Judgement of Line Orientation Test (JLOT; Benton, Varney, & Hamsher, 1978) (e.g., Demaree et al., 1999). Still, both primary visual impairment and secondary perceptual problems may adversely influence processing speed task performance. Due caution must be exercised before interpreting PASAT performance deficits alone as indicative of processing speed impairment.

Perhaps the most significant confound of the PASAT processing speed is working memory (Figure 3.1(b)). In a mixed medical sample, Chiaravalloti, Christodoulou, and colleagues (2003) used factor analysis and found the PASAT to correlate primarily with "complex" processing speed measures, with additional but secondary loadings on a working memory factor as well. This finding should not be surprising because the speed/accuracy confound has long been recognized in the literature (e.g., Salthouse, 1996b): Improved accuracy comes at a cost, namely, slowed speed of processing (and vice versa). Such data call into question the discriminant validity of the traditional PASAT and suggest that it may be impossible to disentangle processing speed from working memory on the PASAT.

To counter this confound, Bruce Diamond developed computerized derivatives of the PASAT and PVSAT called the AT-SAT and VT-SAT, respectively. As previously described, to attain a purer measure of processing speed, these programs were designed to alter the inter-stimulus interval during the task to ensure that each participant achieves a 50% accuracy rate. Using these measures instead of the traditional PASAT, information processing speed (while controlling for working memory) has been shown to be a primary deficit in MS (Demaree et al., 1999), TBI (Madigan et al., 2000) and CFS (DeLuca, Christodoulou et al., 2004). These data are consistent with more recent findings of impaired processing speed without working memory deficits among persons with MS, as indicated by PSI score deficits on the WAIS-III with non-deficient scores on the working memory index (WMI) of the Wechsler Memory Scale—3rd edition (WMS-III; Wechsler, 1997b) (Chelune, 2002; DeLuca, Chelune et al., 2004; Kalmar, Bryant, Tulsky, & DeLuca, 2004). Thus the AT-SAT and VT-SAT appear to be relatively efficient PASAT-like instruments designed to parse information processing speed from working memory. Use of the AT- and VT-SAT is highly recommended for future processing speed research.

Strategic planning is another potential confound of the PASAT (Figure 3.1(c)). One effective strategy to reduce task difficulty is by "chunking" the stimuli presented in the PASAT (Snyder, Aniskiewicz, & Snyder, 1993). Specifically, by adding two numbers and then taking the next digit "off," one is able to effectively reduce processing speed and working memory burdens. Snyder and colleagues (1993) recommended quantifying participant score as the number of correct responses that immediately follow another correct response (termed "dyads"): The higher the number of dyads, the better the participant performed the test in the intended manner. This scoring method has been helpful in terms of quantifying speed/working memory performance while controlling for the use of a "chunking" strategy. For instance, in their comparison of 35 MS patients to 35 matched controls, Fisk and Archibald (2001) found that the standard scoring procedure failed to discriminate patients from controls at the 1.2 and 1.6 s ISI trials. Conversely, use of the dyad scoring procedure revealed impaired performance among MS patients across all four ISI trials. Shucard and colleagues (2004) presented just the two slowest inter-stimulus interval trials (e.g., 2.0 and 2.4 s/digit) to 45 SLE patients and 27 controls. Like Fisk and Archibald (2001), group differences were only observed when using the dyad quantification method. Such an advance in scoring protocol is not only useful in terms of identifying deficits, but may also be invaluable in terms of appreciating true relationships between processing speed and other neurological/neuropsychological measures. As an example of this, Snyder and Cappelleri (2001) used both standard and dyad PASAT scoring procedures to predict total brain lesion volume (TLV) among 41 MS patients (as determined by magnetic resonance imaging, MRI). After adjusting for age, sex, and education, the dyad score correlated significantly with TLV ($r = -.40$, $p = .01$), whereas the traditional (number correct) score did not ($r = .03$, $p = .88$). In fact, each correct dyad response predicted about 364 mm^2 less TLV.

It is important to note that some processing speed tasks appear less confounded than others (e.g., the PASAT). The Sternberg Memory Scanning Test (SMST), for example, which requires participants to determine whether a number was previously presented to them as part of a memory set, provides a particularly good measure of processing speed. In the SMST, set size varies across trials, from 1 to 6. Assuming equal performance accuracy between groups, which is generally the case, the slope of the reaction time (RT) to set size (1 to 6) is a pure measure of scanning speed. The y-intercept of this RT function, which is another dependent variable of interest in individual difference and clinical literatures, reflects a composite of many confounds presented in Figure 3.1, including perceptual and motor processing. Thus, along with the AT- and VT-SAT, SMST slope is considered an attractive measure of processing speed which, if it covaries with other tasks designed to measure other pure neuropsychological constructs, may provide strong evidence of a true neuropsychological relationship. Of note, similar to the PASAT dyad score, SMST slope has been found to predict MRI lesion volume within the posterior fossa brain region (Archibald et al., 2004).

In sum, when conducting processing speed research, it is important to choose as pure a measure as possible and to analyze the data in such a way that maximizes its construct validity.

Methodological problems and future research issues

Several methodological problems limit the conclusions that can be drawn from these studies regarding whether processing speed mediates memory changes in the above clinical populations. These include poor specification of the processing speed and memory constructs, inadequate statistical methods for examining the mediator hypothesis, and failure to examine other potential mediators of memory decline in clinical samples. Each of these problems will be discussed in turn.

The majority of the above studies using clinical samples employed a single task (e.g., PASAT), or several slightly different variations of a measure, to operationalize the construct of processing speed. The exceptions to this were studies in which several different measures were averaged to create a processing speed index. When a single measure or several highly similar measures are used to index processing speed, it is difficult to determine whether results are a result of the particular validity of the measure, the modality of stimulus presentation, and/or behavioral requirements for response. There are no pure measures of processing speed alone. The use of averaged measures or composites only partially obviates this concern, depending on whether all the measures have similar or different modalities of stimulus presentation, require similar or different responses, or place similar emphasis on basic cognitive skills. For example, in the study by Chiaravalloti and colleagues

(2003) information processing ability was operationalized as the average of three scores derived from versions of the PASAT using different modalities of presentation and a digit span task. In this case, averaging may reduce the chance that results were indicative of stimulus modality; however, this average is likely to substantially increase the load on working memory abilities. The use of averaging multiple measures is also less than ideal since not all measures would be expected to contribute equal variance to the measurement of processing speed. The issues of stimulus modality and behavioral response are highly relevant to interpretations of the processing speed index of the WAIS-III (Wechsler, 1997a). This index involves the averaging of two measures, both of which involve visually presented information and motor responses. Additionally, future research should pay more careful attention to the issue of construct validity. Use of more sophisticated statistical approaches, such as structural equation modeling, can help to lessen construct validity concerns by identifying latent processing speed and memory variables using multiple distinct individual measures. When used in this way, structural equation models limit the influence of stimulus and response confounds and yield more generalizable findings. The work of Salthouse (see Salthouse & Madden, chapter 10 in this volume) is a good example of how to use such techniques for processing speed research.

Several of the clinical comparisons reviewed above utilized hierarchical regression or ANCOVA procedures. While these procedures are useful for examining shared and distinct variance among a set of variables, they have less utility for examining complex mediational processes. For example, entering processing speed before schizophrenia status in a hierarchical regression allows the researcher to observe whether processing speed and the dependent variable (e.g., memory) share significant variance, and whether schizophrenia status accounts for incremental variance. However, it does not speak to whether processing speed deficits actually mediated or caused memory deficits. Thus the possibility remains that disease-related memory decline is a function of processing speed, executive functions, working memory, elementary sensory or motor functions, all these functions, or a general common factor influencing all these specific functions. Structural equation models specifying latent variables for each of the sensory, motor, cognitive, or even emotional factors of interest permit greater power of the inferences made regarding which variables mediate memory performance and the strength of the mediation. Another problem with these uses of regression and ANOVA-based procedures is the likely non-equivalence of disease groups on the covariate (for an extended discussion see Miller & Chapman, 2001). This is not a problem for studies examining the relations between processing speed within a single group, such as normal aging studies, but it is a substantial problem for group comparisons. It is recommended that future research use statistical procedures and research designs that can better account for the difficulties in examining mediator/moderator models in clinical groups.

Future directions

The above methodological limitations leave several unanswered questions. Future work examining the relative contributions of processing speed to various aspects of episodic memory is necessary for better specifying the meaning of memory deficits in clinical groups. For example, one would anticipate that if processing speed mediates memory deficits, its influence would be strongest on the encoding and acquisition of information. Alternatively, if executive functioning is the primary mediator, then it might be expected to show the strongest effect for consolidation and retrieval. Future research should also examine whether processing speed only mediates certain aspects of memory (visual vs. verbal, semantic vs. episodic) and should examine procedurally varied, but relatively specific, measures of processing speed. These studies have the potential to greatly increase our understanding of the functional effects of various neurological and psychological processes.

References

Archibald, C. J., & Fisk, J. D. (2000). Information processing efficiency in patients with multiple sclerosis. *Journal of Clinical and Experimental Neuropsychology*, 22 (5), 686–701.

Archibald, C. J., Wei, X., Scott, J. N., Wallace, C. J., Zhang, Y., Metz, L. M., et al. (2004). Posterior fossa lesion volume and slowed information processing in multiple sclerosis. *Brain*, 127, 1526–1534.

Arnett, P. A. (2004). Speed of presentation influences story recall in college students and persons with multiple sclerosis. *Archives of Clinical Neuropsychology*, 19, 507–523.

Arnett, P. A., Higginson, C. I., & Randolph, J. J. (2001). Depression in multiple sclerosis: Relationship to planning ability. *Journal of the International Neuropsychological Society*, 7, 665–674.

Arnett, P. A., Rao, S. M., Grafman, J., Bernadin, L., Luchetta, T., Binder, J. R., et al. (1997). Executive functions in multiple sclerosis: An analysis of temporal ordering, semantic encoding, and planning abilities. *Neuropsychology*, 11, 535–544.

Baddeley, A. (1981). The concept of working memory: A view of its current state and probable future development. *Cognition*, 10, 17–23.

Baddeley, A. (1992). Working memory. *Science*, 255, 556–559.

Baddeley, A. (1997). Working memory. In M. S. Gazzaniga (Ed.), *The cognitive neurosciences* (pp. 755–764). Cambridge, MA: MIT Press.

Baddeley, A. (1998). Recent developments in working memory. *Current Opinion in Neurobiology*, 8, 234–238.

Baddeley, A. D. (1986). *Working memory*. Oxford: Clarendon Press.

Baddeley, A. D., & Hitch, G. (1974). Working memory. In G. H. Bower (Ed.), *The psychology of learning and motivation* (Vol. 8, pp. 47–89). New York: Academic Press.

Baron, R. M., & Kenny, D. A. (1986). The moderator–mediator variable distinction in social psychological research: Conceptual, strategic, and statistical considerations. *Journal of Personality and Social Psychology*, 51 (6), 1173–1182.

Benton, A. L., Hamsher, K., & Sivan, A. B. (1994). *Multilingual aphasia examination*. Iowa City: AJA Associates.
Benton, A. L., Varney, N. R., & Hamsher, K. (1978). Visuospatial judgement: A clinical test. *Archives of Neurology, 35*, 364–367.
Brebion, G., David, A. S., Pilowsky, L. S., & Jones, H. (2004). Recognition of visual stimuli and memory for spatial context in schizophrenic patients and healthy volunteers. *Journal of Clinical and Experimental Neuropsychology, 26* (8), 1093–1102.
Brennan, M., Welsh, M. C., & Fisher, C. B. (1997). Aging and executive function skills: An examination of a community-dwelling older adult population. *Perceptual and Motor Skills, 84*, 1187–1197.
Bryan, J., & Luszcz, M. A. (1996). Speed of information processing as a mediator between age and free recall performance. *Psychology and Aging, 11*, 3–9.
Buschke, H., & Fuld, P. A. (1974). Evaluating storage, retention, and retrieval in disordered memory and learning. *Neurology, 24*, 1019–1025.
Buschke, H., Sliwinski, M., Kuslansky, G., & Lipton, R. B. (1997). Diagnsosis of early dementia by the Double Memory Test: Encoding specificity improves diagnostic sensitivity. *Neurology, 48*, 989–997.
Carroll, J. B. (1993). *Human cognitive abilities: A survey of factor-analytic studies*. New York: Cambridge University Press.
Cerella, J., & Hale, S. (1994). The rise and fall in information-processing rates over the life span. *Acta Psychologica, 86*, 109–197.
Chaytor, N., & Schmitter-Edgecombe, M. (2004). Working memory and aging: A cross-sectional and logitudinal analysis using a self-ordered pointing task. *Journal of the International Neuropsychological Society, 10* (4), 489–503.
Chelune, G. J. (2002). Prevalence and estimated risk of processing speed deficits in multiple sclerosis. *Journal of the International Neuropsychological Society, 8*, 185–186.
Chiaravalloti, N. D., Christodoulou, C., Demaree, H. A., & DeLuca, J. (2003). Differentiating simple versus complex processing speed: Influence on new learning and memory performance. *Journal of Clinical and Experimental Neuropsychology, 25* (4), 489–501.
Chiaravalloti, N. D., Demaree, H. A., & Gaudino, E. A. (2003). Can the repetition effect maximize learning in multiple sclerosis? *Clinical Rehabilitation, 17*, 58–68.
Cicerone, K. D. (1997). Clinical sensitivity of four measures of attention to mild traumatic brain injury. *The Clinical Neuropsychologist, 11* (3), 266–272.
Cirillo, M. A., & Seidman, L. J. (2003). Verbal declarative memory dysfunction in schizophrenia: From clinical assessment to genetics and brain mechanisms. *Neuropsychology Review, 13* (2), 43–77.
Cook, S. E., Nebes, R. D., Halligan, E. M., Burmeister, L. A., Saxton, J. A., Ganguli, M., et al. (2002). Memory impairments in elderly individuals with a mildly elevated serum TSH: The role of processing resources, depression, and cerebrovascular disease. *Aging, Neuropsychology, and Cognition, 9* (3), 175–183.
Corey-Bloom, J., Wiederholt, W. C., Edelstein, S., Salmon, D. P., Cahn, D., & Barrett-Connor, E. (1996). Cognitive and functional status of the oldest old. *Journal of the American Geriatric Society, 44*, 671–674.
Davis, H. P., Bajszar, G. M., & Squire, L. R. (1994). *Colorado neuropsychology tests: Explicit memory, implicit memory, and problem solving*. Colorado Springs: Colorado Neuropsychology Tests Co.

de Jong, P. F., & Das-Smaal, E. A. (1995). Attention and intelligence: The validity of the star counting test. *Journal of Educational Psychology, 87*, 80–92.
Delis, D. C., Kramer, J. H., Kaplan, E., & Ober, B. A. (1987). *California Verbal Learning Test (CVLT) manual.* New York: Psychological Corporation.
DeLuca, J., Barbieri-Berger, S., & Johnson, S. K. (1994). The nature of memory impairments in multiple sclerosis: Acquisition versus recall. *Journal of Clinical and Experimental Neuropsychology, 16* (2), 183–189.
DeLuca, J., Chelune, G. J., Tulsky, D. S., Lengenfelder, J., & Chiaravalloti, N. D. (2004). Is speed of processing or working memory the primary information processing deficit in multiple sclerosis? *Journal of Clinical and Experimental Neuropsychology, 26* (4), 550–562.
DeLuca, J., Christodoulou, C., Diamond, B. J., Rosenstein, E. D., Kramer, N., & Natelson, B. H. (2004). Working memory deficits in chronic fatigue syndrome: Differentiating between speed and accuracy of information processing. *Journal of the International Neuropsychological Society, 10*, 101–109.
DeLuca, J., Gaudino, E. A., Diamond, B. J., Christodoulou, C., & Engel, R. A. (1998). Acquisition and storage deficits in multiple sclerosis. *Journal of Clinical and Experimental Neuropsychology, 20* (3), 376–390.
DeLuca, J., Johnson, S. K., Beldowicz, D., & Natelson, B. H. (1995). Neuropsychological impairments in chronic fatigue syndrome, multiple sclerosis, and depression. *Journal of Neurology, Neurosurgery, and Psychiatry, 58* (1), 38–43.
DeLuca, J., Johnson, S. K., & Natelson, B. H. (1993). Information processing efficiency in chronic fatigue syndrome and multiple sclerosis. *Archives of Neurology, 50* (3), 301–304.
Demaree, H. A., DeLuca, J., Gaudino, E. A., & Diamond, B. J. (1999). Speed of information processing as a key deficit in multiple sclerosis: Implications for rehabilitation. *Journal of Neurology, Neurosurgery, and Psychiatry, 67*, 661–663.
Demaree, H. A., Gaudino, E. A., DeLuca, J., & Ricker, J. H. (2000). Learning impairment is associated with recall ability in multiple sclerosis. *Journal of Clinical and Experimental Neuropsychology, 22* (6), 865–873.
Dempster, F. N. (1981). Memory span: Sources of individual and developmental differences. *Psychological Bulletin, 89*, 63–100.
Dempster, F. N. (1985). Short-term memory development in childhood and adolescence. In C. J. Brainerd & M. Pressley (Eds.), *Basic processes in memory development* (pp. 209–248). New York: Springer.
Dempster, F. N. (1992). The rise and fall of the inhibitory mechanism: Toward a unified theory of cognitive development and aging. *Developmental Review, 12*, 45–75.
Denney, D. R., Lynch, S. G., Parmenter, B. A., & Horne, N. (2004). Cognitive impairment in relapsing and primary progressive multiple sclerosis: Mostly a matter of speed. *Journal of the International Neuropsychological Society, 10*, 948–956.
Diamond, B. J., DeLuca, J., Kim, H., & Kelley, S. M. (1997). The question of disproportionate impairments in visual and auditory information processing in multiple sclerosis. *Journal of Clinical and Experimental Neuropsychology, 19* (1), 34–42.
Diamond, B. J., DeLuca, J., Rosenthal, R. V., Davis, K., Lucas, G., Noskin, O., et al. (2000). Information processing in older versus younger adults: Accuracy versus speed. *International Journal of Rehabilitation and Health, 5*, 55–64.
Dobbs, A. R., & Rule, B. G. (1989). Adult age differences in working memory. *Psychology and Aging, 4*, 500–503.

Duley, J. F., Wilkins, J. W., Hamby, S. L., Hopkins, D. G., Burwell, R. D., & Barry, N. S. (1993). Explicit scoring criteria for the Rey-Osterrieth and Taylor complex figures. *The Clinical Neuropsychologist*, *7*, 29–38.

Fields, R. B. (1998). The dementias. In P. J. Snyder & P. D. Nussbaum (Eds.), *Clinical neuropsychology: A pocket handbook for assessment*. Washington, DC: American Psychological Association.

Fink, A., & Neubauer, A. C. (2001). Speed of information processing, psychometric intelligence and time estimation as an index of cognitive load. *Personality and Individual Differences*, *30*, 1009–1021.

Fink, A., & Neubauer, A. C. (2005). Individual differences in time estimation related to cognitive ability, speed of information processing and working memory. *Intelligence*, *33*, 5–26.

Fisk, J. D., & Archibald, C. J. (2001). Limitations of the Paced Auditory Serial Addition Test as a measure of working memory in patients with multiple sclerosis. *Journal of the International Neuropsychological Society*, *7*, 363–372.

Fisk, J. E., & Warr, P. (1996). Age and working memory: The role of perceptual speed, the central executive, and the phonological loop. *Psychology and Aging*, *11*, 316–323.

Foong, J., Rozewicz, L., Davie, C. A., Thompson, A. J., Miller, D. H., & Ron, M. A. (1999). Correlates of executive function in multiple sclerosis: The use of magnetic resonance spectroscopy as an index of focal pathology. *Journal of Neuropsychiatry and Clinical Neurosciences*, *11*, 45–50.

Fry, A. F., & Hale, S. (1996). Processing speed, working memory, and fluid intelligence: Evidence for a developmental cascade. *Psychological Science*, *7*, 237–241.

Fry, A. F., & Hale, S. (2000). Relationships among processing speed, working memory, and fluid intelligence in children. *Biological Psychology*, *54*, 1–34.

Gathercole, S. E., & Baddeley, A. (1993). *Working memory and language*. Hillsdale, NJ: Lawrence Erlbaum Associates, Inc.

Gaudino, E. A., Chiaravalloti, N. D., DeLuca, J., & Diamond, B. J. (2001). A comparison of memory performance in relapsing–remitting, primary progressive, and secondary progressive multiple sclerosis. *Neuropsychiatry, Neuropsychology, and Behavioral Neurology*, *14*, 32–44.

Gladsjo, J. A., McAdams, L. A., Palmer, B. W., Moore, D. J., Jeste, D. V., & Heaton, R. K. (2004). A six-factor model of cognition in schizophrenia and related psychotic disorders: Relationships with clinical symptoms and functional capacity. *Schizophrenia Bulletin*, *30* (4), 739–754.

Gronwall, D. M. A. (1977). Paced Auditory Serial-Addition Task: A measure of recovery from concussion. *Perceptual and Motor Skills*, *44*, 367–373.

Hale, S. (1990). A global developmental trend in cognitive processing speed. *Child Development*, *61*, 653–663.

Hartlage, S., Alloy, L. B., Vazquez, C., & Dykman, B. (1993). Automatic and effortful processing in depression. *Psychological Bulletin*, *113*, 247–278.

Hicks, R. E., Miller, G. W., & Kinsbourne, M. (1976). Prospective and retrospective judgments of time as a function of amount of information processed. *American Journal of Psychology*, *89*, 719–730.

Hillary, F. G., Chiaravalloti, N. D., Ricker, J. H., Steffener, J., Bly, B. M., Lange, G., et al. (2003). An investigation of working memory rehearsal in multiple sclerosis using fMRI. *Journal of Clinical and Experimental Neuropsychology*, *25* (7), 965–978.

Holthausen, E. A. E., Wiersma, D., Sitskoom, M. M., Dingemans, P. M., Schene, A. H., & van den Bosch, R. J. (2003). Long-term memory deficits in schizophrenia: Primary or secondary dysfunction. *Neuropsychology, 17*, 539–547.

Joy, S., Kaplan, E., & Fein, D. (2003). Speed and memory in the WAIS-III digit symbol-coding subtest across the adult lifespan. *Archives of Clinical Neuropsychology, 19*, 759–767.

Kail, R. (1991). Developmental change in speed of processing during childhood and adolescence. *Psychological Bulletin, 109*, 490–501.

Kail, R. (1992). Processing speed, speech rate, and memory. *Developmental Review, 28*, 899–904.

Kail, R., & Salthouse, T. A. (1994). Processing speed as a mental capacity. *Acta Psychologica, 86*, 199–225.

Kalmar, J. H., Bryant, D., Tulsky, D. & DeLuca, J. (2004). Information processing deficits in multiple sclerosis: Does choice of screening instrument make a difference? *Rehabilitation Psychology, 49*, 213–218.

Kennedy, J. E., Clement, P. F., & Curtiss, G. (2003). WAIS-III processing speed index scores after TBI: The influence of working memory, psychomotor speed and perceptual processing. *The Clinical Neuropsychologist, 17* (3), 303–307.

Keri, S., Szendi, I., Kelemen, O., Benedek, G., & Janka, Z. (2001). Remitted schizophrenia-spectrum patients with spared working memory show information processing abnormalities. *European Archives of Psychiatry and Clinical Neuroscience, 251*, 60–65.

Keys, B. A., & White, D. A. (2000). Exploring the relationship between age, executive abilities, and psychomotor speed. *Journal of the International Neuropsychological Society, 6*, 76–82.

Kieseppa, T., Tuulio-Henriksson, A., Haukka, J., Van Erp, T., Glahn, D., Cannon, T. D., et al. (2005). Memory and verbal learning functions in twins with bipolar-I disorder, and the role of information processing speed. *Psychological Medicine, 35*, 205–215.

Kirasic, K. C., Allen, G. L., Dobson, S. H., & Binder, K. S. (1996). Aging, cognitive resources, and declarative learning. *Psychology and Aging, 11*, 658–670.

Krikorian, R., Bartok, J., & Gay, N. (1994). Tower of London procedure: A standard method and developmental data. *Journal of Clinical and Experimental Neuropsychology, 16*, 840–850.

Kyllonen, P. C., & Christal, R. E. (1990). Reasoning ability is (little more than) working-memory capacity? *Intelligence, 14*, 389–433.

Lengenfelder, J., Bryant, D., Diamond, B. J., Kalmar, J. H., Moore, N. B., & DeLuca, J. (2006). Processing speed interacts with working memory efficiency in multiple sclerosis. *Archives of Clinical Neuropsychology, 21*, 229–238.

Lezak, M. D. (1995). *Neuropsychological assessment.* New York: Oxford University Press.

Madigan, N. K., DeLuca, J., Diamond, B. J., Tramontano, G., & Averill, A. (2000). Speed of information processing in traumatic brain injury: Modality-specific factors. *Journal of Head Trauma Rehabilitation, 15* (3), 943–956.

Marshall, P. S., Forstot, M., Callies, A., Peterson, P. K., & Schenck, C. H. (1997). Cognitive slowing and working memory difficulties in chronic fatigue syndrome. *Psychosomatic Medicine, 59* (1), 58–66.

McClain, L. (1983). Interval estimation: Effect of processing demands on prospective and retrospective reports. *Perception and Psychophysics, 34*, 185–189.

Michiels, V., & Cluydts, R. (2001). Neuropsychological functioning in chronic fatigue syndrome: A review. *Acta Psychiatrica Scandinavica, 103*, 84–93.

Miller, G. A., & Chapman, J. P. (2001). Misunderstanding analysis of covariance. *Journal of Abnormal Psychology, 110*, 40–48.

Miller, L. T., & Vernon, P. A. (1996). Intelligence, reaction time and working memory in 4- to 6-year-old children. *Intelligence, 22*, 155–190.

Minden, S. L., & Schiffer, R. B. (1990). Affective disorders in multiple sclerosis. *Archives of Neurology, 47*, 98–104.

Nebes, R. D., Butters, M. A., Mulsant, B. H., Pollock, B. G., Zmuda, M. D., Houck, P. R., et al. (2000). Decreased working memory and processing speed mediate cognitive impairment in geriatric depression. *Psychological Medicine, 30*, 679–691.

Neubauer, A. C., & Bucik, V. (1996). The mental speed–IQ relationship: Unitary or modular? *Intelligence, 22*, 23–48.

Neubauer, A. C., & Knorr, E. (1998). Three paper-and-pencil tests for speed of information processing: Psychometric properties and correlations with intelligence. *Intelligence, 26*, 123–151.

Perlstein, W. M., Cole, M. A., Demery, J. A., Seignourel, P. J., Dixit, N. K., & Larson, M. J. (2004). Parametric manipulation of working memory load in traumatic brain injury: Behavioral and neural correlates. *Journal of the International Neuropsychological Society, 10* (5), 724–741.

Raven, J. C. (1958). *Advanced progressive matrices*. London: Lewis.

Robertson, I. H., Ward, T., Ridgeway, V., & Nimmo-Smith, I. (1994). *The Test of Everyday Attention*. Bury St. Edmunds, UK: Thames Valley Test Co.

Ruff, R. M. (1988). *Ruff Figural Fluency Test administration manual*. San Diego, CA: Neuropsychological Resources.

Salmond, C. H., Chatfield, D. A., Menon, D. K., Pickard, J. D., & Sahakian, B. J. (2005). Cognitive sequelae of head injury: Involvement of basal forebrain and associated structures. *Brain, 128* (1), 189–200.

Salthouse, T. A. (1994a). The aging of working memory. *Neuropsychology, 8* (4), 535–543.

Salthouse, T. A. (1994b). The nature of the influence of speed on adult age differences in cognition. *Developmental Psychology, 30*, 240–259.

Salthouse, T. A. (1996a). General and specific speed mediation of adult age differences in memory. *Journals of Gerontology: Series B: Psychological and Social Sciences, 51B*, 30–42.

Salthouse, T. A. (1996b). The processing-speed theory of adult differences in cognition. *Psychological Review, 103*, 289–305.

Salthouse, T. A. (2005). Relations between cognitive abilities and measures of executive functioning. *Neuropsychology, 19* (4), 532–545.

Salthouse, T. A., & Coon, V. E. (1993). Influence of task-specific processing speed on age differences in memory. *Journals of Gerontology, 48*, 245–255.

Sharpe, J. A., & Sanders, M. D. (1975). Atrophy of myelinated nerve fibers in the retina of optic neuritis. *The British Journal of Ophthalmology, 59* (4), 229–232.

Sherman, E. M. S., Strauss, E., & Spellacy, F. (1997). Validity of the Paced Auditory Serial Addition Test (PASAT) in adults referred for neuropsychological assessment of head injury. *The Clinical Neuropsychologist, 11*, 34–45.

Shucard, J. L., Parrish, J., Shucard, D. W., McCabe, D. C., Benedict, R. H. B., & Ambrus, J., Jr. (2004). Working memory and processing speed deficits in systemic lupus erythematosus as measured by the Paced Auditory Serial Addition Test. *Journal of the International Neuropsychological Society, 10*, 35–45.

Sliwinski, M., & Buschke, H. (1997). Processing speed and memory in aging and dementia. *Journals of Gerontology: Series B: Psychological and Social Sciences, 52B*, 308–318.

Smith, A. (1982). *Symbol Digit Modalities Test (SDMT) manual (revised)*. Los Angeles: Western Psychological Services.

Snyder, P. J., Aniskiewicz, A. S., & Snyder, A. M. (1993). Quantitative MRI correlates and diagnostic utility of multi-modal measures of executive control in multiple sclerosis. *Journal of Clinical and Experimental Neuropsychology, 15*, 18.

Snyder, P. J., & Cappelleri, J. C. (2001). Information processing speed deficits may be better correlated with the extent of white matter sclerotic lesions in multiple sclerosis than previously suspected. *Brain and Cognition, 46* (1–2), 279–284.

Sternberg, S. (1966). High-speed scanning in human memory. *Science, 153*, 652–654.

Stroop, J. R. (1935). Studies of interference in serial verbal reactions. *Journal of Experimental Psychology, 18*, 643–662.

Tiersky, L. A., Cicerone, K. D., Natelson, B. H., & DeLuca, J. (1998). Neuropsychological functioning in chronic fatigue syndrome and mild traumatic brain injury: A comparison. *The Clinical Neuropsychologist, 12* (4), 503–512.

Tsourtos, G., Thompson, J. C., & Stough, C. (2002). Evidence of an early information processing speed deficit in unipolar major depression. *Psychological Medicine, 32* (2), 259–265.

U.S. Army. (1944). *Army individual test battery manual of directions and scoring*. Washington, DC: Adjutant General's Office.

van der Werf, S. P., de Vree, B., van der Meer, J. W., & Bleijenberg, G. (2002). The relations among body consciousness, somatic symptom report, and information processing speed in chronic fatigue syndrome. *Neuropsychiatry, Neuropsychology, and Behavioral Neurology, 15* (1), 2–9.

Verhaeghen, P., & Salthouse, T. A. (1997). Meta-analyses of age–cognition relations in adulthood: Estimates of linear and nonlinear age effects and structural models. *Psychological Bulletin, 122*, 231–249.

Vink, M., & Jolles, J. (1985). A new version of the Trail Making Test as an information processing task. *Journal of Clinical Neuropsychology, 7*, 162.

Wechsler, D. (1981). *Manual for the Wechsler Adult Intelligence Scale—Revised*. San Antonio, TX: The Psychological Corporation.

Wechsler, D. (1997a). *Wechsler Adult Intelligence Scale—Third Edition*. San Antonio, TX: The Psychological Corporation.

Wechsler, D. (1997b). *Wechsler Memory Scale—Third Edition*. San Antonio, TX: The Psychological Corporation.

Zakay, D., Nitzan, D., & Glicksohn, J. (1983). The influence of task difficulty and external tempo on subjective time estimation. *Perception and Psychophysics, 34*, 451–456.

4 The genetics of information processing speed in humans

Danielle Posthuma and Eco de Geus

Introduction

This chapter reviews the extant twin studies reporting on the heritability of processing speed. In general the heritability of this trait is modest, but its proximity to actual neurobiology (e.g., when operationalized as nerve velocity or electrophysiological recording) makes it a useful endophenotype in the search for genetic variation causing individual differences in general cognitive abilities. Furthermore, indices of impaired processing speed traditionally play a role as biomarkers in disorders like reading disability, autism, and attention-deficit/hyperactivity disorder. For instance, we recently showed in a genome scan for IQ that the genomic regions influencing IQ overlap with areas previously implicated in these disorders. Heritability of processing speed, therefore, can be expected to overlap with heritability for these disorders and, with this chapter, we aim to encourage gene hunters for these afflictions to add measures of processing speed to their gene finding efforts.

What is processing speed? Speed of (information) processing is the speed with which subjects can perform basic cognitive operations, including, but not limited to, perception, allocation of attention, chunking, rehearsal, long-term memory retrieval, response selection, and long-term memory storage. Differences in speed of processing are thought to depend critically on structural aspects of neural wiring, like nerve diameter, integrity of myelin sheathing, the number of ion channels, and the efficiency of synaptic neurotransmission. Faster processing speed may allow more information to be processed before it is lost through decay or interference, and is therefore more efficient (Jensen, 1993). Faster speed of rehearsal may allow the maintenance of a larger amount of information in working memory (Baddeley, 1986). Consistent with this view, working memory and processing speed are correlated measures (e.g., Fry & Hale, 2000; Vernon & Weese, 1993), although they can be separable (DeLuca, Chelune, Tulsky, Lengenfelder, & Chiaravalloti, 2004). Both working memory and processing speed play a crucial role in the "neural speed and efficiency" hypothesis of intelligence, which states that the speed with which basic cognitive operations are carried out is predictive of general cognitive ability (Jensen, 1982; Vernon, 1983, 1987).

How do we measure processing speed? Processing speed has been operationalized at various levels from the measurement of peripheral nerve conduction to a higher order factor obtained from the timed subscales of general intelligence tests. In the field of behaviour genetics, processing speed is mostly operationalized "in between"; that is, as the time it takes to make a correct discrimination between two stimuli, the time it takes to generate a meaningful waveform in an electroencephalographic recording, or the time it takes for a subject to press a button in response to a given stimulus. Below we briefly introduce the exact measures and paradigms that have been used in twin studies so far, as we discuss the evidence for a genetic contribution to this trait. We start with a brief introduction to heritability estimation in behaviour genetics, and more specifically the twin design.

Methods in behaviour genetics

Studies in human behaviour genetics describe the decomposition of observed, phenotypic variance into sources of genetic origin and sources of environmental origin. Sources of environmental origin are usually separated into sources that are shared between family members (such as diet, rearing style, socioeconomic status), and sources that are not shared between family members and are unique to an individual (such as sports participation, lifestyle, or accidents). These sources of variance can be separated using a design that includes subjects of different degrees of genetic relationship, such as adoption designs, family designs or twin designs. Resemblance between relatives is a function of the degree to which phenotypic expression is determined by shared genes, shared environmental, and non-shared environmental factors (Lynch & Walsh, 1998).

In an *adoption design* the resemblance between the adopted child and his or her adoptive parents is compared with the resemblance between the adopted child and the biological parents. This provides information on genetic influences on a trait. One particularly strong design is that in which resemblance between identical (monozygotic, MZ) twins reared apart is compared with resemblance between MZ twins reared together. If the resemblance in these two different groups is similar, it can only be ascribed to a sharing of genes in MZ twins, and not to the sharing of environmental influences. Adoption designs, however, are often criticized for unrepresentativeness due to selective placements.

In the *family design*, resemblance on a trait within families is compared with resemblance between families. In other words, the clustering of traits within families is investigated. As family members do not only share genes but also share environmental influences, resemblance between family members can be ascribed to both these sources. Family studies thus provide information on the *familial* influences on a trait, but do not allow the separation of genetic influences from shared environmental influences.

The most widely used design in behaviour genetics is the *twin design*. This is based on a comparison of the phenotypic resemblance on a certain trait between MZ twins with the phenotypic resemblance on that trait between fraternal (dizygotic, DZ) twins. Since MZ twins living at home share 100% of their family environment and 100% of their genes (but see Martin, Boomsma, & Machin, 1997), any resemblance between them is attributed to these two sources of resemblance. The extent to which MZ twins do not resemble each other is ascribed to factors that MZ twins do not share; that is, the unique or non-shared environmental factors, which also include measurement error. Resemblance between DZ twins is also ascribed to the sharing of the family environment, and to the sharing of genes. However, DZ twins share on average only 50% of their segregating genes, so any resemblance between them as a result of genetic influences will be lower than for MZs. The extent to which DZ twins do not resemble each other is a result of non-shared environmental factors and non-shared genetic influences.

Resemblance between MZ twins and between DZ twins on a certain trait can be quantified in a correlation. For MZ twins this correlation is a function of the sharing of additive genetic influences (A) and a function of the sharing of shared, or common, environmental influences (C). The DZ twin correlation is a function of .5A (as they share 50% of their genes) and C. A first estimate of the proportion of additive genetic influences on a trait is therefore given by twice the difference between the MZ and DZ correlations. An estimate of the proportional contribution of the shared environmental influences to the trait variation is given by subtracting the MZ correlation from twice the DZ correlation. The proportional contribution of the non-shared environmental influences can be obtained by subtracting the MZ correlation from 1. It should be noted that the total genetic variance can be decomposed into additive genetic variance and dominant genetic influences (denoted by D). As genetic dominance is hard to detect (Posthuma & Boomsma, 2000), and as the estimate of D is confounded with the estimate of C in a twin design, we here only discuss ACE models. In behaviour genetic studies, results are often reported in terms of the heritability of a trait. The heritability is the proportion of the genetic variance relative to the phenotypic variance.

Although the correlational method described above is intuitive and simple, there are several inherent problems. It does not allow for calculation of standard errors, confidence intervals or *p*-values for the effect of genetic or environmental influences on a trait, it does not easily generalize to the multivariate case or to extended twin families, it does not allow for ascertainment correction, and it handles missing values quite inefficiently (Neale, 2003). In behaviour genetic studies, it is therefore common to use structural equation modelling implemented in statistical software such as LISREL (Jöreskog & Sörbom, 1986), EQS (Bentler, 1995), Amos (Arbuckle, 1994) or Mx (Neale, 1997). A structural equation model is a linear regression model that describes relationships between observed values of latent variables. Based on the known relations for MZ and DZ twins between their latent genes (A) and environmental factors (C or E), structural equations for the expected covariance matrices for MZ and DZ twins can be derived. Effect sizes of the latent, unmeasured parameters (A, C, or E) can then be estimated using several different estimation algorithms. A widely used algorithm is Maximum Likelihood, which uses numerical optimization to find those parameter values that make the observed data most likely (Neale & Cardon, 1992). Structural relations between measured variables (traits) and unmeasured variables (sources of variance) are often graphically represented in a path diagram, which is a mathematically complete description of a structural equation model. A common path diagram for univariate twin data is provided in Figure 4.1.

An index of how well a structural equation model describes the observed data is the goodness-of-fit statistic of a model. Several nested models can be compared on this statistic, to provide a test of the relative importance of additive genetic or (non-)shared environmental influences to the trait of interest. As behaviour geneticists investigate components of variance, as opposed to mean differences between groups, sample sizes need to be relatively high (i.e., between 200 and 1000 twin pairs depending on the effect sizes and multivariate nature of a trait) to draw sensible conclusions on the relative contributions of genes and environmental factors to variation in a trait.

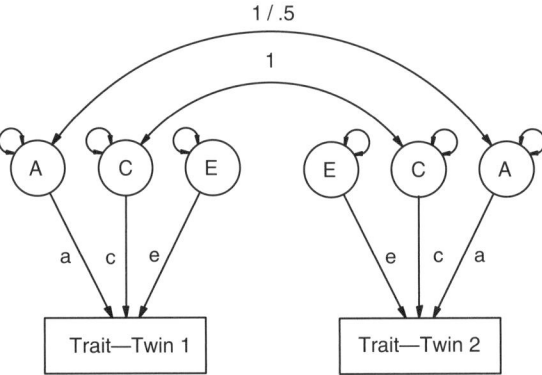

Figure 4.1 Typical path diagram for a univariate ACE twin model. Measured variables are presented in boxes (trait of twin 1 and twin 2), latent variables are denoted by circles. The variance is decomposed into sources of additive genetic variance (A), shared environmental variance (C), and unique or non-shared environmental variance (E). The path coefficients represent the standard deviation of the additive genetic influences (a), shared environmental influences (c), and non-shared environmental influences (e). The correlation between the shared environmental influences of two members of a twin pair is 1, while the correlation between the genetic influences is 1 for MZ pairs and .5 for DZ pairs. The variance of the trait is derived as $a^2 + c^2 + e^2$. The covariance for MZ pairs is $a^2 + c^2$, whereas the covariance for DZ pairs is $.5a^2 + c^2$.

Genetics of processing speed

The genetic architecture of processing speed has been tested at several different levels. Below, we follow a "bottom-up" approach, from low-level neurophysiological measures, such as peripheral nerve conduction velocity, to complex behavioural measures, such as the speed with which an intelligence test is performed.

Peripheral nerve conduction velocity

Peripheral nerve conduction velocity (PNCV) is a measure of the speed with which action potentials travel the length of the axons in the peripheral nervous system. The speed of nerve conduction is a function of the nerve diameter and the degree of myelination.

Only one study to date has investigated the genetic architecture of PNCV (Rijsdijk, Boomsma, & Vernon, 1995). In this study, PNCV was measured twice in a non-clinical sample of 16-year-old (18 at the second measurement occasion) twins. Rijsdijk et al. (1995) determined the PNCV for the wrist–elbow segment of the median nerve of the right arm for 213 16-year-old twin pairs. Using structural equation modelling, they found that at age 16, 76% of the observed variance in PNCV was a result of genetic variance, whereas at age 18 this was 66%. Thus a substantial part of the observed variation in PNCV is due to variation at a genetic level.

In the above study, PNCV was assumed to be a proxy for *central* NCV. According to the "neural speed and efficiency" hypothesis of intelligence (Jensen, 1982; Vernon, 1983, 1987), faster central NCV allows rapid processing of information and should be related to more efficient *cognitive* information processing and higher intelligence. A second paper (Rijsdijk & Boomsma, 1997) therefore specifically investigated the relation between PNCV and intelligence. They found a small correlation of .15 between PNCV and intelligence at age 18, which was completely ascribed to a genetic factor that influences both.

Although the study of Rijsdijk et al. (1995) applies to variation in PNCV in the normal range, these findings may also be of interest to clinical samples. For example, persons that are genetically predisposed to have a slow PNCV—although still in the normal range—may suffer earlier and more severely from the effects of neuropathological diseases, such as Guillain-Barré syndrome, multiple sclerosis, Charcot-Marie-Tooth disease, or chronic inflammatory conditions resulting from diabetes or alcoholism (Weber, 1990).

Inspection time

Inspection time is a measure of central nervous system processing and is defined as the minimum display time a subject needs for making an accurate perceptual discrimination on an obvious stimulus. There is no need to make this discrimination quickly; all that is required is an accurate response. It is therefore distinct from reaction time since it does not involve a speeded response. Visual inspection time can easily be measured using a computerized version of the so-called Π-paradigm. In this paradigm subjects are asked to decide which leg of the Greek letter Π is longest. Visual inspection time is generally thought to reflect speed of apprehension or perceptual speed, and is part of the early stages of information processing. Shorter (i.e., faster) inspection time is related to higher scores on intelligence tests (Luciano, Smith, Wright, Geffen, Geffen, & Martin, 2001; Posthuma, de Geus, & Boomsma, 2001).

The early stage of information processing measured by the inspection time task appears to be compromised in Alzheimer's disease and Korsakoff's psychosis (Deary, Hunter, Langan, & Goodwin, 1991), hypoglycaemia (McCrimmon, Deary, Huntly, MacLeod, & Frier, 1996), Williams syndrome (Rae et al., 1998), Parkinson's disease (Johnson, Almeida, Stough, Thompson, Singarayer, & Jog, 2004; Phillips, Schiffter, Nicholls, Bradshaw, Iansek, & Saling, 1999; Shipley, Deary, Tan, Christie, & Starr, 2002), and schizophrenia (Badcock, Dragovic, Waters, & Jablensky, 2005).

To date, two large twin studies have investigated the heritability of inspection time, in non-clinical twin samples (Luciano, Smith, et al., 2001; Posthuma, de Geus, et al., 2001). Using 184 monozygotic (MZ) pairs and 206 dizygotic (DZ) pairs Luciano, Smith, et al. (2001) found a heritability estimate of inspection time of 36% at age 16. Posthuma, de Geus, et al. (2001) reported a heritability estimate of inspection time of 46% in a sample of 102 MZ pairs and 525 DZ/sib pairs belonging to two age cohorts (mean ages 26 and 50).

Variation in inspection time is thus moderately heritable, and shows increasing heritability from late adolescence to middle age.

Electrophysiological measures

Electroencephalographic (EEG) recording is a non-invasive technique to measure electrical activity of the brain. EEG activity can be analysed in the time domain as well as in the frequency domain. Within the time domain several so-called event related potentials (ERPs) can be distinguished, such as the N1(100), P2(00), P3(00) or the lateralized readiness potential (LRP). Within the frequency domain, several frequency bands can be distinguished that correspond to the rhythmic activity that derives from the summed synchronized synaptic activity of large populations of neurons (Steriade, Gloor, Llinás, Lopes da Silva, & Mesulam, 1990).

EEG frequency

A frequency spectrum of EEG activity is obtained when a Fourier transformation is performed on an EEG time series. Generally five frequencies are distinguished in the EEG power spectrum: delta (0.5–4 cycles per second), theta (4–8 cycles per second), alpha (8–13 cycles per second), beta (13–30 cycles per second), and gamma (> 30 cycles per second). Over the last decade the underlying biological mechanisms of the different frequencies, especially the alpha and beta rhythms, have become well understood.

The dominant frequency in an adult human EEG spectrum lies in the alpha range and averages about 10 cycles per second. Large individual differences in the alpha peak frequency are found however, and a substantial number of subjects can have an alpha frequency as low as 7 Hz or as high as 13 Hz. Alpha waves have been shown to be generated in thalamo-cortical feedback loops of excitatory and inhibitory nerve cells (Lopes da Silva, 1991; Steriade et al., 1990). In the visual cortex the alpha rhythm can also be generated by cortico-cortical networks involving layer V pyramidal neurons (Lopes da Silva & Storm van Leeuwen, 1977; Steriade et al., 1990). The specific alpha peak frequency of an individual is determined by the intrinsic membrane properties of the thalamic neurons projecting to the cortex (Steriade et al., 1990).

Although alpha peak frequency did not reflect general intelligence in two large studies (Anokhin & Vogel, 1996; Posthuma, Neale, Boomsma, & de Geus, 2001), it has been found to correlate positively to working memory performance in a number of studies (Angelakis, Lubar, & Stathopoulou, 2004; Ellingson & Lathrop, 1973; Klimesch, 1997; Richard-Clark et al., 2004). In a review of his work, Klimesch (1999), concluded that the alpha peak frequency of good working memory performers lies about 1 Hz higher than that of bad working memory performers. Using a continuous measure of working memory performance, Richard-Clark et al. (2004) in a large study of 550 normal subjects aged between 11 and 70 years, showed that each 1 Hz increase in frequency was associated with a 0.21 increase in reverse digit span score. They also showed that alpha peak frequency slowed with ageing, corroborating similar findings by others (Klimesch, 1999; Köpruner, Pfurtscheller, & Auer, 1984). Age-related slowing may reflect a decrease in the speed of processing in thalamocortical loops (Steriade et al., 1990) but can also arise by a relative shift in power from the lower band, related to attentional processing, to the upper band, related to semantic memory (Klimesch, 1999; Kolev, Yordanova, Basar-Eroglu, & Basar, 2002). The normal age-related slowing of alpha frequency appears to be enhanced by neurodegeneration. A study by Lehtovirta et al. (1996) compared Alzheimer patients to controls and found that alpha peak frequency of Alzheimer patients was significantly lower than that of controls.

Results from a few small twin studies have suggested that alpha peak frequency is strongly influenced by genetic factors (e.g., Christian, Morzorati, Norton, Williams, O'Connor, & Li, 1996; Hume, 1973; Propping, 1977; Stassen et al., 1999; Young, Lader, & Fenton, 1972). Lykken, Tellegen, and Iacono (1982) further showed that intrapair resemblance of MZ twins adopted in different families was as large as the resemblance of those raised in the same family. High heritability of this trait was confirmed in full by Posthuma, Neale, et al. (2001) who conducted the first large twin study on the alpha peak frequency, using a sample of 271 twin-sibling families. In young adults (mean age 26 years) heritability was estimated at 71%, and in older adults (mean age 50 years) at 83%. This places alpha peak frequency among the most heritable human traits known.

Thus studies examining EEG frequencies have found that the alpha peak frequency is highly heritable and might be related to cognitive slowing in age-related diseases.

P3

First reported by Sutton, Braren, Zubin, and John (1965) and Desmedt, Debecker, and Manil (1965), the P3 event-related potential is typically elicited in an oddball task where a low probability target stimulus (the oddball) is easily discriminated from a frequent non-target. The classical P3 component or P3b, which peaks 300–600 ms after the target stimulus in such oddball paradigms has a mainly parietal distribution on the scalp. It has been linked to the cognitive processes of context updating, context closure, and event categorization (Dien, Spencer, & Donchin, 2004; Donchin & Coles, 1988; Kok, 2001; Verleger, 1988). The slightly earlier P3a, which has a fronto-central distribution, has mainly been associated with the orienting response (Friedman, Cycowicz, & Gaeta, 2001). For the P3 to occur it is necessary that the stimulus is relevant to the task at hand, and that the subject is conscious of this task-relevancy: on missed target trials, such as in experiments on the attentional blink, the P3 is absent (Vogel & Luck, 2002; Vogel, Luck, & Shapiro, 1998).

Like other ERP components, the P3 is characterized by large individual differences and this applies to both amplitude and latency. These individual differences may be meaningful as markers of differences in mental health (Polich & Herbst, 2000). The P3 latency reflects the time needed to fully evaluate and classify a stimulus. In normal ageing, P3 latency has been found to increase as cognitive processing slows down (Pfefferbaum, Ford, Wenegrat, Roth, & Kopell, 1984), although the ability of the P3 to differentiate between normal ageing and dementia resulting from neural degenerative disorders such as Alzheimer's disease is still inconclusive (e.g., Cohen, O'Donnell, Meadows, Moonis, Stone, & Drachman, 1995; Pfefferbaum, Ford, & Kraemer, 1990; Polich, 1998). As an index of neural speed, the P3 latency would mainly reflect the speed with which attentional resources are allocated for the processing of a relevant stimulus.

A number of studies have reported that P3 is delayed in children with learning disabilities and ADHD (Frank, Seiden, & Napolitano, 1996, 1998; Sunohara, Malone, Rovet, Humphries, Roberts, & Taylor, 1999; Sunohara, Voros, Malone, & Taylor, 1997; Taylor, Voros, Logan, & Malone, 1993). This delay in processing speed is normalized by medication in ADHD

(Sunohara et al., 1997; Taylor et al., 1993). A significant link between P3 latency and psychometric IQ has been reported in many studies (Egan, Chiswick, Brettle, & Goodwin, 1992; Ertl & Schafer, 1969; Howard & Polich, 1985; Jausovec & Jausovec, 2000; McGarry-Roberts, Stelmack, & Campbell, 1992; O'Donnell, Friedman, Swearer, & Drachman, 1992; Polich, Ladish, & Burns, 1990; Polich & Martin, 1992; Robaey, Cansino, Dugas, & Renault, 1995; Shucard & Horn, 1972; Wright, Scott, Richardson, Rai, & Exton-Smith, 1988) but other studies could not confirm the link between P3 latency and IQ (Engel & Henderson, 1973; Gevins & Smith, 2000; Katsanis, Iacono, McGue, & Carlson, 1997; Nittono, Nageishi, Nakajima, & Ullsberger, 1999; Pelosi, Holly, Salde, Hayward, Barrett, & Blumhardt, 1992; Wright, Luciano, Hansell, Geffen, Geffen, & Martin, 2002). The exact reason for these discrepancies might be the use of different cognitive tasks to tap IQ; the relation between IQ and PS is reviewed in more depth in chapter 1 of this volume.

Twin and family studies indicate moderate to high heritability of the average P3 latency on target trials (e.g., Almasy et al., 1999; Katsanis et al., 1997; Polich & Burns, 1987; Rogers & Deary, 1991; Rust, 1975; Surwillo, 1980; van Baal, de Geus, & Boomsma, 1998; Wright, Hansell, Geffen, Geffen, Smith, & Martin, 2001), although in one study heritability also failed to reach significance (O'Connor, Morzorati, Christian, & Li, 1994). Van Beijsterveldt and van Baal (2002) pooled published twin correlations across six of the larger studies and reported a "meta"-heritability of 51% for P3 latency. Two large studies have been published since. Hansell, Wright, Luciano, Geffen, Geffen, and Martin (2005) collected data from 252 MZ and 297 DZ twin pairs aged 16, and measured the P3 latency during a working memory task. They found a heritability of between 38% and 43% of P3 latency at parietal and frontal leads. Another recent large twin study by Smit, Posthuma, Boomsma, and de Geus (in press) on 665 adult twins and siblings from 292 families reported a heritability for P3 latency in a visual oddball task of 27% at the central frontal (Fz) lead, 42% at the central (Cz) lead and 46% at the central parietal (Pz) lead. A single genetic factor was sufficient to explain genetic variance in P3 latency across the entire midline of the scalp, suggesting a central timing mechanism of the P3.

On the grounds of multiple sources of evidence, Nieuwenhuis, Aston-Jones, and Cohen (2005) have suggested that the central pacemaker in P3 generation may be in the noradrenergic locus coeruleus (LC). They hypothesized that the LC is recruited by input from cortical afferent projections that monitor the motivational aspects of a stimulus. The activated LC then modulates cortical activation and information processing via coeruleo-cortical noradrenergic projections in a pathway from anterior to posterior areas. If the LC indeed plays a key role in P3 generation, then genetic influences on the timing of the stimulus-locked phasic LC bursting could underlie the common genetic factor found to influence P3 latency across the scalp.

N1 and P2

The oddball paradigm also elicits a large negative component, N1, that partly reflects early automatic processing of sensory events, including the type of rapid feature extraction that is also indexed by the inspection time (Naatanen & Picton, 1987). In the context of the oddball task, the P2 component may represent inhibition of other channels competing for attention and further processing (Hansen & Hillyard, 1988). These earlier latencies have only rarely been subjected to genetic analyses in twin samples. Results have been mixed. Significant heritability was found for the N1 or the P2 during auditory oddball tasks by some (Polich & Burns, 1987; Rust, 1975; O'Connor et al., 1994) but not by others (Surwillo, 1980). In a visual oddball paradigm that required mental rotation on half of the target task in either easy (no rotation) or difficult (rotation) trials, no genetic effects were found on N1 and P2 latency in either easy or difficult condition (Katsanis et al., 1997).

The lateralized readiness potential (LRP)

The latency of the lateralized readiness potential (LRP) reflects the speed of (pre-)motor selective response activation. The LRP is mathematically derived from the *Bereitschaftspotential* or readiness potential (RP; Körnhuber & Deecke, 1965), which is an evoked EEG potential observed preceding limb movements. During the preparation of a motor response, an initially symmetrical slow negative potential occurs in the EEG bilaterally over the premotor cortex. This negative potential then lateralizes to the hemisphere contralateral to the limb with which the response needs to be given. At this instant, the largest difference between the EEG of the two hemispheres is recorded above the motor cortex. The point in time at which activity in the motor cortex contralateral to the (intended) response limb becomes larger than activity in the motor cortex in the ipsilateral hemisphere marks the time at which either the left or the right limb has been selected for responding (Kutas & Donchin, 1980). This measure is denoted as the LRP onset, and measures the speed of response selection (Coles, 1989; Hackley & Valle-Inclan, 2003). The time of maximal LRP amplitude, LRP peak latency, is thought to additionally reflect central motor processes that take place after response selection has taken place (Falkenstein, Hohnsbein, & Hoormann, 1994).

To date, only one large genetically informative study has examined the heritability of LRP onset and peak latency (Posthuma, Mulder, Boomsma, & de Geus, 2002). Using a sample of 271 adult twin-sibling families they found that variation in the onset of the LRP was moderately heritable (54–62% depending on stimulus congruency and age cohort). Variation in LRP peak latency was slightly less heritable and ranged from 39 to 45% depending on stimulus congruency. These results clearly indicate that the speed of response selection and ensuing motor preparation is partly influenced by genetic factors.

Reaction times

Reaction time has been the most studied behavioural correlate of processing speed, especially in studies relating processing speed to intelligence. By combining reaction times from tasks of different complexity, up to 50% of the variance in test intelligence scores can be explained (Vernon, 1989). Slowed reaction times are also used as biomarkers in ADHD and reading disorders in children (e.g., Kuntsi, Andreou, Ma, Borger, & van der Meere, 2005; Sigmundsson, 2005), and in Parkinson's and Huntington's diseases (Gauntlett-Gilbert & Brown, 1998).

Several different paradigms to assess reaction times can be employed. The most commonly used are the simple reaction time, the choice reaction time and the recognition or distraction reaction time paradigms. In a simple reaction time paradigm a subject is required to react as fast as possible to the occurrence of a stimulus. There is only one stimulus. In a choice reaction time task the required reaction depends on making a choice induced by different stimuli. For example, a left-handed button press is indicated when the presented stimulus is a letter, while a right-handed response is indicated if a number is presented. In a recognition or distraction paradigm certain stimuli should be responded to, whereas others should be ignored. It has been known for over a century that reaction time increases with increasing task difficulty (i.e., speed/accuracy trade-off) (Donders, 1868). Several small-scale studies (Baker, Vernon, & Ho, 1991; Boomsma & Somsen, 1991; McGue, Bouchard, Lykken, & Feuer, 1984; McGue & Bouchard, 1989) and large-scale studies (Luciano, Wright, et al., 2001; Neubauer, Spinath, Riemann, Angleitner, & Borkenau, 2000; Petrill, Thompson, & Detterman, 1995; Posthuma et al., 2002; Rijsdijk, Vernon, & Boomsma, 1998) have investigated the heritability of reaction time. For an extensive review including the small-scale studies we refer to Spinath and Borkenau (2000). Here we focus on the five largest studies, including the two studies that have been published since 2000.

Petrill et al. (1995) used a sample of 149 MZ twins and 138 same-sex DZ twins aged 6–13. They found that variation in reaction time was a result of variation in shared and non-shared environmental factors, but not variation at the genetic level. Rijsdijk et al. (1998) conducted a genetic analysis on reaction time data using 213 Dutch twin pairs measured at ages 16 and 18. The heritability of simple reaction time at age 16 was 64%, and decreased to 48% at the age of 18. For two-choice reaction time the heritability was 62% at age 16, which decreased to 49% at the age of 18. Similar results in 16-year-olds were found in an Australian sample of 166 MZ pairs and 190 DZ pairs (Luciano, Wright, et al., 2001). Luciano, Wright, et al. (2001) reported a heritability of 52% for two-choice reaction time, 60% for four-choice reaction time and 34% for eight-choice reaction time. Posthuma et al. (2002) used a sample of 271 adult twin-sibling families from two age cohorts. They used an Eriksen Flanker Task, in which the stimulus set included both target stimuli and distractor stimuli (Eriksen & Eriksen, 1974). A heritability of 33% was found for reaction time in the young adult cohort (mean age 26 years), whereas the heritability was 48% in the middle-aged cohort (mean age 50 years).

Neubauer et al. (2000) used two tasks to assess reaction time in a sample of 169 MZ twins and 131 DZ twins aged between 18 and 70 years: a Sternberg Memory Scanning task (Sternberg, 1969) and a Posner Letter Matching task (Posner & Mitchell, 1967). The Sternberg Memory Scanning task assesses the speed of access to short-term memory. Subjects are presented with a random sequence of one to five digits that have to be stored in memory. After a warning signal the target digit is shown, after which subjects are required to respond as quickly as possible by pressing a "yes" button if the target was part of the sequence and pressing a "no" button if it was not. The mean latencies of correct responses are regressed on the size of the random sequence (i.e., the memory set). The slope of this regression line indicates the time required to retrieve a single item from short-term memory, whereas the intercept reflects the speed of encoding and (pre-)motoric response processes. The heritability of reaction time was zero for a memory set of one, 45% for a memory set of three, and 47% for a memory set of five. The intercept showed a heritability of 23%, whereas the heritability of the slope was even lower, at 11%.

The Posner Letter Matching task requires subjects to compare simultaneously presented letters and respond by pressing one of two buttons. The letters to be compared can be *same name–physically same* (e.g., "AA"), *same name–physically different* (e.g., "Aa") or *different name–physically different* (e.g., "Ab"). Subjects have to judge either the physical identity or the name identity. Physical identity measures visual discrimination ability only, whereas name identity measures access to highly overlearned material stored in long-term memory. The difference between the physical and the name identity reaction times is, therefore, thought to reflect the speed with which information from long-term memory is retrieved (Hunt, 1980). The heritability of the difference between the physical and the name identity reaction times was 22%.

In summary, results from twin studies suggest that the heritability of reaction time increases from childhood to adulthood, as well as with increasing task difficulty. At most, the heritability of reaction is around 50%.

Processing speed from intelligence tests

The third version of the Wechsler Adult Intelligence Scale (WAIS-III) includes calculation of four dimensions of IQ. One of these dimensions is the *Processing Speed Index* (PSI), which consists of the subtests Digit Symbol Coding and Symbol Search (Wechsler, 1997). In the Digit Symbol Coding subtest the subject is presented with an array of numbers with matched abstract symbols as a key and multiple empty boxes with numbers below. Subjects are required to fill out the empty boxes below the numbers with the corresponding symbol as fast as possible within 120 seconds. This subtest assesses visual-motor coordination, and motor and mental speed. During Symbol Search the subject is presented with a target symbol and a set of symbols from which the target needs to be identified as fast as possible. This subtest assesses visual perception and speed.

PSI decreases with normal ageing and the test serves as a screening instrument for neuropsychological dysfunction (Joy, Kaplan, & Fein, 2004). PSI is lower in pre-term children compared to full-term children (Rose & Feldman, 1996), and a lower PSI is associated with a smaller white matter volume in adults (Posthuma, Baaré, Hulshoff Pol, Kahn, Boomsma, & de Geus, 2003). PSI is lower in patients with multiple sclerosis, which results from the immune system breaking down and attacking the myelinated sheath around nerve axons (DeLuca et al., 2004; Demaree, DeLuca, Gaudino, & Diamond, 1999).

Only Posthuma et al. (2003) explicitly looked at the heritability of the PSI measured with the Dutch version of the revised WAIS-III. In a sample of 688 adult subjects from 271 extended twin families they reported a heritability of 63% for PSI, confirming the well-known genetic contribution to test intelligence, and more specifically the heritability of processing speed.

Conclusion

As shown in Table 4.1, the heritability of processing speed ranges from very low (reaction times in the Sternberg Memory Scanning task) to very high (alpha peak frequency), depending on the actual measure, task complexity and age of the sample.

Normal cognitive functioning is strongly dependent on genetic make-up. Scores on a variety of psychometric IQ tests are highly heritable from young adulthood onwards, up to age 80 and over (Boomsma & van Baal, 1998; Bouchard & McGue, 1981; Cherny & Cardon, 1994; Plomin, Pedersen, Lichtenstein, & McClearn, 1994; Posthuma, de Geus, et al., 2001; Posthuma, Neale, et al., 2001). The actual genes, however, have eluded us so far. Finding these genes may be directly relevant to our understanding of abnormal cognitive functioning, which often shows a substantial genetic component. Heritability of reading disability, for instance, is estimated at 46% (Wadsworth, Olson, Pennington, & DeFries, 2000), that of autism at 90% (Santangelo & Tsatsanis, 2005) and that of ADHD at 75% or higher (Price et al., 2005; Price, Simonoff, Waldman, Asherson, & Plomin, 2001; Rietveld, Hudziak, Bartels, van Beijsterveldt, & Boomsma, 2004). We recently showed in a genome scan for IQ that the genomic regions influencing IQ overlap with areas previously implicated in these disorders (Posthuma et al., 2005). This supports the idea that trait variation within the normal range of cognitive abilities might be used to detect genes for disorders that are accompanied by cognitive impairment.

Because processing speed is considered a crucial component of higher

Table 4.1 Heritability estimates from twin studies reporting a significant contribution of genes to processing speed

Measure	Range of heritability estimates (%)
Peripheral nerve conduction velocity	66–76
Inspection time	36–46
EEG—alpha peak frequency	71–83
EEG—P3 latency	27–51
EEG—N1 latency	19–57
EEG—LRP, onset latency	54–62
EEG—LRP, peak latency	39–45
Reaction time—simple	48–64
Reaction time—2-choice	49–62
Reaction time—4 choice	60
Reaction time—8 choice	34
Sternberg task—slope	11
Sternberg task—intercept	23
Reaction time—Posner	22
IQ test—Processing Speed Index	63

cognitive ability, finding genetic variation underlying its heritability might be used to identify genes for disorders like reading disability, autism and ADHD. Hence, many of the twin studies reviewed above specifically aimed to develop processing speed into a biomarker (or endophenotype) that could support gene finding (de Geus, 2002; de Geus, Wright, Martin, & Boomsma, 2001). This has already met with a few small successes. Inspection time, for instance, is correlated with IQ and that correlation reflects genes shared by both traits (Luciano, Smith, et al., 2001; Posthuma, de Geus, et al., 2001). Disappointing results, however, have also been found. The index of processing speed can fail to show heritability, as regards P2 latency (Katsanis et al., 1997), or show that it is not systematically related to IQ, as regards peak alpha frequency (Posthuma, Neale, et al., 2001), or that the relationship between processing speed and IQ is not mediated by shared genes, as regards P3 latency (Wright et al., 2002). Such variability should serve to remind us that the genes influencing cognition do not necessarily always do so through their effects on processing speed. Fast and accurate behaviour (such as a high score on an IQ test or neuropsychological tests) can emerge from a neural network for a variety of reasons, including sheer size of the network (i.e., brain size), its complexity, signalling reliability, neural adaptability, and local and regional connectivity (Deary & Caryl, 1997). Each of these traits may be influenced by sets of genes that are largely independent of the genes at play in processing speed.

References

Almasy, L., Porjesz, B., Blangero, J., Chorlian, D. B., O'Connor, S. J., Kuperman, S., et al. (1999). Heritability of event-related brain potentials in families with a history of alcoholism. *American Journal of Medical Genetics, 88*, 383–390.

Angelakis, E., Lubar, J. F., & Stathopoulou, S. (2004). Electroencephalographic peak alpha frequency correlates of cognitive traits. *Neuroscience Letters, 371* (1), 60–63.

Anokhin, A. P., & Vogel, F. (1996). EEG alpha rhythm frequency and intelligence in normal adults. *Intelligence, 23*, 1–14.

Arbuckle, J. L. (1994) AMOS: Analysis of moment structures. *Psychometrika, 59*, 135–137.

Badcock, J. C., Dragovic, M., Waters, F. A., & Jablensky, A. (2005). Dimensions of intelligence in schizophrenia: Evidence from patients with preserved, deteriorated and compromised intellect. *Journal of Psychiatric Research, 39*, 11–19.

Baddeley, A. D. (1986) *Working memory*. Oxford, UK: Oxford University Press.

Baker, L. A., Vernon, P. A., & Ho, H. Z. (1991). The genetic correlation between intelligence and speed of information processing. *Behavior Genetics, 21*, 351–367.

Bentler, P. M. (1995). *EQS Structural Equations Program manual*. Encino, CA: Multivariate Software, Inc.

Boomsma, D. I., & Somsen, R. J. M. (1991). Reaction times measured in a choice reaction time and a double task condition: A small twin study. *Personality and Individual Differences, 12*, 519–522.

Boomsma, D. I., & van Baal, G. C. M. (1998). Genetic influences on childhood IQ in 5- and 7-year-old Dutch twins. *Developmental Neuropsychology, 14*, 115–126.

Bouchard, T. J., Jr., & McGue, M. (1981). Familial studies of intelligence: A review. *Science, 212*, 1055–1059.

Cherny, S., & Cardon, L. (1994). General cognitive ability. In J. DeFries, R. Plomin, & D. Fulker (Eds.), *Nature and nurture during middle childhood* (pp. 46–56). Oxford, UK: Blackwell Publishers.

Christian, J. C., Morzorati, S., Norton, J. A., Jr., Williams, C. J., O'Connor, S., & Li, T. K. (1996). Genetic analysis of the resting electroencephalographic power spectrum in human twins. *Psychophysiology, 33*, 584–591.

Cohen, R. A., O'Donnell, B. F., Meadows, M. E., Moonis, M., Stone, W. F., & Drachman, D. A. (1995). ERP indices and neuropsychological performance as predictors of functional outcome in dementia. *Journal of Geriatric Psychiatry and Neurology, 8*, 217–225.

Coles, M. G. (1989). Modern mind-brain reading: Psychophysiology, physiology, and cognition. *Psychophysiology, 26* (3), 251–269.

Deary, I. J., & Caryl, P. G. (1997). Neuroscience and human intelligence differences. *Trends in Neurosciences, 20* (8), 365–371.

Deary, I. J., Hunter, R., Langan, S. J., & Goodwin, G. M. (1991). Inspection time, psychometric intelligence and clinical estimates of cognitive ability in pre-senile Alzheimer's disease and Korsakoff's psychosis. *Brain, 114*, 2543–2554.

de Geus, E. J. (2002). Introducing genetic psychophysiology. *Biological Psychology, 61* (1–2), 1–10.

de Geus, E. J., Wright, M. J., Martin, N. G., & Boomsma, D. I. (2001). Genetics of brain function and cognition. *Behavior Genetics, 31* (6), 489–495.

DeLuca, J., Chelune, G. J., Tulsky, D. S., Lengenfelder, J., & Chiaravalloti, N. D. (2004). Is speed of processing or working memory the primary information processing deficit in multiple sclerosis? *Journal of Clinical and Experimental Neuropsychology, 26*, 550–562.

Demaree, H. A., DeLuca, J., Gaudino, E. A., & Diamond, B. J. (1999). Speed of information processing as a key deficit in multiple sclerosis: Implications for rehabilitation. *Journal of Neurology, Neurosurgery, and Psychiatry, 67* (5), 661–663.

Desmedt, J. E., Debecker, J., & Manil, J. (1965). Demonstration of a cerebral electric sign associated with the detection by the subject of a tactile sensorial stimulus. The analysis of cerebral evoked potentials derived from the scalp with the aid of numerical ordinates. *Bulletin et Memoires de l'Academie Royale de Medecine de Belgique, 5* (11), 887–936.

Dien, J., Spencer, K. M., & Donchin, E. (2004). Parsing the late positive complex: Mental chronometry and the ERP components that inhabit the neighborhood of the P300. *Psychophysiology, 41* (5), 665–678.

Donchin, E., & Coles, M. (1988). Is the P300 component a manifestation of context updating? *Behavioral and Brain Sciences, 11*, 357–427.

Donders, F. C. (1868). On the speed of mental processes (trans. W. G. Koster, 1969). *Acta Psychologica, 30*, 412–431.

Egan, V. G., Chiswick, A., Brettle, R. P., & Goodwin, G. M. (1992). The Edinburgh cohort of HIV-positive drug users: The relationship between auditory P3 latency, cognitive function and self-rated mood. *Psychological Medicine, 23*, 613–622.

Ellingson, R. J., & Lathrop, G. H. (1973). Intelligence and frequency of the alpha rhythm. *American Journal of Mental Deficiency, 78*, 334–338.

Engel, R., & Henderson, N. B. (1973). Visual evoked responses in IQ scores at school age. *Developmental Medicine and Child Neurology, 15* (2), 136–145.

Eriksen, B. A., & Eriksen, C. W. (1974). Effects of noise letters upon the identification of a target letter in a nonsearch task. *Perception and Psychophysics, 16*, 143–149.

Ertl, J. P., & Schafer, E. W. P. (1969) Neural efficiency and human intelligence. *Nature, 223*, 421–423

Falkenstein, M., Hohnsbein, J., & Hoormann, J. (1994). Effects of choice complexity on different subcomponents of the late positive complex of the event-related potential. *Electroencephalography and Clinical Neurophysiology, 92*, 148–160.

Frank, Y., Seiden, J., & Napolitano, B. (1996). Visual event related potentials and reaction time in normal adults, normal children, and children with attention deficit hyperactivity disorder: Differences in short-term memory processing. *International Journal of Neuroscience, 88* (1–2), 109–24.

Frank, Y., Seiden, J. A., & Napolitano, B. (1998). Electrophysiological changes in children with learning and attentional abnormalities as a function of age: event-related potentials to an "oddball" paradigm. *Clinical Electroencephalography, 29* (4), 188–193.

Friedman, D., Cycowicz, Y. M., & Gaeta, H. (2001). The novelty P3: An event-related brain potential (ERP) sign of the brain's evaluation of novelty. *Neuroscience and Biobehavioral Reviews, 25* (4), 355–373.

Fry, A. F., & Hale, S. (2000). Relationships among processing speed, working memory, and fluid intelligence in children. *Biological Psychology, 54* (1–3), 1–34.

Gauntlett-Gilbert, J., & Brown, V. J. (1998). Reaction time deficits and Parkinson's disease. *Neuroscience and Biobehavioral Reviews, 22* (6), 865–881.

Gevins, A., & Smith, M. E. (2000). Neurophysiological measures of working memory and individual differences in cognitive ability and cognitive style. *Cerebral Cortex*, *10*, 829–839.

Hackley, S. A., & Valle-Inclan, F. (2003).Which stages of processing are speeded by a warning signal? *Biological Psychology*, *64* (1–2), 27–45.

Hansell, N. K., Wright, M. J., Luciano, M., Geffen, G. M., Geffen, L. B., & Martin, N. G. (2005). Genetic covariation between event-related potential (ERP) and behavioral non-ERP measures of working-memory, processing speed, and IQ. *Behavior Genetics*, *35* (6), 695–706.

Hansen, J. C., & Hillyard, S. A. (1988). Temporal dynamics of human auditory selective attention. *Psychophysiology*, *25*, 316–329.

Howard, L., & Polich, J. (1985). P300 latency and memory span development. *Developmental Psychology*, *21*, 283–289.

Hume, W. (1973). Physiological measures in twins. In G. Claridge, S. Canter, and W. Hume (Eds.), *Personality differences and biological variations: A study of twins* (pp. 87–114). Oxford & New York: Pergamon.

Hunt, E. (1980). Intelligence as an information processing concept. *British Journal of Psychology*, *71*, 449–474.

Jausovec, N., & Jausovec, K. (2000). Correlations between ERP parameters and intelligence: A reconsideration. *Biological Psychology*, *55* (2), 137–154.

Jensen, A. R. (1982). Reaction times and psychometric *g*. In H. J. Eysenck (Ed.), *A model for intelligence*. Berlin: Springer-Verlag.

Jensen, A. R. (1993). Why is reaction time correlated with psychometric *g*? *Current Directions in Psychological Science*, *2*, 53–56.

Johnson, A. M., Almeida, Q. J., Stough, C., Thompson, J. C., Singarayer, R., & Jog, M. S. (2004). Visual inspection time in Parkinson's disease: Deficits in early stages of cognitive processing. *Neuropsychologia*, *42* (5), 577–583.

Jöreskog, K., & Sörbom, D. (1986). *LISREL: Analsysis of linear structural relationships by the method of maximum likelihood*. Chicago: National Education Resources.

Joy, S., Kaplan, E., & Fein, D. (2004). Speed and memory in the WAIS-III Digit Symbol-Coding subtest across the adult lifespan. *Archives of Clinical Neuropsychology*, *19* (6), 759–767.

Katsanis, J., Iacono, W. G., McGue, M. K., & Carlson, S. R. (1997). P300 event-related potential heritability in monozygotic and dizygotic twins. *Psychophysiology*, *34* (1), 47–58.

Klimesch, W. (1997). EEG-alpha rhythms and memory processes. *International Journal of Psychophysiology*, *26*, 319–340.

Klimesch, W. (1999). EEG alpha and theta oscillations reflect cognitive and memory performance: A review and analysis. *Brain Research. Brain Research Reviews*, *29* (2–3), 169–195.

Kok, A. (2001). On the utility of P3 amplitude as a measure of processing capacity. *Psychophysiology*, *38* (3), 557–577.

Kolev, V., Yordanova, J., Basar-Eroglu, C., & Basar, E. (2002). Age effects on visual EEG responses reveal distinct frontal alpha networks. *Clinical Neurophysiology*, *113* (6), 901–910.

Köpruner, V., Pfurtscheller, G., & Auer, L. M. (1984). Quantitative EEG in normals and in patients with cerebral ischemia. *Progress in Brain Research*, *62*, 29–50.

Kornhuber, H. H., and Deecke, L. (1965). Hirnpotentialänderungen bei Willkürbewegungen und passiven Bewegungen des Menschen. Bereitschaftspotential und reafferente Potentiale. *Pflügers Archiv*, *284*, 1–17.

Kuntsi, J., Andreou, P., Ma, J., Borger, N. A., & van der Meere, J. J. (2005). Testing assumptions for endophenotype studies in ADHD: Reliability and validity of tasks in a general population sample. *BMC Psychiatry, 5*, 40.

Kutas, M., & Donchin, E. (1980). Preparation to respond as manifested by movement-related brain potentials. *Brain Research, 202* (1), 95–115.

Lehtovirta, M., Partanen, J., Kononen, M., Soininen, H., Helisalmi, S., Mannermaa, A., et al. (1996). Spectral analysis of EEG in Alzheimer's disease: Relation to apolipoprotein E polymorphism. *Neurobiology of Aging, 17*, 523–526.

Lopes da Silva, F. H. (1991). Neural mechanisms underlying brain waves: From neural membranes to networks. *Electroencephalography and Clinical Neurophysiology, 79*, 81–93.

Lopes da Silva, F. H., & Storm van Leeuwen, W. (1977). The cortical source of alpha rhythm. *Neuroscience Letters, 6*, 237–241.

Luciano, M., Smith, G. A., Wright, M. J., Geffen, G. M., Geffen, L. B., & Martin, N. G. (2001). On the heritability of inspection time and its covariance with IQ: A twin study. *Intelligence, 29* (6), 443–457.

Luciano, M., Wright, M. J., Smith, G. A., Geffen, G. M., Geffen, L. B., & Martin, N. G. (2001). Genetic covariance amongst measures of information processing speed, working memory and IQ. *Behavior Genetics, 31* (6), 581–592.

Lykken, D. T., Tellegen, A., & Iacono, W. G. (1982). EEG spectra in twins: Evidence for a neglected mechanism of genetic determination. *Physiological Psychology, 10*, 60–65.

Lynch, M., & Walsh, B. (1998). *Genetics and analysis of quantitative traits.* Sunderland, MA: Sinauer Associates.

Martin, N. G., Boomsma, D. I., & Machin, G. (1997). A twin pronged attack on complex traits. *Nature Genetics, 17*, 387–392.

McCrimmon, R. J., Deary, I. J., Huntly, B. J., MacLeod, K. J., & Frier, B. M. (1996). Visual information processing during controlled hypoglycaemia in humans. *Brain, 119* (4), 1277–1287.

McGarry-Roberts, P. A., Stelmack, R. M., & Campbell, K. B. (1992). Intelligence, reaction time, and event-related potentials. *Intelligence, 16*, 289–313.

McGue, M., & Bouchard, T. J. (1989). Genetic and environmental determinants of information processing and special mental abilities: A twin analysis. In R. J. Sternberg (Ed.), *Advances in the psychology of human intelligence* (Vol. 5, pp. 7–45). Hillsdale, NJ: Lawrence Erlbaum Associates, Inc.

McGue, M., Bouchard, T. J., Jr., Lykken, D. T., & Feuer, D. (1984). Information processing abilities in twins reared apart. *Intelligence, 8*, 239–258.

Naatanen, R., & Picton, T. (1987). The N1 wave of the human electric and magnetic response to sound—a review and an analysis of the component structure. *Psychophysiology, 24* (4), 375–425.

Neale, M. C. (1997). *Mx: Statistical modeling* (3rd ed.). Box 980126 MCV, Richmond, VA 23298.

Neale, M. C. (2003). Twin studies: Software and algorithms. In D. N. Cooper (Ed.), *Encyclopedia of the human genome.* New York: Macmillian Publishers Ltd, Nature Publishing Group.

Neale, M. C., & Cardon, L. R. (1992). *Methodology for genetic studies of twins and families.* Dordrecht, The Netherlands: Kluwer Academic Publishers.

Neubauer, A. C., Spinath, F. M., Riemann, R., Angleitner, A., & Borkenau, P. (2000). Genetic and environmental influences on two measures of speed of information processing and their relation to psychometric intelligence: Evidence from the German observational study of adult twins. *Intelligence, 28* (4), 267–289.

Nieuwenhuis, S., Aston-Jones, G., & Cohen, J. A. (2005). Decision making, the P3, and the locus coeruleus-norepinephrine system. *Psychological Bulletin, 131* (4), 510–532.

Nittono, H., Nageishi, Y., Nakajima, Y., & Ullsberger, P. (1999). Event-related potential correlates of individual differences in working memory capacity. *Psychophysiology, 36*, 745–754.

O'Connor, S., Morzorati, S., Christian, J. C., & Li, T. K. (1994). Heritable features of the auditory oddball event-related potential: Peaks, latencies, morphology and topography. *Electroencephalography and Clinical Neurophysiology, 92* (2), 115–125.

O'Donnell, B. F., Friedman, S., Swearer, J. M., & Drachman, D. A. (1992). Active and passive P3 latency and psychometric performance: Influence of age and individual differences. *International Journal of Psychophysiology, 12*, 187–195.

Pelosi, L., Holly, M., Slade, T., Hayward, M., Barrett, G., & Blumhardt, L. D. (1992). Wave form variations in auditory event-related potentials evoked by a memory-scanning task and their relationship with tests of intellectual function. *Electroencephalography and Clinical Neurophysiology, 84*, 344–352.

Petrill, S. A., Thompson, L. A., & Detterman, D. K. (1995). The genetic and environmental variance underlying elementary cognitive tasks. *Behavior Genetics, 25*, 199–209.

Pfefferbaum, A., Ford, J. M., & Kraemer, H. C. (1990). Clinical utility of long latency "cognitive" event-related potentials (P3): The cons. *Electroencephalography and Clinical Neurophysiology, 76*, 6–12.

Pfefferbaum, A., Ford, J. M., Wenegrat, B. G., Roth, W. T., & Kopell, B. S. (1984). Clinical application of the P3 component of event-related potentials. I. Normal aging. *Electroencephalography and Clinical Neurophysiology, 59* (2), 85–103.

Phillips, J. G., Schiffter, T., Nicholls, M. E., Bradshaw, J. L., Iansek, R., & Saling, L. L. (1999). Does old age or Parkinson's disease cause bradyphrenia? *Journal of Gerontology A: Biological Science and Medical Science, 54* (8), M404–M409.

Plomin, R., Pedersen, N. L., Lichtenstein, P., & McClearn, G. E. (1994). Variability and stability in cognitive abilities are largely genetic later in life. *Behavior Genetics, 24*, 207–215.

Polich, J. (1998). P300 clinical utility and control of variability. *Journal of Clinical Neurophysiology, 15* (1), 14–33.

Polich, J., & Burns, T. (1987). P300 from identical twins. *Neuropsychologia, 25* (1B), 299–304.

Polich, J., & Herbst, K. L. (2000). P300 as a clinical assay: Rationale, evaluation, and findings. *International Journal of Psychophysiology, 38* (1), 3–19.

Polich, J., Ladish, C., & Burns, T. (1990). Normal variation of P300 in children: Age, memory span, and head size. *International Journal of Psychophysiology, 9*, 237–248.

Polich, J., & Martin, S. (1992). P300, cognitive capability, and personality: A correlational study of university undergraduates. *Personality and Individual Differences, 13*, 533–543.

Posner, M. J., & Mitchell, R. F. (1967). Chronometric analysis of classification. *Psychological Review, 74*, 392–409.

Posthuma, D., Baaré, W. F. C., Hulshoff Pol, H. E., Kahn, R. S., Boomsma, D. I., & de Geus, E. J. C. (2003). Genetic correlations between brain volumes and the

WAIS-III dimensions of verbal comprehension, working memory, perceptual organization and processing speed. *Twin Research, 6* (6), 131–139.

Posthuma, D., & Boomsma, D. I. (2000). A note on the statistical power in extended twin designs. *Behavior Genetics, 30,* 147–158.

Posthuma, D., de Geus, E. J. C., & Boomsma, D. I. (2001). Perceptual speed and IQ are associated through common genetic factors. *Behavior Genetics, 31* (6), 593–602.

Posthuma, D., Luciano, M., de Geus, E. J. C., Wright, M. J., Slagboom, P. E., Montgomery, G. W., et al. (2005). A genome-wide scan for intelligence identifies quantitative trait loci on 2q and 6p. *American Journal of Human Genetics, 77* (2), 318–326.

Posthuma, D., Mulder, E. J. C. M., Boomsma, D. I., & de Geus, E. J. C. (2002). Genetic analysis of IQ, processing speed and stimulus-response incongruency effects. *Biological Psychology, 61,* 157–182.

Posthuma, D., Neale, M. C., Boomsma, D. I., & de Geus, E. J. C. (2001). Are smarter brains running faster? Heritability of alpha peak frequency, IQ and their interrelation. *Behavior Genetics, 31* (6), 567–579.

Price, T. S., Simonoff, E., Asherson, P., Curran, S., Kuntsi, J., Waldman, I., et al. (2005). Continuity and change in preschool ADHD symptoms: Longitudinal genetic analysis with contrast effects. *Behavior Genetics, 35* (35), 121–132.

Price, T. S., Simonoff, E., Waldman, I., Asherson, P., & Plomin, R. (2001). Hyperactivity in preschool children is highly heritable. *Journal of the American Academy of Child and Adolescent Psychiatry, 40* (12), 1362–1364.

Propping, P. (1977). Genetic control of ethanol action on the central nervous system. An EEG study in twins. *Human Genetics, 35* (3), 309–334.

Rae, C., Karmiloff-Smith, A., Lee, M. A., Dixon, R. M., Grant, J., Blamire, A. M., et al. (1998). Brain biochemistry in Williams syndrome: Evidence for a role of the cerebellum in cognition? *Neurology, 51* (1), 33–40.

Richard-Clark, C., Veltmeyer, M. D., Hamilton, R. J., Simms, E., Paul, R., Hermens, D., et al. (2004). Spontaneous alpha peak frequency predicts working memory performance across the age span. *International Journal of Psychophysiology, 53* (1), 1–9.

Rietveld, M. J., Hudziak, J. J., Bartels, M., van Beijsterveldt, C. E., & Boomsma, D. I. (2004). Heritability of attention problems in children: Longitudinal results from a study of twins, age 3 to 12. *Journal of Child Psychology and Psychiatry, 45* (3), 577–588.

Rijsdijk, F. V., & Boomsma, D. I. (1997). Genetic mediation of the correlation between peripheral nerve conduction velocity and IQ. *Behavior Genetics, 27* (2), 87–98.

Rijsdijk, F. V., Boomsma, D. I., & Vernon, P. A. (1995). Genetic analysis of peripheral nerve conduction velocity in twins. *Behavior Genetics, 25* (4), 341–348.

Rijsdijk, F. V., Vernon, P. A., & Boomsma, D. I. (1998). The genetic basis of the relation between speed-of-information-processing and IQ. *Behavioural Brain Research, 95* (1), 77–84.

Robaey, P., Cansino, S., Dugas, M., & Renault, B. (1995). A comparative study of ERP correlates of psychometric and Piagetian intelligence measures in normal and hyperactive children. *Electroencephalography and Clinical Neurophysiology, 96* (1), 56–75.

Rogers, T. D., & Deary, J. (1991). The P300 component of the auditory event-related potential in monozygotic and dizygotic twins. *Acta Psychiatrica Scandinavica, 83*, 412–416.

Rose, S. A., & Feldman, J. F. (1996). Memory and processing speed in preterm children at eleven years: A comparison with full-terms. *Child Development, 67* (5), 2005–2021.

Rust, J. (1975). Genetic effects in the cortical auditory evoked potential: A twin study. *Electroencephalography and Clinical Neurophysiology, 39* (4), 321–327.

Santangelo, S. L., & Tsatsanis, K. (2005). What is known about autism: Genes, brain, and behavior. *American Journal of Pharmacogenomics, 5* (2), 71–92.

Shipley, B. A., Deary, I. J., Tan, J., Christie, G., & Starr, J. M. (2002). Efficiency of temporal order discrimination as an indicator of bradyphrenia in Parkinson's disease: The inspection time loop task. *Neuropsychologia, 40* (8), 1488–1493.

Shucard, D., & Horn, J. L. (1972). Evoked cortical potentials and measurement of human abilities. *Journal of Comparative Physiology and Psychology, 78*, 59–68.

Sigmundsson, H. (2005). Do visual processing deficits cause problem on response time task for dyslexics? *Brain and Cognition, 58* (2), 213–216.

Smit, D. J. A., Posthuma, D., Boomsma, D. I., & de Geus, E. J. C. (in press). Genetic contribution to the P3 in young and middle-aged adults. *Twin Research and Human Genetics*.

Spinath, F. M., & Borkenau, P. (2000). Genetic and environmental influences on reaction times: Evidence from behavior-genetic research. *Psychologische Beiträge, 42*, 58–69.

Stassen, H. H., Coppola, R., Gottesman, I. I., Torrey, E. F., Kuney, S., Rickler, C., et al. (1999). EEG differences in monozygotic twins discordant and concordant for schizophrenia. *Psychophysiology, 26*, 109–117.

Steriade, M., Gloor, P., Llinás, R. R., Lopes da Silva, F. H., & Mesulam, M. M. (1990). Basic mechanisms of cerebral rhythmic activities. *Electroencephalography and Clinical Neurophysiology, 76*, 481–508.

Sternberg, S. (1969). Memory-scanning: Mental processes revealed by reaction-time experiments. *American Scientist, 57*, 421–457.

Sunohara, G. A., Malone, M. A., Rovet, J., Humphries, T., Roberts, W., & Taylor, M. J. (1999). Effect of methylphenidate on attention in children with attention deficit hyperactivity disorder (ADHD): ERP evidence. *Neuropsychopharmacology, 21* (2), 218–228.

Sunohara, G. A., Voros, J. G., Malone, M. A., & Taylor, M. J. (1997). Effects of methylphenidate in children with attention deficit hyperactivity disorder: A comparison of event-related potentials between medication responders and non-responders. *International Journal of Psychophysiology, 27* (1), 9–14.

Surwillo, W. W. (1980). Cortical evoked potentials in monozygotic twins and unrelated subjects: Comparison of exogenous and endogenous components. *Behavior Genetics, 10*, 201–209.

Sutton, S., Braren, M., Zubin, J., & John, E. R. (1965). Evoked-potential correlates of stimulus uncertainty. *Science, 150* (700), 1187–1188.

Taylor, M. J., Voros, J. G., Logan, W. J., & Malone, M. A. (1993). Changes in event-related potentials with stimulant medication in children with attention deficit hyperactivity disorder. *Biological Psychology, 36* (3), 139–156.

van Baal, G. C. M., de Geus, E. J. C., & Boomsma, D. I. (1998). Longitudinal study of genetic influences on ERP-P3 during childhood. *Developmental Neuropsychology, 14* (1), 19–45.

Van Beijsterveldt, C. E., & van Baal, G. C. (2002). Twin and family studies of the human electroencephalogram: A review and a meta-analysis. *Biological Psychology, 61* (1–2), 111–138.
Verleger, R. (1988). Event-related potentials and cognition: A critique of the context updating hypothesis and an alternative interpretation of P3. *Behavioral and Brain Sciences, 11*, 343–427.
Vernon, P. A. (1983). Speed of information processing and general intelligence. *Intelligence, 7*, 53–70.
Vernon, P. A. (Ed.). (1987). *Speed of information-processing and intelligence*. Norwood, NJ: Ablex.
Vernon, P. A. (1989). The heritability of measures of speed of information processing. *Personality and Individual Differences, 10*, 573–576.
Vernon, P. A., & Weese, S. E. (1993). Predicting intelligence with multiple speed of information-processing tests. *Personality and Individual Differences, 14* (3), 413–419.
Vogel, E. K., & Luck, S. J. (2002). Delayed working memory consolidation during the attentional blink. *Psychonomic Bulletin and Review, 9* (4), 739–743.
Vogel, E. K., Luck, S. J., & Shapiro, K. L. (1998). Electrophysiological evidence for a postperceptual locus of suppression during the attentional blink. *Journal of Experimental Psychology. Human Perception and Performance, 24* (6), 1656–1674.
Wadsworth, S. J., Olson, R. K., Pennington, B. F., & DeFries, J. C. (2000). Differential genetic etiology of reading disability as a function of IQ. *Journal of Learning Disability, 33* (2), 192–199.
Weber, G. A. (1990). Nerve conduction studies and their clinical applications. *Clinics in Podiatric Medicine and Surgery, 7* (1), 151–178.
Wechsler, D. (1997). *WAIS-III Wechsler Adult Intelligence Scale*. San Antonio, TX: Psychological Corporation.
Wright, G. M., Scott, L. C., Richardson, C. E., Rai, G. S., & Exton-Smith, A. N. (1988). Relationship between the P300 auditory event-related potential and automated psychometric tests. *Gerontology, 34*, 134–138.
Wright, M. J., Hansell, N. K., Geffen, G. M., Geffen, L. B., Smith, G. A., & Martin, N. G. (2001). Genetic influence on the variance in P3 amplitude and latency. *Behavior Genetics, 31* (6), 555–565.
Wright, M. J., Luciano, M., Hansell, N. K., Geffen, G. M., Geffen, L. B., & Martin, N. G. (2002). Genetic sources of covariation among P3(00) and online performance variables in a delayed-response working memory task. *Biological Psychology, 61* (1–2), 183–202.
Young, J. P., Lader, M. H., & Fenton, G. W. 1972. A twin study of the genetic influences on the electroencephalogram. *Journal of Medical Genetics, 9* (1), 13–16.

5 Speed of processing in childhood and adolescence: Nature, consequences, and implications for understanding atypical development

Robert V. Kail

In 1884–85, Francis Galton established an Anthropometric Laboratory at the International Health Exhibition in London, where he measured many human responses, including simple response time (RT). The participants, which included nearly 1600 boys between the ages of 5½ and 20½ years, pressed a key as soon as they saw a light (Koga & Morant, 1923). Roughly 100 years later, I (Kail, 1991b) administered an updated task—participants now pushed a button on a joystick when they saw asterisks on a computer monitor—to nearly 200 7½- to 21-year-olds. The results of both studies, shown in Figure 5.1, demonstrate the developmental profile that has been revealed in countless other developmental studies: time to respond declines substantially

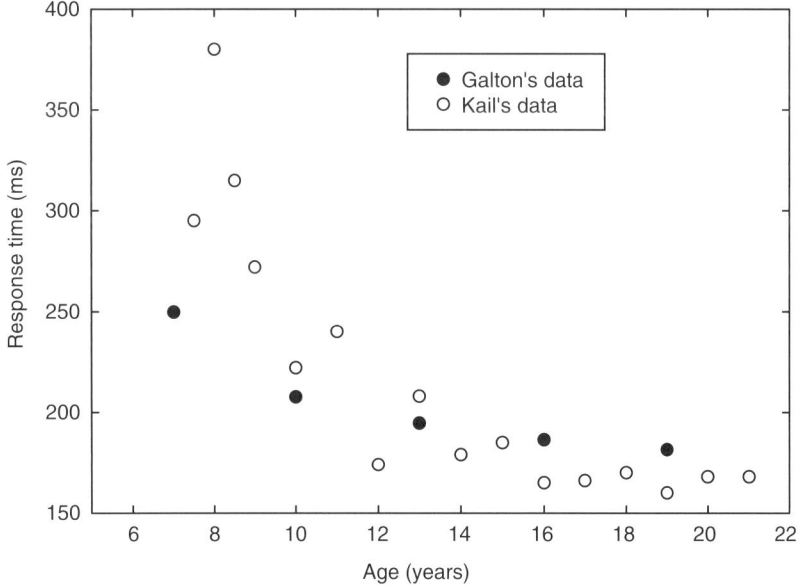

Figure 5.1 Change in simple response time (RT) as a function of chronological age in years, separately for data published by Koga and Morant (1923) and by Kail (1991b).

throughout childhood and adolescence. Furthermore, the pattern of developmental change is nonlinear: RT declines rapidly during childhood and continues to decline, but much more slowly, during adolescence.

It may be tempting to dismiss these age differences as reflecting change in perceptual and motor systems, and therefore not relevant to the study of cognitive development in childhood and adolescence. Nothing could be further from the truth. In this chapter, I show that the differences in Figure 5.1 are due to fundamental changes in the child's developing information processing system, changes that have important implications for children's ability to perform "higher-order" cognitive processes such as reading and problem-solving, as well as implications for understanding atypical development.

The nature of developmental change in speed of processing

The age differences illustrated in Figure 5.1 for simple RT are also seen in tasks with a stronger cognitive component. Figure 5.2 shows the factor by which 8-year-olds respond more slowly than adults on four cognitive tasks. The differences are nontrivial, ranging from 1.4 for memory scanning to 1.8 for mental rotation. Generalizing from the data in Figures 5.1 and 5.2, substantial age differences in speed of response are the rule whenever participants are encouraged to respond rapidly.

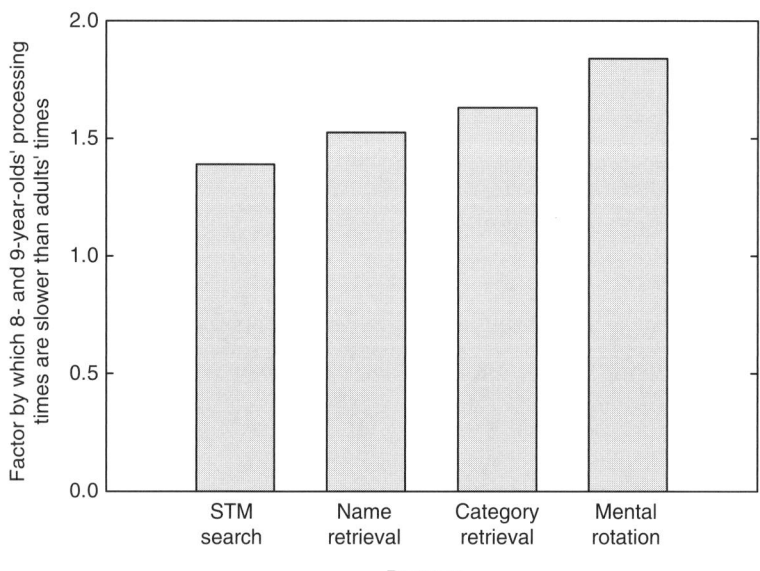

Figure 5.2 Factor by which 8- and 9-year-olds' processing times exceed adults' processing times. STM denotes short-term memory. After Figure 1 in Kail (1986). Copyright 1986 by the Society for Research in Child Development; reprinted with permission.

What factors might contribute to this age-related increase in speed of processing? One view is that this change reflects the impact of practice and experience. Compared to adults, young children are far less experienced in most domains and this lack of experience is thought to lead to slower processing. Said differently, the typical correlation between age and processing speed is thought to be a byproduct of two other correlations—the correlation between age and experience and the correlation between experience and speed (e.g., Chi, 1977).

Illustrating this view would be theories in which increased processing speed with practice is represented as a shift from performance based on algorithms, which are relatively slow, to performance based on rapid, direct retrieval of the appropriate response (e.g., Rickard, 1997). That is, individuals initially respond using an algorithm (e.g., in the case of addition, a counting algorithm). However, each time a task is performed, the stimulus and the person's response are stored in long-term memory. Repeated task performance increases the number and strength of these representations, such that ultimately the presentation of a problem leads to automatic retrieval of the response. According to these theories, change in RT associated with practice should be negatively decelerated: Early phases of practice produce substantial change, but later phases produce relatively modest change.

Consistent with this view, children's processing speed improves dramatically following practice: Park and I (Kail & Park, 1990) found that after more than 3000 trials of practice, 11-year-olds' rate of mental rotation of letters surpassed that of unpracticed 19-year-olds. Furthermore, practice-related changes in rate of mental rotation were negatively decelerated, as predicted by the view that initial responses reflect algorithms (which are slow) but responses quickly begin to reflect retrieval of answers (which is much faster).

Also consistent with an experience-oriented account are studies of expertise. When people acquire expertise in a domain, their knowledge in that domain is more elaborate, providing multiple paths by which task-relevant information can be accessed more rapidly. Applied to developmental change in processing speed, the prediction is that age differences in processing speed should be eliminated if children and adults have the same expertise. Described in terms of correlations between age, experience, and speed, if the age–speed correlation is actually an artifact of large age–experience and experience–speed correlations, then setting the age–experience correlation at 0 should result in an age–speed correlation of 0.

In the sole test of this prediction with children and adolescents, Roth (1983) tested 11-year-olds and adults on a task in which they compared pairs of chessboards that had 10–26 pieces per board placed in game-like positions. On some trials the boards were identical; on other trials, one piece was placed in a different location on the two boards. The comparisons of interest involve children who were chess experts—they were winners of local chess tournaments—with child and adult chess novices who had no experience with chess. Relative to search times for adult novices, times were greater by 1.58 for

11-year-old chess novices but by only 1.23 for 11-year-old chess experts. Thus when children have more task-relevant experience than adults (i.e., greater chess knowledge), age differences in processing speed are much reduced.

An alternate view is that age-related change in processing time reflects systemic or global change. More rapid responding with age is seen as a fundamental property of the developing information-processing system. That is, just as technological change has resulted in personal computers with ever-faster central processing units, developmental change results in steadily faster cognitive processing times.

This view does not deny the impact of task-specific practice or expertise on processing speed. Instead, it simply claims that practice and experience cannot provide a complete account of age-related change in processing speed. Consistent with this view, in the study by Roth (1983) described previously, age differences in processing speed were reduced when children had greater task-relevant knowledge, but they were not eliminated or reversed (as might be expected from a strong form of the expertise hypothesis). Thus findings like these suggest that expertise alone does not provide a sufficient explanation for age-related change in processing speed.

If, in fact, a common, global mechanism contributes to age-related change in processing time, then age differences in processing time should be pervasive and, more specifically, they should be quantitatively similar across tasks. The most compelling evidence for this pattern of age differences comes from studies based on a method used widely in studies of cognitive aging; namely, Brinley plots (Brinley, 1965). The rationale for this method is as follows. Suppose adults' response time (RT_a) on a task involves several processes:

$$RT_a = f + g + h + \ldots \quad (5.1)$$

where f is the time to execute process F, g is the time for process G, and so on. If children at age j execute each process more slowly than adults, by the same factor, then the corresponding equation for children would be:

$$RT_j = m_j f + m_j g + m_j h \ldots = m_j(f + g + h \ldots) \quad (5.2)$$

where m_j denotes the factor by which children at age j respond more slowly than adults. Rewriting Equation 5.2 to express children's RTs as a function of adults' RTs yields:

$$RT_j = m_j RT_a \quad (5.3)$$

As shown in Figure 5.3, Equation 5.3 leads to the prediction that RTs for children at age j should increase linearly as a function of adults' RTs from the same experimental conditions, and the slope of this function, which estimates m_j, should decrease with increasing age.

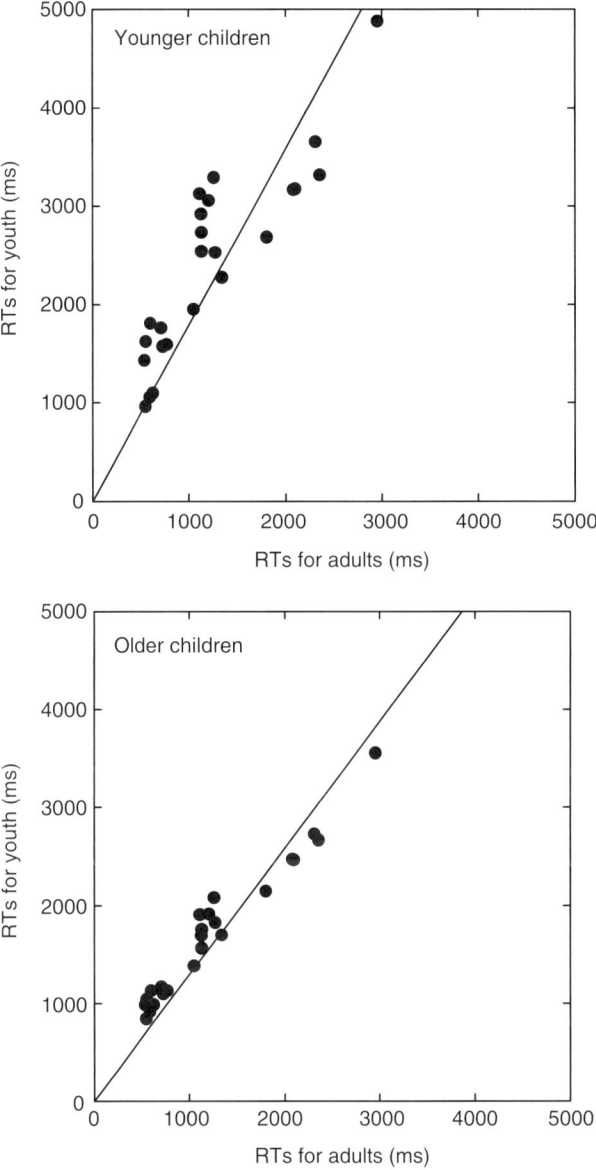

Figure 5.3 Hypothetical data showing the predictions of Equation 5.3. Each point depicts the mean RT for adults in an experimental condition, paired with the mean RT for children from the same condition. Equation 5.3 predicts that such points should be linked by a straight line and the slope of that line estimates m_j, the amount by which children respond more slowly than adults.

In one of the first uses of this method in the child-development literature, Hale (1990) tested 10-year-olds, 12-year-olds, 15-year-olds, and adults on four speeded tasks (e.g., choice RT, letter matching) that included a total of eight different experimental conditions. Mean RTs in each condition were calculated for all four age groups, and then the means for the three groups of children and adolescents were fitted separately to Equation 5.3, along with the adults' RTs. The fit was excellent ($R^2 = .987$), and the slope the linear function (which estimates m_j, the factor by which children respond more slowly than adults) decreased with age.

Perhaps the most compelling evidence for global developmental change comes from a meta-analysis that I conducted of 72 studies of speeded performance in children and adolescents (Kail, 1991a). The studies were selected without regard to the specific cognitive, perceptual, or motor task that was used; the only criteria were that (a) the data were collected under instructions that emphasized responding rapidly, and (b) the sample included adults and children. The studies included 1826 pairs of youth–adult mean RTs (i.e., each data point consisted of a mean RT for young adults paired with a mean RT for youths from the same experimental condition). The data were divided into 11 sets based on the age of the youths and separately fitted to Equation 5.3. Replicating the main results of Hale (1990), the fits were excellent at all ages ($R^2s = .90$) and the value of m_j decreased with age.

Also noteworthy is the pattern of developmental change in m_j, the factor by which children respond more slowly than adults. In the meta-analysis (Kail, 1991a), this change was nonlinear: m_j decreased in childhood and continued to decrease in early adolescence, but more slowly. That is, increase in processing speed is not steady throughout childhood and adolescence but, instead, is much more pronounced during childhood. In fact, this pattern of change was well characterized by the exponential function:

$$m_j = 1 + be^{-cj} \qquad (5.4)$$

where 1 is the asymptotic value of m_j, e is the base of natural logarithms, $1 + b$ is the intercept, c is a "decay" parameter that determines how rapidly the function approaches the asymptotic value of 1, and j denotes age. With $b = 5.16$ and $c = .21$, Equation 5.4 accounted for 77% of the variance in m_j values. Subsequent studies in which these analyses were applied to new (rather than archival) data and applied to data from individuals instead of groups (Fry & Hale, 1996; Kail & Park, 1992; Luna, Garver, Urban, Lazar, & Sweeney, 2004; Miller & Vernon, 1997; Weiler, Forbes, Kirkwood, & Waber, 2003) have confirmed the finding of exponential change in global processing speed and yielded estimates of b and c that resemble those obtained in the meta-analysis. Taken together, these data show that across many tasks children respond more slowly than adults by a constant factor (m_j), and that this factor decreases rapidly in childhood and more slowly in adolescence.

Longitudinal evidence

The evidence described thus far has been derived entirely from cross-sectional studies, and consequently provides no information concerning the shape of the developmental functions for individuals. There are, in fact, three studies that have reported relevant longitudinal data. Canfield, Smith, Brezsnyak, and Snow (1997) tested 13 infants monthly from 2 to 9 months and again at 12 months. The task was a visual expectancy paradigm in which infants' eye movements were recorded as targets appeared. Developmental change in RTs, determined from infants' eye movements, declined substantially in the first year of life and this decline was well characterized by Equation 5.3, accounting for an average of 94% of the variance in RT for individual infants. Canfield et al. (1997) also discovered that RTs were slightly better characterized by a modified version of Equation 5.3 in which processing speed was assumed to reach a local minimum at 12 months.

Because of the ages of the participants, the Canfield et al. (1997) findings are of limited value in determining the shape of the function that characterizes growth of processing speed in childhood and adolescence. More informative for this purpose are the findings of McCardle, Ferrer-Caja, Hamagami, and Woodcock (2002), who studied lifespan changes in cognitive functioning by examining performance on different tests from the Woodcock–Johnson Psycho-Educational Battery—Revised (WJ-R). Two of the tests that were studied—Visual Matching and Cross Out—define a processing speed construct on the WJ-R and, in fact, have been used frequently to estimate processing speed in developmental work (e.g., Kail, Hall & Caskey, 1999). The sample included 1193 individuals ranging in age from 2 to 95 years who were adminstered the WJ-R tests twice over an average interval of about 2.5 years. McCardle et al. (2002) explored many different growth models and determined that growth in processing speed during childhood and adolescence was nonlinear, changing rapidly early in childhood, but more slowly thereafter. Although these data do not provide direct evidence for exponential growth in processing speed, they clearly indicate the pattern of decelerating growth that typifies exponential functions.

Ferrer and I (Kail & Ferrer, 2004) reported similar findings from a sample of 132 children, each of whom completed the Visual Matching and Cross Out tasks twice. This sample consisted of five subsamples, based on the age of the participant at the time of testing and the interval between tests. There were 46 5- and 6-year-olds tested 4 years later as 9- and 10-year-olds, as well as 8-, 9-, 10-, and 11-year-olds tested 15 months later as 9-, 10-, 11-, and 12-year-olds ($n = 22, 18, 25,$ and 21, respectively).

Scores on the two tasks were fitted to a linear growth model as well as to an exponential model of the form:

$$Y = a - be^{-c*age} \tag{5.5}$$

where *a* represents asymptotic performance, *a* + b is the intercept, *e* is the base of natural logarithms, and *c* is a "growth" parameter indicating the rate with which performance approaches asymptotic value. For Visual Matching and Cross Out, developmental change was well characterized by the exponential function.

It is also worth noting that McCardle et al. (2002) found that, beginning with the school-age years, individuals' relative processing speeds are quite stable. Stability indices over approximately 1.5 years for a composite index of processing speed (aggregated across the Visual Matching and Cross Out tasks) were only .30 for 2- to 5-year-olds but .71 for 6- to 10-year-olds and .75 for 11- to 19-year-olds. Similarly, Kail and Ferrer (2004) reported stability indices for 8-, 9-, 10-, and 11-year-olds tested 15 months later of .71–.79 for Visual Matching and .58–.88 for Cross Out. Corresponding values for 6-year-olds retested as 10-year-olds were .53 and .67. By the school-age years, then, processing speed seems to be a moderately stable characteristic of individual children.

Extending the model

The view that processing speed reflects global or systematic change receives additional support from findings that Equation 5.3 can account for other important phenomena associated with speeded processing (Kail, 1995). To illustrate, consider the trade-off between speed and accuracy. Children and adults can regulate response speed, emphasizing accuracy at the cost of speed, or speed at the cost of accuracy (Brewer & Smith, 1989). The impact of these different emphases can be incorporated into Equations 5.1–5.3 by introducing additional constants to both children's and adults' RTs. Emphasizing accuracy might increases RTs by a factor of 1.2 over RTs in a neutral condition, whereas emphasizing speed might decrease RTs by a factor of .8. Assuming these constants are the same for children and adults, the result is that across various speed and accuracy conditions, children's RTs should be greater than adults' RTs by m_j, and this result has been obtained (Kail, 1995).

A similar analysis can be made for the impact of practice. As described previously, children (and adults) respond more rapidly with practice and this change can be represented as a shift from algorithmic solutions to direct retrieval of answers. Consequently, when applied to practice data, Equation 5.3 must be expanded to included two types of responses: relatively slow responses that reflect the use of an algorithm, and relatively rapid responses that reflect retrieval. However, assuming that the proportion of algorithmic solutions is approximately the same for children and adults at comparable phases of practice, then Equation 5.3 still holds. Consistent with this prediction, a single function relates youths' mean RTs before and after practice to adults' RTs before and after practice (Kail, 1995). Both groups respond more rapidly with practice, but times before and after practice differ by the same multiplicative constant, m_j.

An exception to global change

Research designed to examine developmental change in processing speed during childhood and adolescence typically has contrasted the possibility of global developmental change with task-specific developmental change. That is, the hypothesis that speeds of all processes develop at the same rate has been contrasted with the hypothesis that the speed of each process develops at a unique rate. Of course, global developmental change need not be the only alternative to task-specific change in processing speed. Change in processing speed could be consistent *within* a domain of processes but vary *across* such domains. For example, speed of perceptual processes might develop at a common constant rate that differs from the rate with which speed of cognitive processes develops. Domain-specific change in processing would mean that developmental change in processing speed would entail more than the single rate parameter of the global model but fewer rate parameters than a task-specific account of processing speed.

Among older adults, age-related slowing is greater on visual-spatial tasks than on verbal tasks (Jenkins, Myerson, Joerding, & Hale, 2000; Lawrence, Myerson, & Hale, 1998; Lima, Hale, & Myerson, 1991). For example, Lawrence et al. (1998) tested younger and older adults on verbal tasks (e.g., lexical decision, category membership) and visual-spatial tasks (e.g., shape classification, line-length discrimination). Within each domain, older adults' RTs increased linearly as a function of younger adults' RTs, but the slope was much steeper for the visual-spatial domain than for the verbal domain. Values of m_j were 3.29 and 1.43, respectively, for 70- to 79-year-olds, indicating that older adults responded approximately three times more slowly than young adults on visual-spatial tasks but only half again more slowly on verbal tasks. Similarly, Jenkins et al. (2000) found a steeper slope for visual-spatial tasks, 2.56, than for verbal tasks, 1.22. Thus age-related slowing that occurs during adulthood is consistent with a model that includes separate speeds for the visual-spatial and verbal domains, with speed in the former domain changing more with age than speed in the latter domain.

Miller and I (Kail & Miller, 2006) examined possible change in processing speed during childhood and adolescence that was specific to the language domain. We administered a battery of tasks to adults and to children at age 9 and then again at age 14. The battery included tasks assessing a range of language skills (e.g., phonological, lexical, and grammatical skills) as well as tasks assessing nonlanguage skills (e.g., motor, cognitive); the latter were viewed as representative of the broad range of perceptual-motor and cognitive tasks used previously and were used to estimate global processing speed.

To evaluate domain-specific characterizations of age-related change in processing speed, the data from the six language tasks and the four nonlanguage tasks were fitted separately to Equation 5.3. Values of m_j became smaller with age (indicating faster processing), but more rapidly on nonlanguage tasks because m_j was significantly greater for nonlanguage tasks than for language tasks at age 9. In other words, as shown in Figure 5.4, language processing speed was faster than global processing speed at age 9 but not at age 14.

Thus in childhood, as in middle and old age, processing speed is faster in the language domain than global processing speed. Evidently processing speed within the language domain follows a unique developmental trajectory, reaching mature levels more rapidly and maintaining those levels longer. And there may be other entrenched domains in which processing speed develops at a unique rate. However these findings are not inconsistent with the hypothesized global mechanism: When tasks do not tap entrenched domains, global processing speed would regulate the time needed for children to execute cognitive processes.

The nature of the global mechanism

Previously, I suggested that processing speed may be analogous to the operating speed of the central processing unit (CPU) of a personal computer (Kail, 1996). This speed is, for all practical purposes, fixed for a given CPU and, consequently, is considered a part of the architecture of the computer in which it is installed. Differences between CPUs in rate of processing are explained at a lower level of analysis, in terms of differences in their

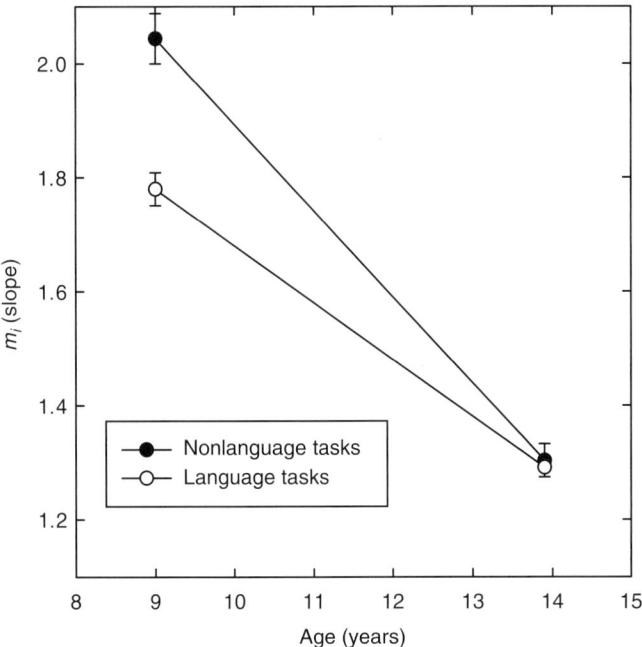

Figure 5.4 Processing speed as a function of age, separately for language and nonlanguage tasks. Data from Kail and Miller (2006).

circuitry. Similarly, developmental differences in processing speed would be linked to neural functioning. In fact, there is a scant literature that links processing speed to neural development and function; the evidence is often indirect and sometimes speculative but, in aggregate, provides an intriguing picture.

Change in neural architecture

There are important neural changes occurring during childhood and adolescence, periods when processing speed changes so dramatically. During this time there are age-related changes in the number of transient connections in the central nervous system (e.g., Huttenlocher, 1979) as well as age-related increases in myelinization (e.g., Yakovlev & Lecours, 1967). Furthermore, research relying on diffusion tensor imaging has linked white matter change to more rapid processing. For example, Mabbott, Laughlin, Noseworthy, Rockel, and Bouffet (2005) reported that age-related change in speed of visual search between 6 and 17 years of age was associated with increases in parietal white matter.

Studies of children with central nervous system (CNS) insults

If processing speed reflects, in part, changes in underlying neural functioning, a straightforward prediction is that children with impairments to the CNS should have slower processing speed. This prediction has been confirmed many times in studies from different groups of atypical children, including, for example, children with mental retardation (Nettelbeck & Wilson, 1997) and children with closed head injury (Capruso & Levin, 1992). I review this literature in more detail in the concluding section of this chapter.

Also relevant here are studies of children afflicted with acute lymphoblastic leukemia (ALL). Treatment for these children often involves substantial amounts of radiation to the skull and spine, which typically damages myelin (e.g., Hertzberg et al., 1997). Not surprisingly, many investigators have found slower processing speed in long-term survivors of childhood ALL who received radiation therapy (Cousins, Ungerer, Crawford, & Stevens, 1991; Schatz, Kramer, Ablin, & Matthay, 2000, 2004).

Association with physical maturity

Adolescence is a time of continued brain development. For example, volume of white matter increases steadily in most brain regions. In contrast, volume of gray matter increases, then decreases, at rates that vary by region (e.g., Giedd, 2004). These and other structural changes taking place in the CNS during adolescence lead to the hypothesis that youths who enter adolescence early should have a more adult-like CNS (i.e., faster processing) than youths who enter adolescence later. Thus the prediction is that early-maturing youths should have faster processing speed than late-maturing youths.

This hypothesis has been tested directly only once, by Eaton and Ritchot (1995). They identified groups of early- and later-maturing 9- and 10-year-old boys and girls who were then tested on a battery of three speeded tasks. Early-maturing boys had substantially faster processing speed than did later-maturing boys. A similar trend was evident for girls but was not significant, in part because even the later-maturing girls were relatively mature (e.g., they were more physically mature than the early-maturing boys).

Considered separately, none of these lines of evidence would make an airtight case. Collectively, however, work on (a) neuroanatomical changes, (b) children with CNS insult, and (c) links between speed and maturation makes it plausible to consider processing speed as a basic parameter of the child's developing cognitive architecture, one that is based in part on underlying biological processes.

Summary

Collectively, the findings of these studies converge on the conclusion that some sort of global, biologically driven mechanism limits the speed with which children process information. These results are not readily explained in terms of experiences and practice that are specific to particular processes or tasks, and thus suggest that experience- and practice-based mechanisms are not sufficient to account for age-related change in speed of cognitive processing.

Cognitive consequences of age-related change in processing speed

Several theorists have proposed that processing speed is a mechanism that could drive cognitive development in other domains. Flavell (1992), for example, wrote that "Developmentalists have long searched for a maturational process that could serve as a kind of universal regulator and pacesetter for cognitive growth, thereby making for similarities among all of the cognitive-developmental courses. [Processing speed] might be one such process" (p. 1002).

Developmental regularity is one reason why processing speed is a plausible mechanism for cognitive growth. Another reason is that much cognitive processing is subject to important temporal limits: Processing must occur within a finite window of time or it fails. Consequently, global developmental change in processing speed might influence the quality of cognitive processing whenever a number of cognitive processes must be completed in a fixed period of time. In this situation, younger children's slower processing speed may result in reduced performance because they cannot complete all components of task performance in the time available.

In fact, substantial evidence now reveals an important role for processing speed in developmental changes in other cognitive processes. One process that should be particularly sensitive to age-related change in processing speed would be working memory. One reason to expect a link is the fact that speed and working memory have a similar developmental profile (Dempster, 1981; Siegel, 1994): both change nonlinearly with age and approach asymptotic values in early adolescence (Kail, 2005). Moreover, models of working memory suggest a role for processing speed. In the model proposed by Baddeley (1996; Baddeley & Logie, 1999), for example, information is lost rapidly from the articulatory loop unless it is refreshed by rehearsal. Rate of rehearsal determines the amount of information that can be refreshed per unit of time; consequently, it is not surprising that age-related change in rehearsal rate predicts change in working memory (e.g., Hitch, Halliday, & Littler, 1989; Hulme & Tordoff, 1989).

Drawing on findings like these, Fry and Hale (1996) proposed a model of developmental cascade in which processing speed typically affects cognitive processes such as reasoning and problem solving indirectly, by increasing the functional capacity of working memory, and directly, by facilitating more rapid retrieval of task-relevant information. This model is a useful heuristic for organizing an emerging literature on the impact of processing speed on cognitive development. This research has addressed two components of the cascade model: the impact of processing speed on working memory and on the complex cognitive processes that are involved in academic skills. I review each literature in turn.

Processing speed and working memory

As described previously, theoretical accounts of working memory and extant research on rehearsal speed suggest that developmental change in processing speed should influence the growth of working memory. Hitch et al. (1989), for example, showed that age differences in word span were accurately predicted by the equation:

$$\text{span} = 1.2(\text{articulation rate}) + 1.14 \qquad (5.6)$$

where articulation rate was defined as the rate with which children could pronounce the words they were to remember. Hitch et al. suggested that age-related change in span is linked specifically to age-related increases in articulation rate, which reflect the rate with which information is refreshed in the articulatory loop of working memory. A more general view is that articulation rate itself is a reflection of global developmental change in processing speed. That is, increased processing speed with age would yield more rapid articulation, which, in turn, would yield more accurate retention.

In a series of studies designed to test this hypothesis (Kail, 1992, 1997a; Kail & Park, 1994), we assessed processing speed (with psychometric measures), the speed with which individuals could name digits and letters aloud, and, finally, digit span and letter span. As predicted, age-related increases in processing speed were associated with change in speech rate, which, in turn was associated with increases in span. In addition, later studies (Kail, 1997a; Ferguson & Bowey, 2005) have shown that age-related increases in processing speed enhance working memory through an independent path—by allowing more rapid retrieval of phonological information from long-term memory. That is, measures of children's phonological skill (e.g., identifying one word from a set of three words that did not rhyme with the other two) were predicted by age-related change in processing speed, and in turn predicted memory span. These effects were interpreted as reflecting age-related increases in the speed with which phonological information is retrieved from long-term memory during rehearsal and retrieval.

A subsequent study (Kail, 1997b) was designed to determine whether parallel changes mediated developmental change in spatial memory. That is, on tasks that require recalling the positions of objects (e.g., dots in a matrix), age differences in recall are typical (Pickering, 2001). This age difference might be linked to the visual-spatial sketchpad of working memory. Just as information is lost rapidly from the articulatory loop but loss can be avoided by rehearsing, image-based information is lost rapidly from the visual-spatial sketchpad but this loss can be avoided by regenerating images (Baddeley, 1996; Juhel, 1991). Presumably, processing speed would affect spatial memory indirectly by limiting the speed with which individuals can regenerate images.

Kail (1997b) provided an initial test of this hypothesis. The participants, 8- to 20-year-olds, were administered psychometric measures of processing speed along with "spatial span" tasks analogous to conventional span tasks (e.g., remembering marked cells in a matrix, beginning with two marked cells). Speed at refreshing visual images was estimated from two tasks. In one, participants learned to draw three upper-case letters in a 4×5 matrix; then they were shown a lower-case letter and a matrix with one cell marked. Participants judged, as rapidly as possible, whether the marked cell was part of the upper-case version of the specified letter; RT was presumed to reflect the time needed to generate the upper-case version of the letter and compare it with the single marked cell. In the second task, each trial had three phases: participants (a) first studied two line segments appearing on a computer screen that connected two points in an implicit 4×4 matrix, (b) studied two more line segments, and (c) judged whether a stimulus presented was a composite of the two previous sets of line segments.

Consistent with the developmental cascade model, age-related increases in processing speed were associated with speed at refreshing images in the visual-spatial sketchpad, which was, in turn, associated with greater spatial memory span. Furthermore, Chuah and Maybery (1999) assessed children's verbal and visual span and found that links to processing speed were approximately the same for both types of span task. Thus these findings suggest parallel developments in verbal (digit, letter, and word) span and spatial span: in both domains, developmental changes are mediated, in part, by the speed with which individuals can refresh information, which is driven, in part, by age-related change in global processing speed.

Strictly speaking, the studies described thus far demonstrate the influence of processing speed on short-term memory. Theoretically, short-term memory is often considered a subcomponent of working memory. For example, Engle, Kane, and Tuholski (1999) argued that working memory consists of "(a) a store in the form of long-term memory traces active above threshold, (b) the processes for achieving and maintaining that activation, and (c) controlled attention" (p. 104). Operationally, short-term memory is assessed with simple span tasks like those described previously (e.g., digit span, letter span); working memory is assessed with complex span tasks in which participants recall information while simultaneously performing other cognitive operations requiring manipulation of the information. In the prototypic span task, reading span (Daneman & Carpenter, 1980), participants read sets of sentences and concurrently remember the last word from each sentence in the set.

Consequently, Kail and Hall (2001) examined links from processing speed to working memory. In two studies 8- to 12-year-olds were administered measures of processing speed (the Visual Matching and Cross Out tasks described previously) as well as complex span tasks (e.g., reading span). Age-related change in processing speed was consistently related to change in working memory; we suggested that age-related change in speed "results in more efficient controlled processing. That is, more rapid processing makes it possible to direct attention more readily between the competing demands of complex span tasks" (p. 8).

Collectively, the studies in this series show that age-related change in processing speed consistently influences working memory. Furthermore, longitudinal studies also point to a connection between increased processing speed and greater working memory capacity. Demetriou, Christou, Spanoudis, and Platsidou (2002) found that over a 2-year period, 8- to 14-year-olds' processing efficiency (a composite of processing speed and processing "control") predicted working memory capacity. The nature of this influence is typically indirect, by enabling more rapid execution of processes that refresh information in the slave systems of working memory. Of course, more rapid refreshing of information driven by change in processing speed is not the sole explanation of age-related change in short-term and working memory. In particular, Cowan and his colleagues (Cowan, Wood, Wood, Keller, Nugent, & Keller, 1998; Cowan et al., 2003) have described the importance of other processes in the development of short-term and working memory. Nevertheless, increased processing speed is clearly one process that contributes to more efficient use of working memory, which can have widespread impact on cognitive performance.

Processing speed and academic skills

Academic skills such as reading and arithmetic are cognitively rich. Consequently, age-related improvements in these skills are likely to have multiple causes. In fact, studies of reading and arithmetic skill both show the influence of processing speed. Here I describe two studies that illustrate this influence, one for reading and one for arithmetic.

McBride-Chang and I (McBride-Chang & Kail, 2002) examined links between processing speed, naming, and word decoding in the context of other cognitive skills known to predict reading. That is, phonological awareness (defined as awareness of and access to sounds of letters, syllables, and words) is a critical skill in early reading in alphabetic and non-alphabetic languages (Goswami, 1999; McBride-Chang & Ho, 2000). In addition, the visual skills required to perceive and interpret visual forms have been shown to predict reading in Chinese (e.g., Ho & Bryant, 1997), evidently because Chinese characters contain more visual information than do English letters (but not all studies find that visual skill predicts reading in Chinese, e.g., Hu & Catts, 1998). McBride-Chang and Kail (2002) hypothesized that processing speed would influence age-related change in reading skill indirectly, by enhancing phonological awareness, naming, and visual skills. In fact, in two studies—one conducted with 4- to 6-year-olds from Hong Kong learning to read Chinese and the other conducted with 6- and 7-year-olds from the US learning to read English—age-related change in processing speed was consistently related to phonological awareness, to naming, and to visual skill. However, in both samples, only phonological skill uniquely predicted word decoding skill. Evidently, increased processing speed results in more rapid access to the phonological codes that are crucial in early reading.

A similar influence of processing speed is evident in studies of children's ability to solve arithmetic word problems. Children solve such problems more accurately over the elementary-school years (Morales, Shute, & Pellegrino, 1985), and explanations of this improvement have emphasized the contributions of domain-specific factors, such as knowledge of the underlying arithmetic operations and recognizing different forms of word problems (Morales et al., 1985; Zentall, 1990). Nevertheless, Hall and I (Kail & Hall, 1999) argued that global skills probably contribute to the accuracy with which children solve such problems. Increased processing speed might contribute, for example, by allowing more rapid retrieval of schemata for different types of problems. In addition, increased working memory might contribute by facilitating understanding of the problem (i.e., facilitating reading comprehension) and facilitating storage of problem facts during problem solving. We (Kail & Hall, 1999, Study 2) tested 8- to 12-year-olds on measures of processing speed, knowledge of addition and subtraction, working memory, reading comprehension, and word problem solving accuracy. Analyses showed that global measures (processing speed, working memory) and domain-specific measures (knowledge of addition and subtraction facts) both predicted accuracy on word problems.

These studies illustrate that developmental change in two important academic skills—word decoding and solving arithmetic word problems—cannot be explained solely in terms of domain-specific skills. Instead, systemic changes in processing speed and working memory allow the developing cognitive system to operate more efficiently on a wide range of tasks.

Studies of processing speed in atypical children

If processing speed is a fundamental element of the developing child's cognitive architecture, we would expect processing speed to be slower in children for whom that architecture is not intact. As I mentioned previously, this prediction has been documented numerous times with many groups of children. In this section, I briefly describe relevant research from two groups of atypical children: those with mental retardation and those with closed-head injury. These groups are instructive because they represent very different forms of atypical development—individuals with mental retardation have atypical development from very early in life whereas individuals with closed-head injury experience typical development until their injury. Thus these groups afford an opportunity to examine the generality of claims regarding the role of processing speed in cognitive development.

Consider first mental retardation. Nettelbeck and Wilson (1997) provide a comprehensive review of the literature on speed of cognitive processes in adolescents and adults with mental retardation. They note that there is an extensive literature dating from the 1960s. The aim of much of the initial work was to determine whether slowing could be isolated in a particular stage of information processing (e.g., perceptual encoding, central processing, response selection); in fact, there was evidence for slower processing at each stage. They also note that the slower mean rate of processing by individuals with mental retardation is usually associated with greater variability in response speed, and with more frequent errors. They suggest that the slower processing associated with mental retardation is partially due to attentional, motivational, and task-specific limits (e.g., use of inefficient strategies), but also reflects fundamental limits in the cognitive structures of individuals with mental retardation.

Next, consider children with closed-head injury. Slower processing speed is a common consequence of closed-head injury (Dennis & Levin, 2004). For example, Bawden, Knights, and Winogron (1985) tested 9-year-old children who had experienced head injuries ranging in severity from mild (i.e., lost consciousness for 20 minutes or less) to severe (i.e., in coma when admitted to the hospital and remained unconscious for 11 days or more). Children were tested approximately 1 year after their injury on a variety of speeded tasks, including the Coding subtest of the WISC-R (in which children draw lines based on a simple code) and a pegboard task (in which children move pegs from one row to another). The pattern of results on these two tasks typified the entire battery, in that children who experienced severe head injury had substantially lower scores than children who had experienced mild or moderate injury (who did not differ from one another). Similarly, Brookshire, Levin, Song, and Zhang (2004) tested children at 3 and 36 months after head injury. On both occasions, children with severe head injury had significantly lower scores on a composite speed score than children with mild or moderate head injury.

Thus processing speed is substantially slower in children with mental retardation, as well as children with closed-head injury. Furthermore, in both cases, the degree of slowing is related to the degree of impairment: Processing speed is particularly slow in children with IQs below 65 and in children with severe head injury.

A straightforward prediction from the research reviewed previously on typically developing children is that these deficits in processing speed should mediate impaired cognitive functioning in children with mental retardation and children with closed-head injury. Here there is much less research. On the one hand, impaired cognitive functioning and reduced academic achievement are well established for both groups of children. On the other hand, the contribution of processing speed to these deficits is not well established. There is, for example, indirect evidence that processing speed may contribute to impaired reading in children with closed-head injury. Ewing-Cobbs, Barnes, Fletcher, Levin, Swank, and Song (2004) reported that word decoding skill in children with closed-head injury was predicted by their ability to rapidly name familiar objects, which is known to be highly correlated with global processing speed (e.g., Kail et al., 1999). Unfortunately, reports like this one are few and far between. We clearly need studies that probe the link between slower processing speed and reduced academic performance in atypical children. Such work will test the generality of claims regarding the impact of processing speed, and also provide a clearer picture of the factors that contribute to delayed cognitive growth in atypical children.

Conclusions

The research reviewed in this chapter documents that processing speed changes substantially in childhood and adolescence, and that these changes are important determinants of developmental change in other memory and cognitive processes. One way to put these findings into proper perspective is by considering two goals common to much research and theory in cognitive development: one is to describe age-related differences in cognitive functioning; another is to explain how children move from less to more skilled functioning. Historically, cognitive developmentalists have invested more effort on the first (and easier) goal, but in the past quarter century they have vigorously attacked the problem of developmental mechanisms. The result is a handful of plausible mechanisms that propel growth—the modern equivalents of Piaget's assimilation and accommodation. Processing speed is one of these plausible mechanisms—a basic process that can help explain regularities of developmental change across a broad range of tasks.

Given the popular view that atypical development is often a delayed or slower form of typical development, processing speed is likely to be among those basic processes that contribute to atypical development. There is clearly evidence of this in the literature reviewed here, in which slower processing speed is a consistent and nontrivial manifestation of mental retardation and closed-head injury. However, we are only beginning to specify the links between these basic processes and clinically relevant outcomes for these children. There is clearly a need for longitudinal studies of atypical children that combine detailed diagnostic information, careful specification of basic processes such as processing speed, and meaningful outcome measures. Such research might help to identify the need for cognitive remediation focusing on processing speed in children with disabilities. If, for example, it were shown that many cognitive impairments in atypical children were byproducts of slower processing speed, then the goal of remediation would be to increase processing speed; such remediation should improve the functioning of all downstream cognitive processes, such as working memory.

References

Baddeley, A. D. (1996). The concept of working memory. In S. E. Gathercole (Ed.), *Models of short-term memory*. Hove, UK: Psychology Press.

Baddeley, A. D., & Logie, R. (1999). Working memory: The multiple component model. In A. Miyake & P. Shah (Eds.), *Models of working memory: Mechanisms of active maintenance and executive control* (pp. 28–61). New York: Cambridge University Press.

Bawden, H. N., Knights, R. M., & Winogron, H. W. (1985). Speeded performance following head injury in children. *Journal of Clinical and Experimental Neuropsychology, 7*, 39–54.

Brewer, N., & Smith, G. A. (1989). Developmental changes in processing speed: Influence of speed–accuracy regulation. *Journal of Experimental Psychology: General, 118*, 298–310.

Brinley, J. F. (1965). Cognitive sets, speed, and accuracy of performance in the elderly. In A. T. Welford & J. E. Birren (Eds.), *Behavior, aging, and the nervous system* (pp. 114–149). Springfield, IL: Charles C. Thomas.

Brookshire, B., Levin, H. S., Song, J. X., & Zhang, L. (2004). Components of executive function in typically developing and head-injured children. *Developmental Neuropsychology, 25*, 61–83.

Canfield, R. L., Smith, E. G., Brezsnyak, M. P., & Snow, K. L. (1997). Information processing through the first year of life: A longitudinal study using the Visual Expectation Paradigm. *Monographs of the Society for Research in Child Development, 62* (Serial No. 250).

Capruso, D. X., & Levin, H. S. (1992). Cognitive impairment following closed head injury. *Neurologic Clinics, 10*, 879–893.

Chi, M. T. H. (1977). Age differences in the speed of processing: A critique. *Developmental Psychology, 13*, 543–544.

Chuah, Y. M. L., & Maybery, M. T. (1999). Verbal and spatial short-term memory: Common sources of developmental change? *Journal of Experimental Child Psychology, 73*, 7–44.

Cousins, P., Ungerer, J. A., Crawford, J. A., & Stevens, M. M. (1991). Cognitive effects of childhood leukemia therapy: A case for four specific deficits. *Journal of Pediatric Psychology, 16*, 475–488.

Cowan, N., Towse, J. N., Hamilton, Z., Saults, J. S., Elliott, E. M., Lacey, J. F., et al. (2003). Children's working-memory processes: A response-timing analysis. *Journal of Experimental Psychology: General, 132*, 113–132.

Cowan, N., Wood, N. L., Wood, P. K., Keller, T. A., Nugent, L. D., & Keller, C. V. (1998). Two separate verbal processing rates contributing to short-term memory span. *Journal of Experimental Psychology: General, 127*, 141–160.

Daneman, M., & Carpenter, P. A. (1980). Individual differences in working memory and reading. *Journal of Verbal Learning and Verbal Behavior, 19*, 450–466.

Demetriou, A., Christou, C., Spanoudis, G., & Platsidou, M. (2002). The development of mental processing: Efficiency, working memory, and thinking. *Monographs of the Society for Research in Child Development, 67* (Serial No. 268).

Dempster, F. N. (1981). Memory span: Sources of individual and developmental differences. *Psychological Bulletin, 89*, 63–100.

Dennis, M., & Levin, H. S. (2004). New perspectives on cognitive and behavioral outcomes after childhood closed head injury. *Developmental Neuropsychology, 25*, 1–3.

Eaton, W. O., & Ritchot, K. F. M. (1995). Physical maturation and information-processing speed in middle childhood. *Developmental Psychology, 31*, 967–972.

Engle, R. W., Kane, M. J., & Tuholski, S. W. (1999). Individual differences in working memory capacity and what they tell us about controlled attention, general fluid intelligence, and functions of the prefrontal cortex. In A. Miyake & P. Shah (Eds.), *Models of working memory* (pp. 102–134). Cambridge: Cambridge University Press.

Ewing-Cobbs, L., Barnes, M., Fletcher, J. M., Levin, H. S., Swank, P. R., & Song, J. (2004). Modeling of longitudinal academic achievement scores after pediatric traumatic brain injury. *Developmental Neuropsychology, 25*, 107–133.

Ferguson, A. N., & Bowey, J. A. (2005). Global processing speed as a mediator of developmental changes in children's auditory memory span. *Journal of Experimental Child Psychology, 91*, 89–112.

Flavell, J. H. (1992). Cognitive development: Past, present, and future. *Developmental Psychology, 28*, 998–1005.

Fry, A. F., & Hale, S. (1996). Processing speed, working memory, and fluid intelligence: evidence for developmental cascade. *Psychological Science, 7*, 237–241.

Giedd, J. (2004). Structural magnetic resonance imaging of the adolescent brain. *Annals of the New York Academy of Science, 1021*, 77–85.

Goswami, U. (1999). The relationship between phonological awareness and orthographic representation in different orthographies. In M. Harris & G. Hatano (Eds.), *Learning to read and write: A cross-linguistic perspective* (pp. 134–156). New York: Cambridge University Press.

Hale, S. (1990). A global developmental trend in cognitive processing speed in children. *Child Development, 61*, 653–663.

Hertzberg, H., Huk, W. J., Ueberall, M. A., Langer, T., Meier, W., Dopfer, R., et al. (1997). CNS late effects after ALL therapy in childhood. Part I: Neuroradiological findings in long-term survivors of ALL—an evaluation of the inferences between morphology and neuropsychological performance. *Medical and Pediatric Oncology, 28*, 387–400.

Hitch, G. J., Halliday, M. S., & Littler, J. E. (1989). Item identification and rehearsal rate as predictors of memory span in children. *Quarterly Journal of Experimental Psychology, 41A*, 321–337.

Ho, C. S.-H., & Bryant, P. (1997). Phonological skills are important in learning to read English and Chinese. *Developmental Psychology, 33*, 946–951.

Hu, C.-F., & Catts, H. W. (1998). The role of phonological processing in early reading ability: What we can learn from Chinese. *Scientific Studies of Reading, 2*, 55–79.

Hulme, C., & Tordoff, V. (1989). Working memory development: The effects of speech rate, word length, and acoustic similarity on serial recall. *Journal of Experimental Child Psychology, 47*, 72–87.

Huttenlocher, P. R. (1979). Synaptic density in human frontal cortex—Developmental changes and effects of aging. *Brain Research, 163*, 195–205.

Jenkins, L., Myerson, J., Joerding, J. A., & Hale, S. (2000). Converging evidence that visuospatial cognition is more age-sensitive than verbal cognition. *Psychology and Aging, 15*, 157–175.

Juhel, J. (1991). Spatial abilities and individual differences in visual information processing. *Intelligence, 15*, 117–137.

Kail, R. (1986). Sources of age differences in speed of processing. *Child Development, 57*, 969–987.

Kail, R. (1991a). Developmental change in speed of processing during childhood and adolescence. *Psychological Bulletin, 109*, 490–501.

Kail, R. (1991b). Processing time declines exponentially during childhood and adolescence. *Developmental Psychology, 27*, 259–266.

Kail, R. (1992). Processing speed, speech rate, and memory. *Developmental Psychology, 28*, 899–904.

Kail, R. (1995). Processing speed, memory, and cognition. In W. Schneider & F. E. Weinert (Eds.), *Memory development: State of the art and future directions*. Hillsdale, NJ: Lawrence Erlbaum Associates, Inc.

Kail, R. (1996). Nature and consequences of developmental change in speed of processing. *Swiss Journal of Psychology, 55*, 133–138.

Kail, R. (1997a). Phonological skill and articulation time independently contribute to the development of memory span. *Journal of Experimental Child Psychology, 67*, 57–68.

Kail, R. (1997b). Processing time, imagery, and spatial memory. *Journal of Experimental Child Psychology, 64*, 67–78.

Kail, R. V. (2005). *Memory span develops exponentially*. Paper presented at the biennial meeting of the Society for Research in Child Development, Atlanta, GA.

Kail, R., & Ferrer, E. (2004). *Exponential developmental change in processing speed: Longitudinal evidence*. Paper presented at the annual meeting of the American Psychological Society, Chicago.

Kail, R., & Hall, L. K. (1999). Sources of developmental change in children's word problem performance. *Journal of Educational Psychology, 91*, 660–668.

Kail, R., & Hall, L. K. (2001). Distinguishing short-term memory from working memory. *Memory & Cognition, 29*, 1–9.

Kail, R., Hall, L. K., & Caskey, B. J. (1999). Processing speed, exposure to print, and naming speed. *Applied Psycholinguistics, 20,* 303–314.

Kail, R. V., & Miller, C. A. (2006). Developmental change in processing speed: Domain specificity and stability during childhood and adolescence. *Journal of Cognition and Development, 7,* 119–137.

Kail, R., & Park, Y. (1990). Impact of practice on speed of mental rotation. *Journal of Experimental Child Psychology, 49,* 227–244.

Kail, R., & Park, Y. (1992). Global developmental change in processing time. *Merrill-Palmer Quarterly, 38,* 525–541.

Kail, R., & Park, Y. (1994). Processing time, articulation time, and memory span. *Journal of Experimental Child Psychology, 57,* 281–291.

Koga, Y., & Morant, G. M. (1923). On the degree of association between reaction times in the case of different senses. *Biometrika, 15,* 346–372.

Lawrence, B., Myerson, J., & Hale, S. (1998). Differential decline of verbal and visuo-spatial processing speed across the adult life span. *Aging, Neuropsychology, and Cognition, 5,* 129–146.

Lima, S. D., Hale, S., & Myerson, J. (1991). How general is general slowing? Evidence from the lexical domain. *Psychology and Aging, 6,* 416–425.

Luna, B., Garver, K. E., Urban, T. A., Lazar, N. A., & Sweeney, J. A. (2004). Maturation of cognitive processes from late childhood to adulthood. *Child Development, 75,* 1357–1372.

Mabbott, D. J., Laughlin, S., Noseworthy, M., Rockel, C., & Bouffet, E. (2005). *Age related changes in DTI measures of white matter and processing speed.* Paper presented at the annual meeting of the Organization for Human Brain Mapping, Toronto, Canada.

McBride-Chang, C., & Ho, C. S.-H. (2000). Developmental issues in Chinese children's character acquisition. *Journal of Educational Psychology, 92,* 50–55.

McBride-Chang, C., & Kail, R. V. (2002). Cross-cultural similarities in the predictors of reading acquisition. *Child Development, 73,* 1392–1407.

McCardle, J. J., Ferrer-Caja, E., Hamagami, F., & Woodcock, R. W. (2002). Comparative longitudinal structural analyses of the growth and decline of multiple intellectual abilities over the life span. *Developmental Psychology, 38,* 115–142.

Miller, L. T., & Vernon, P. A. (1997). Developmental changes in speed of information processing in young children. *Developmental Psychology, 33,* 544–548.

Morales, R. V., Shute, V. J., & Pellegrino, J. W. (1985). Developmental differences in understanding and solving simple mathematics word problems. *Cognition and Instruction, 2,* 41–57.

Nettelbeck, T., & Wilson, C. (1997). Speed of information processing and cognition. In W. E. MacLean Jr. (Ed.), *Ellis' handbook of mental deficiency, psychological theory and research* (3rd ed., pp. 245–274). Mahwah, NJ: Lawrence Erlbaum Associates, Inc.

Pickering, S. J. (2001). The development of visuo-spatial working memory. *Memory, 9,* 423–432.

Rickard, T. C. (1997). Bending the power law: A CMPL theory of strategy shifts and the automatization of cognitive skills. *Journal of Experimental Psychology: General, 126,* 288–311.

Roth, C. (1983). Factors affecting developmental changes in the speed of processing. *Journal of Experimental Child Psychology, 35,* 509–528.

Schatz, J., Kramer, J. H., Ablin, A., & Matthay, K. K. (2000). Processing speed, working memory, and IQ: A developmental model of cognitive deficits following cranial radiation therapy. *Neuropsychology, 14*, 189–200.

Schatz, J., Kramer, J. H., Ablin, A., & Matthay, K. K. (2004). Visual attention in long-term survivors of leukemia receiving cranial radiation therapy. *Journal of the International Neuropsychological Society, 10*, 211–220.

Siegel, L. S. (1994). Working memory and reading: A life-span perspective. *International Journal of Behavioral Development, 17*, 109–124.

Weiler, M. D., Forbes, P., Kirkwood, M., & Waber, D. (2003). The developmental course of processing speed in children with and without learning disabilities. *Journal of Experimental Child Psychology, 85*, 178–194.

Yakovlev, P. I., & Lecours, A. R. (1967). The myelogenetic cycles of regional maturation of the brain. In A. Minkowski (Ed.), *Regional development of the brain in early life*. Oxford, UK: Blackwell.

Zentall, S. S. (1990). Fact-retrieval automatization and math problem solving by learning disabled, attention-disordered, and normal adolescents. *Journal of Educational Psychology, 82*, 856–865.

6 Processing speed and the Digit Symbol Substitution Test in schizophrenia

Dwight Dickinson and James M. Gold

Introduction

In 1998, Heinrichs and Zakzanis published an exhaustive meta-analysis of 204 studies from the cognitive deficit literature in schizophrenia (Heinrichs & Zakzanis, 1998). The analyses provided some evidence of a selective deficit in verbal memory performance compared with other cognitive domains, but against the backdrop of a broadly based impairment in cognitive functioning. A contemporaneous meta-analysis of 70 studies by Aleman and colleagues (Aleman, Hijman, de Haan, & Kahn, 1999) also emphasized the verbal memory deficit in this illness. Notable for its absence from either review was the Digit Symbol Substitution Test (DSST) from the Wechsler Adult Intelligence Scale (Wechsler, 1997). The omission is significant because the DSST is perhaps the most widely known and used measure of information processing speed, a dimension of cognitive performance that has received growing attention in the field in recent years, and has been a focus of research in our group (Bellack, Gold, & Buchanan, 1999; Dickinson & Coursey, 2002; Dickinson, Iannone, Wilk, & Gold, 2004; Gold, Goldberg, McNary, Dixon, & Lehman, 2002; Gold, McMahon, Wilk, Thaker, Bellack, & Buchanan, in preparation).

Many people with schizophrenia are noticeably slow in engaging with the environment, responding to inquiries and events, and initiating and completing tasks. This slowing is a central characteristic of schizophrenia, especially among patients with negative symptomatology and syndromes (Andreasen, 1985; Andreasen & Olsen, 1982; Crow, 1980a, 1980b; Kirkpatrick & Buchanan, 1990; Kirkpatrick, Buchanan, McKenney, Alphs, & Carpenter, 1989; Liddle, 1987). It appears to involve a broad range of sensory, cognitive, and motor processes and poses obvious challenges for functioning in the everyday world. Driving a car, operating machinery, following programming on television, and participating fluently in conversation are just a few examples of ordinary activities that require a degree of alacrity in understanding, thought, and/or action. Anecdotally, these are all areas of difficulty for patients with schizophrenia.

Information processing speed

Information processing speed is the cognitive construct most closely aligned with these clinical and functional observations. As used here, the term simply refers to the speed with which different cognitive operations can be executed (Salthouse, 1996). Psychometrically, processing speed is typically indexed by the time taken to complete relatively simple operations. For example, the DSST reflects speeded performance of a number of simple scanning, matching, and motor operations. Despite the narrow measurement approach, we believe that this performance dimension represents a very general constraint on cognitive processing (Salthouse, 1996). That is, many higher cognitive operations—including perceptual processes, encoding and retrieval operations, transformation of information held in active memory, and decision processes—involve internal dynamics that are speed-dependent to an important extent. Thus the Letter Number Sequencing task from the Wechsler Adult Intelligence Scale requires individuals to reorganize and report a string of numbers and letters. The task is untimed. However, mental speed is needed to quickly perform the necessary reorganization between rehearsals of the original stimuli. As this example illustrates, an individual who performs slowly on the DSST may, for related reasons, show impairments on a wide variety of cognitive tasks, including many that are not overtly speeded tasks.

The apparent link of information processing speed to other higher and lower order cognitive functions likely explains, in part, the hesitation of the field to embrace it as a main focus of cognitive research in schizophrenia. Following the Salthouse definition, processing speed does not appear to be associated with particular regional or functional brain systems but, rather, is a characteristic of many such systems. Not surprisingly, given the general nature of the construct, performance in this area seems to be a sensitive marker of cognitive functioning across many developmental and clinical contexts, but not a *specific* marker in any of these contexts. Indeed, cognitive slowing similar to that of schizophrenia is observed in normal aging (Birren & Fisher, 1995) and in a variety of non-psychiatric clinical populations (e.g., multiple sclerosis, Denney, Lynch, Parmenter, & Horne, 2004). Among psychiatric conditions, this slowing is probably more closely associated with depression than schizophrenia. Impaired processing speed performance in unipolar and bipolar depression, and its relationship to disease course and symptomatology, has been reviewed extensively (Colbert & Harrow, 1967; Goodwin & Jamison, 1990; Miller, 1975; Sackheim & Steif, 1988; Widlocher, 1983). As one depression researcher concluded, "cognitive slowing seems a constant dimension in depression and, probably, its core" (Widlocher, 1983, p. 36). At the same time, depression researchers have recognized that processing speed impairment is not specific to depression but is more likely to mark illness severity (Goodwin & Jamison, 1990).

Despite the lack of specificity, there has been increasing recognition of the importance of information processing speed in schizophrenia. Various reports have documented modestly disproportionate deficits on processing speed measures in the illness (including Stroop word and color conditions and Trail Making Test, form A, along with the DSST), in the context of generalized cognitive impairment (Bellack et al., 1999; Dickerson, Boronow, Ringel, & Parente, 1996; Dickinson et al., 2004; Gladsjo, McAdams, Palmer, Moore, Jeste, & Heaton, 2004; Mohamed, Paulsen, O'Leary, Arndt, & Andreasen, 1999). Processing speed is also emerging as an important correlate of functional status for patients (Bellack et al., 1999; Brekke, Raine, Ansel, Lencz, & Bird, 1997; Dickinson & Coursey, 2002; Gladsjo et al., 2004; J. Gold, Iannone, McMahon, & Buchanan, 2001; J. M. Gold et al., in preparation; Jaeger et al., 2005). Bilder and colleagues (2002) have provided initial evidence of a genetic association to the processing speed domain (see also chapter 4 in this volume). Some recent reports even raise the possibility that such speeded tasks may show disproportionate benefit from new generation antipsychotics (Galletly, Clark, McFarlane, & Weber, 2000; Keefe et al., 2004) or adjunctive medication strategies targeting cognitive and negative symptoms in schizophrenia (Buchanan, Summerfelt, Tek, & Gold, 2003).

The Digit Symbol Substitution Test

The DSST has been perhaps the most widely used index of processing speed in schizophrenia research and more generally. Early versions of the task were used in the screening of non-English speaking immigrants at Ellis Island in the early 1900s and army recruits during World War I (Richardson, 2003). The DSST was included in the first and all subsequent editions of Wechsler's intelligence battery (Wechsler, 1955, 1981, 1997). The longevity and popularity of the DSST and similar substitution tests trace to a number of characteristics. In healthy populations, they are strongly associated with general cognitive ability or intelligence (DSST r = .61 with Full Scale IQ in the WAIS-III; The Psychological Corporation, 1997). As might be expected, they are sensitive markers of brain dysfunction across a wide spectrum of neuropsychiatric conditions. For example, in a series of special group validity studies published in the WAIS-III/WMS-III Technical Manual, the WAIS-III processing speed index (comprising the DSST and Symbol Search subtests) showed the greatest impairment among all WAIS/WMS indexes in schizophrenia, Huntington's disease, Parkinson's disease, traumatic brain injury, and attention-deficit/hyperactivity disorder (ADHD) samples, and was lowest but for selected memory indexes in Korsakoff's syndrome, chronic alcohol abuse, and Alzheimer's disease (The Psychological Corporation, 1997; see also Carey et al., 2004, HIV-related cognitive impairment; Frazier, Demaree, & Youngstrom, 2004, ADHD; Pier, Hulstijn, & Sabbe, 2004, unmedicated major depression). The DSST and its variants also have a variety of desirable measurement properties. They are relatively culture-fair (Laux & Lane, 1985). One recent large scale meta-analysis showed the DSST to be independent of educational level in non-clinical groups (Hoyer, Stawski, Wasylyshyn, &

Verhaeghen, 2004). These tests can be administered and scored quickly and reliably—in 5 minutes or less in the case of the DSST. Average test–retest reliability for DSST in the 2450-person WAIS-III normative sample was .84, with limited variation across the 13 age groups (range .81 to .87; The Psychological Corporation, 1997). These results also highlight that substitution measures are appropriate for repeated assessment.

Meta-analysis

Study and variable selection

We conducted a focused meta-analysis to illustrate the importance of information processing speed, and of the DSST in particular, in schizophrenia. Articles considered for inclusion were identified through searches of MEDLINE with keyword combinations of *schizophrenia, cognitive tests, digit symbol,* and *neuropsychological*. To avoid overlap with the substantial meta-analyses of Heinrichs and Aleman, we limited our search to the time period since 1998. Additional studies were identified from the bibliographies of identified studies and from an issue-by-issue review of the *American Journal of Psychiatry, Archives of General Psychiatry, and Schizophrenia Research* for the second half of 2004 and the first months of 2005, in case relevant articles were not yet available in computerized databases. We set demanding criteria for inclusion in this analysis. As an initial matter, each study needed to compare the cognitive test performance of healthy control subjects with individuals well-diagnosed with schizophrenia or schizoaffective disorder. Because of inconsistencies in cognitive domain composites across studies, we only included studies reporting means and standard deviations for individual cognitive tests from which effect sizes could be calculated.

Given our focus on processing speed, we considered only studies incorporating the Digit Symbol and/or Trails A measures, which have been more widely used in cognitive research on schizophrenia patients than other processing speed measures. To obtain the most reliable information most efficiently, we limited inclusion to *major* studies judged along two dimensions. *First*, we required that the processing speed measures had been administered as part of broad test batteries addressing dimensions of cognition that have been consistently implicated in studies of cognitive impairment in schizophrenia. Thus, in addition to the processing speed measures, we included only studies where data were reported for one or more individual tests in at least four of the following additional categories: (1) executive functioning (e.g., Wisconsin Card Sort, Trails B, Stroop); (2) declarative memory (Logical Memory, list learning, Visual Reproduction); (3) verbal fluency (letters, categories); (4) working memory (Digit Span (total score), Arithmetic); (5) premorbid/verbal ability (Vocabulary, WRAT Reading); and (6) motor speed (Finger Tapping, Grooved Pegboard). Obviously, there is no definitive assignment of individual tests to cognitive domains. Rather, we grouped the tests into domains on the basis of literature, expert consensus, and our experience with the various tasks (Mishara & Goldberg, 2004). *Second*, we required that the studies have schizophrenia samples of at least 45 subjects. Smaller samples yield effect size estimates that are systematically upwardly biased, but this bias becomes negligible as within-study sample sizes approach 50 (Hedges & Olkin, 1985). When we identified different studies in which data from the same or overlapping groups of subjects were reported, only one of the studies was included in the analysis to avoid data duplication. We identified seven studies meeting these criteria and added data from our own study of good and poor vocational outcomes in schizophrenia, which also met all study selection criteria (Bilder et al., 2000; Egan et al., 2001; Gold et al., in preparation; Hill, Schuepbach, Herbener, Keshavan, & Sweeney, 2004; Hoff, Svetina, Maurizio, Crow, Spokes, & DeLisi, 2005; Hughes et al., 2003; Mohamed et al., 1999; Seidman, Kremen, Koren, Faraone, Goldstein, & Tusang, 2002). Although this stringent study selection process resulted in a small number of studies for the meta-analysis, we believe that they are of uniformly high quality (Moher et al., 1999), and the sample sizes associated with different effect size estimates are substantial. Table 6.1 provides summary information about each of these eight studies.

Test batteries varied substantially from one study to the next. However, 17 variables, all of which have been commonly included in schizophrenia cognitive research test batteries, were reported with some consistency across the different studies. Table 6.2 identifies these tests, groups them by cognitive domains, and indicates which of the selected studies included each test. As the table shows, each test was included in at least four studies, with the exceptions of the WAIS Arithmetic (two studies), categorical fluency (three studies), and Grooved Pegboard (three studies). We retained these measures, nevertheless, because of their association with important and under-represented cognitive domains. The reader should note that, even with the Arithmetic results, our working memory category is less informative than would be ideal. The Digit Span results reflect total scores across forward and backward conditions, and thus confound immediate and working memory. As noted, we selected studies that reported test results for individual measures and separately analyzed the results for each of the measures across studies. We made a number of exceptions. First, one of the studies used the Symbol Digit Modalities Test (SDMT; written version) rather than the Digit Symbol Substitution Test (Hoff et al., 2005) and another used the National Adult Reading Test instead of WRAT Reading (Hughes et al., 2003). We decided a priori to include the divergent data points on the assumption that, in both cases, the tests tap very similar abilities. Second, for the same reason, we grouped different verbal list learning tasks (California Verbal Learning Test, Rey Auditory Verbal Learning Test, Hopkins Verbal Learning Test, and Word Lists from the Wechsler Memory Scale) into a single category. Similarly, we grouped letter fluency results although some studies used different letter cues, and categorical fluency results although studies used different

Table 6.1 Studies included in meta-analysis

	HCn Age (SD) Ed. (SD)	SZn Age (SD) Ed. (SD)	Patient sample notes
Bilder et al. (2000)	36 25.3 (6.5) 14.9 (1.5)	~94 25.7 (6.3) 13.1 (2.3)	1st psychotic episode; <12 weeks cumulative medications
Egan et al. (2001)	43 33.3 (8.8) 15.1 (2.3)	120 35.9 (8.2) 13.4 (2.3)	History of SZ, stable clinical course and medications, family study; SZ sample 83% male
Gold et al. (in preparation)	44 37.4 (10.1) 14.1 (1.8)	~77 40.2 (5.9) 13.0 (2.5)	Chronic outpatients, stable clinical course and medications
Hill et al. (2004)	33 23.5 (5.3) 14.9 (1.7)	45 26.1 (8.1) 13.7 (3.3)	Unmedicated 1st episode patients, baseline data used in current analyses; patients and controls retested longitudinally
Hoff et al. (2005)	74 30.2 (9.3) N.R.	51 38.1 (8.8) N.R.	History of SZ, family study
Hughes et al. (2003)	25 34.9 (13.0) 15.2 (3.3)	62 37.7 (10.3) 12.8 (2.5)	SZ outpatients with incomplete response to conventional APs
Mohamed et al. (1999)	~305 25.5 (5.7) 14.1 (1.9)	~94 26.1 (8.1) 12.8 (1.9)	1st episode patients, 73 never medicated at testing, 21 medicated briefly
Seidman et al. (2002)	94 42.3 (15.2) 13.5 (2.5)	87 43.3 (11.7) 12.1 (2.3)	History of SZ, family study

Notes: HCn = number of healthy controls in study; SZn = number of schizophrenia patients in study; Ed. = education in years; SD = standard deviation; SZ = schizophrenia; ~ = individual tests where samples varied below total sample size; APs = antipsychotics; N.R. = not reported.

category prompts. Variants of the continuous performance test (CPT) have been important assays of attention in schizophrenia. Three of the included studies reported CPT results. However, fundamental differences in the nature of the tasks and the variables reported (Gordon's CPT, Mohamed et al., 1999, vs. Identical Pairs CPT, Gold et al., in preparation, vs. an auditory detection CPT, Seidman et al., 2002) led us to exclude these data from the analysis.

Data analysis

We calculated an effect size comparing schizophrenia patients with healthy controls for each of the 87 separate cognitive effects identified in Table 6.2 (i.e., for each neuropsychological variable reported for each study). The effect

Table 6.2 Cognitive variables compiled from each study and domain groupings

	Bilder	Egan	Gold	Hill	Hoff	Hughes	Moha.	Seid.
Processing speed								
Digit Symbol (DSST)	X		X	X	X*	X	X	X
Trails A	X	X		X	X	X		X
Executive functioning								
WCST Categories		X	X			X	X	X
WCST Perseverative Errors	X	X	X	X		X	X	X
Trails B	X	X		X	X	X		X
Stroop Color–Word			X	X	X		X	
Declarative memory								
Logical Memory I	X	X	X		X	X	X	X
List Learning (AVLT, CVLT, HVLT, WMS)	X	X	X	X	X	X	X	
Visual Reproduction I	X	X		X	X	X		
Working memory								
Digit Span (total score)	X		X	X			X	X
Arithmetic	X		X					
Verbal fluency								
Letter Fluency	X	X	X	X	X	X	X	
Category Fluency	X	X	X					
Premorbid/verbal ability								
WRAT Reading	X	X	X		X	X**		X
Vocabulary	X		X				X	X
Motor speed								
Finger Tapping	X			X	X	X	X	
Grooved Pegboard	X			X	X			

Notes: * Symbol Digit Modalities Test (written version); **National Adult Reading Test; Moha. = Mohamed; Seid. = Seidman; WCST = Wisconsin Card Sorting Test; AVLT = Auditory Verbal Learning Test; CVLT = California Verbal Learning Test; HVLT = Hopkins Verbal Learning Test; WMS = Wechsler Memory Scale; WRAT = Wide Range Achievement Test.

size was Cohen's *d* (also called Hedges' *g*), calculated as the difference between the means of the schizophrenia group and the comparison group divided by the pooled standard deviation (Hedges & Olkin, 1985; Shaddish & Haddock, 1994). The sign of the effect size was positive if healthy controls performed better than schizophrenia patients. Because we required large within-study sample sizes, it was not necessary to make any correction for upward bias in effect size estimates (Hedges & Olkin, 1985).

We then combined the individual effect sizes across studies for each of the 17 neuropsychological variables. These results are essentially mean effect sizes across studies for the control/patient differences on each variable. There was one adjustment. Prior to combination, each effect size was weighted using standard methodology to give greatest weight to the studies with largest sample sizes, given that such studies tend to produce the most reliable estimates of population effects (Hedges & Olkin, 1985; Shaddish & Haddock, 1994). We also calculated 95% confidence intervals for the weighted mean effect size estimates. Apart from indicating the precision with which current estimates were made, the confidence intervals also serve as significance tests for the performance differences between patients and controls (i.e., if the 95% confidence intervals do not overlap zero, the difference is significant at $p < .05$, Cumming & Finch, 2005), as well as for significant differences in magnitude between effect sizes for different variables (i.e., if the 95% confidence intervals for two variables do not overlap one another, the difference is significant at least at $p < .05$). We also calculated a "homogeneity" test statistic, Q, which follows a chi square distribution. A significant result for Q indicates a degree of heterogeneity among the individual effect sizes for a given variable greater than would be expected on the basis of random sampling variation alone (Shaddish & Haddock, 1994). In other words, heterogeneity signals real between-study differences for individual variables and raises a question whether the weighted mean effect size for a given variable should be assumed to reflect a common population effect size, or simply the mean of the observed individual effect sizes. In such cases, a more conservative "random effects" meta-analytic model should be used in the place of the more commonly used "fixed effects" model. Weighted mean effect sizes, 95% confidence intervals, and Q statistics for each variable are reported in Table 6.3. Also reported are cumulative sample sizes for schizophrenia and healthy control participants, and the number of effect sizes that contributed in the calculation of each weighted effect size.

Results and discussion of meta-analysis

Table 6.3 displays the results of the meta-analyses of schizophrenia patients and healthy control group differences in performance on a range of "typical" cognitive measures addressing information processing speed, executive functioning, declarative memory, working memory, premorbid/verbal ability, and motor speed. As the Q statistics were largely non-significant, weighted effect sizes are based on a fixed effects model. Although not exhaustive in the Heinrichs and Zakzanis sense, the current analyses provide a substantial survey of large-scale cognitive assessment studies from the time period since the Heinrichs work. Samples of schizophrenia patients for most of the variables range between 459 and 575, with comparable numbers of comparison subjects. The schizophrenia and control samples were matched across studies in terms of age (schizophrenia $M = 34.1$, $SD = 7.1$; control $M = 31.5$, $SD = 6.2$; t (14 $d.f.$) = 0.76; n.s.). However, as expected in this illness, the patients had lower levels of education (schizophrenia $M = 13.0$, $SD = 0.5$; control $M = 14.5$, $SD = 0.6$; t (12 $d.f.$) = 5.03; $p < .001$). Not surprisingly, the results show a consistent, significant impairment in the schizophrenia group on each variable (i.e., none of the 95% confidence intervals overlaps zero). Cohen's guidelines—0.20 for a small effect, 0.50 for a medium effect, and 0.80 for a large effect—provide a rough guide to interpretation of effect sizes (Cohen, 1988). The grand mean of the weighted effect sizes was 0.99 ($SD = 0.24$), a "large" effect by the Cohen's standards and very close to the grand mean

Table 6.3 Meta-analysis of effect sizes for selected cognitive measures

	HCn	SZn	k	Wtd d	95% CI	Q
Processing speed						
Digit Symbol (DSST)	554	503	7	1.50	1.32–1.67	5.57
Trails A	305	459	6	1.03	.84–1.21	7.37
Executive functioning						
WCST Categories	430	429	5	1.13	.87–1.39	6.23
WCST Perseverative Errors	497	568	7	.98	.83–1.13	6.78
Trails B	305	459	6	1.17	.96–1.37	6.15
Stroop Color–Word	390	251	4	.99	.68–1.30	2.80
Declarative memory						
Logical Memory I	540	575	7	1.24	1.03–1.45	5.90
List Learning (AVLT, CVLT, HVLT, WMS)	479	524	7	1.13	.95–1.31	13.82*
Visual Reproduction I	211	372	5	.99	.80–1.19	3.86
Working memory						
Digit Span (total score)	455	390	5	.72	.57–.88	3.69
Arithmetic	80	171	2	.97	.63–1.31	1.00
Verbal fluency						
Letter Fluency	495	533	7	.80	.64–.96	5.02
Category Fluency	123	290	3	1.29	1.02–1.57	3.34
Premorbid/verbal ability						
WRAT Reading	316	490	6	.49	.26–.72	7.18
Vocabulary	422	345	4	.89	.56–1.22	2.98
Motor speed						
Finger Tapping (average)	377	330	5	.44	.15–.73	6.45
Grooved Pegboard (average)	113	210	3	.99	.85–1.13	1.64

Notes: HCn = number of healthy controls for variable; SZn = number of schizophrenia cases; k = number of effect sizes combined per variable; Wtd d = sample-weighted mean effect size; 95% CI = 95% confidence interval; Q = homogeneity statistic; WCST = Wisconsin Card Sorting Test; AVLT = Auditory Verbal Learning Test; CVLT = California Verbal Learning Test; HVLT = Hopkins Verbal Learning Test; WMS = Wechsler Memory Scale; WRAT = Wide Range Achievement Test. * = $p < .10$.

derived from the earlier, more extensive review of cognitive performance (0.92, Heinrichs, 2005). Homogeneity statistics indicated that differences in effect sizes across studies were no more than would be expected on the basis of random sampling variation. Thus, with the exception of the verbal list learning variable, the combined effects can be regarded as population effect sizes, rather than simply means across studies. It is notable that the list learning variable is the one variable for which we combined effects obtained using several different measures and this could be a source of non-random variation.

The main point that the current analyses make—not addressed in the prior meta-analyses of Heinrichs or others—is that, among the cognitive measures most widely used in schizophrenia research, the 5-minute DSST best discriminates between schizophrenia patients and healthy controls. Across the eight large-scale studies analyzed, the schizophrenia deficit in DSST performance was the largest. The weighted mean effect size of 1.50 is nearly double Cohen's guideline for a "large" effect (Cohen, 1988). To give another index of magnitude, these effect sizes can be translated into the percentile standing of the average schizophrenia participant relative to the control group distribution using normal distribution principles. An effect size of 0.0 would indicate that the average patient was performing at exactly the 50th percentile of the comparison group. Given that positive effect sizes signal better control performance, an effect size of 0.8 (Cohen's "large" effect) would mean that the typical schizophrenia patient was performing near the 21st percentile of the comparison group. The 1.50 effect size found for DSST in the current analysis indicates that the typical schizophrenia patient is performing below the 7th percentile of healthy comparison subjects on this measure.

It is also instructive to contrast the schizophrenia DSST effect with those observed in other psychiatric conditions. For example, in a meta-analysis of studies contrasting neuropsychological performance in ADHD patients and controls, the DSST effect size (combining results from 15 studies in the same manner as here) was 0.82, among the largest reported across all the measures analyzed (Frazier et al., 2004). In a recent study of chronic alcoholism (mean 16 years of alcohol dependence), the DSST effect size was 1.24 (calculated from reported means and standard deviations; Ratti, Bo, Giardini, & Soragna, 2002). Another recent study examined DSST performance in major depressive disorder (Pier et al., 2004). The effect size of the DSST impairment was 1.04 (calculated from reported means and standard deviations), despite the fact that these patients were unmedicated at the time of testing. In an earlier study from the same group, DSST performance of inpatients with acute depression (9/20 untreated) and stable schizophrenia (all 20 treated) were contrasted with controls (van Hoof, Jogems-Kosterman, Sabbe, Zitman, & Hulstijn, 1998). The effect size for the DSST impairment was 0.87 in depression and 1.45 in schizophrenia (in both cases, calculated from reported means and standard deviations), similar to the effect size noted in the current analysis. Only one of these comparisons is a formal meta-analysis. However, the effect sizes reported in or calculated from the studies provide some indication that the typical DSST impairment in schizophrenia is larger than the impairments seen in other psychiatric conditions.

Further, examination of the confidence intervals in Table 6.3 indicates that DSST performance was significantly more impaired than performance on 12 of the 16 other individual measures (i.e., the 95% confidence intervals do not overlap, thus the difference between means is significant at least at $p < .05$; Cumming & Finch, 2005). The exceptions were WCST Categories, Trails B, Logical Memory, and Category Fluency. Of these, effect size differences for WCST Categories and Trails B approached significance. Thus the DSST discriminates between healthy and schizophrenia populations significantly better than widely used executive, visual memory, premorbid intellectual ability, working memory, and motor speed measures, and at least as well as story memory and category fluency measures.

Association with risk, illness, and disability

This DSST signal is not confined to individuals with a confirmed diagnosis of schizophrenia. In the Hoff study (2005) that was included in the meta-analysis, 37 first-degree relatives showed impaired substitution test performance compared with healthy controls (this study used the SDMT rather than the DSST). Laurent and colleagues (2000) also found that scores on the DSST (along with scores on measures of fluency and Trails B) were lower in 47 first-degree relatives of schizophrenia probands than in healthy controls with no psychiatric family history. Cosway et al. (2000) found impaired DSST performance (along with intellectual, verbal memory, and executive deficits) in 78 young adults from the Edinburgh High Risk Study group, which persisted across two assessment points separated by 18 months to 2 years. Focusing on the processing speed construct somewhat more broadly, Egan et al. (2001) (from the meta-analysis) found relative as well as proband impairment on the Trails A task, while Cannon et al. (1994) and Mirsky and colleagues (Mirsky, Yardley, Jones, Walsh, & Kendler, 1995) found relative deficits in attention composites that included the DSST and Trails A with other measures. Niendam and colleagues (2003) pushed the relative risk findings a step further. Drawing subjects from the Philadelphia cohort of the National Collaborative Perinatal Project, these investigators identified 32 adults with schizophrenia and 25 of their unaffected siblings for whom Wechsler intelligence test results from age 7 were available. Long before the onset of proband illness, both the probands and their unaffected siblings showed specific impairments in cognitive functioning. Of seven Wechsler subtests administered, performance on the DSST, vocabulary, and picture arrangement subtests was impaired relative to non-psychiatric comparison subjects. These findings in relatives, high risk, and pre-onset groups suggest that DSST performance may be a heritable and/or premorbid indicator of schizophrenia risk (see also chapter 4 for more on the genetics of processing speed).

At the same time, it is clear that DSST performance is also differentially associated with occurrence of the illness itself. In each of the studies cited above, not only did the relatives of schizophrenia probands perform significantly more poorly on the DSST than controls, but the probands performed significantly worse than their unaffected relatives. In this regard, the Niendam finding is perhaps the most remarkable. In that study, based on premorbid testing conducted at age 7, the DSST and two other Wechsler subtests differentiated probands and their unaffected siblings from controls. However, only DSST performance distinguished individuals who would go on to develop schizophrenia years later, from their own siblings who would not develop the disease (Niendam et al., 2003).

Importantly, the DSST does not only index risk and illness, but also the degree of functional disability that results from illness. Thus Brekke et al. (1997) found DSST, verbal fluency and Stroop performance related to independent living. Stratta and colleagues (Stratta, Daneluzzo, Prosperini, Bustini, Mattei, & Rossi, 1997) found the DSST and Wisconsin Card Sort variables associated with scores on a scale measuring the level of performance in expected community roles. Moreover, the DSST relationship to functioning and outcome has proved to be differentially discriminating in comparison to other cognitive measures in some studies. In the Gold study included in the meta-analysis (Gold et al., in preparation), the DSST was the single best discriminator, from an extensive battery, between schizophrenia patients who worked competitively and those who did not. Jaeger et al. (2005) recently reported that the DSST and certain attention variables were the only cognitive measures associated longitudinally with improved community functioning in 250 schizophrenia patients after discharge from acute hospitalization. Dickinson and Coursey (2002) showed that the Wechsler processing speed factor (comprising the DSST and Symbol Search subtests) was differentially associated with clinician-rated community functioning chronic outpatients relative to other factors from the WAIS. Gladsjo and colleagues reported that, among six broad cognitive factors, a processing speed factor (comprising DSST, Trail Making Test variables, letter fluency, grooved pegboard, and digit vigilance) was most highly associated ($r = .64$) with a performance-based assessment of everyday functional skills (Gladsjo et al., 2004). Thus information processing speed, indexed by the DSST, has a graded relationship with illness risk and severity in schizophrenia. This marker differentiates people with schizophrenia from healthy controls, relatives of people with schizophrenia from healthy controls, and also, unaffected relatives from schizophrenia probands. Further, it appears to index functional disability within the patient group.

Association of DSST with other cognitive measures

The meta-analysis shows that the information processing speed deficit reflected in DSST performance is large and reliable compared with deficits represented by most other cognitive measures examined. This is not to say, however, that the impairment is independent of other cognitive impairments. Indeed, as indicated earlier, we believe that many cognitive operations have inherent speed demands. This proposition draws support from an extensive literature documenting the so-called "positive manifold," the common finding that diverse cognitive measures are positively correlated (Carroll, 1993; Jensen, 1998). Many researchers accept that this network of correlations is characterized by a hierarchical factorial structure in which individual cognitive measures are related to certain cognitive domains, such as information processing speed or episodic memory, which in turn intercorrelate because of an underlying general cognitive ability, often referred to as "psychometric g" (Carroll, 1993; Deary, 2001; Jensen, 1998).

In earlier work, we investigated these issues in schizophrenia using structural equation modeling techniques. We first demonstrated that individual measures sort into the same broad cognitive domains in schizophrenia as in healthy groups (Dickinson, Iannone, & Gold, 2002; Dickinson, Ragland, Caulkins, Gold, & Gur, 2006), consistent with the recent report of Gladsjo and colleagues (2004). In further work, we addressed the question whether schizophrenia imparts domain-specific deficits in processing speed or other cognitive domains, or whether the schizophrenia deficit is generalized across the domains (Dickinson et al., 2004). We used single common factor analysis (SCFA) (Salthouse, 1998; Salthouse & Becker, 1998) to partition Wechsler subtest performance differences between 87 schizophrenia patients and 97 healthy controls into *shared* (i.e., statistically overlapping with differences on other variables) and *independent* (i.e., non-overlapping) components.

Figure 6.1 and its caption provide details of the analysis. The most important contrast in Figure 6.1 is between the parenthesized path coefficient values on the right, representing the effects of diagnosis on cognitive performance insofar as mediated through the common factor, and the path coefficient values on the left, indicating diagnosis effects on cognition independent of the common factor. In short, the SCFA showed that the effect of diagnosis on the Wechsler subtest scores was largely mediated through a common cognitive factor. By comparison, the *independent* associations of group status with the subtest scores were selective and considerably smaller in magnitude. The mean magnitude of the few significant independent diagnosis–subtest performance associations was 0.17 (using absolute values), roughly half the mean path coefficient of 0.32 for the diagnosis associations through the common factor.

Independent associations of diagnosis with Vocabulary, Information, Block Design, DSST, and Family Pictures (I and II) were significant. The path coefficients for direct relations from group status to Vocabulary, Information and Block Design were negatively weighted, indicating that the common factor overestimated impairment on these variables among individuals with schizophrenia, relative to controls. On the other hand, the positive direct associations with the DSST and visual memory subtests demonstrated that, while most of the variance in these measures was associated with the common factor, a small but significant portion was independently associated with diagnosis. It is important to note that the finding of a partly independent association of diagnosis to the DSST does not necessarily imply that this part of the association is different in kind from the part of the association mediated through the common factor. It seems more likely that the DSST is simply a more sensitive and general measure of the range of cognitive impairments in schizophrenia than are other common cognitive measures.

The summarized work supports two conclusions of particular relevance to the current chapter. First, it appears that cognitive impairments in schizophrenia are generalized to a substantial degree. When an individual is impaired in performance on one cognitive measure, he or she is likely to

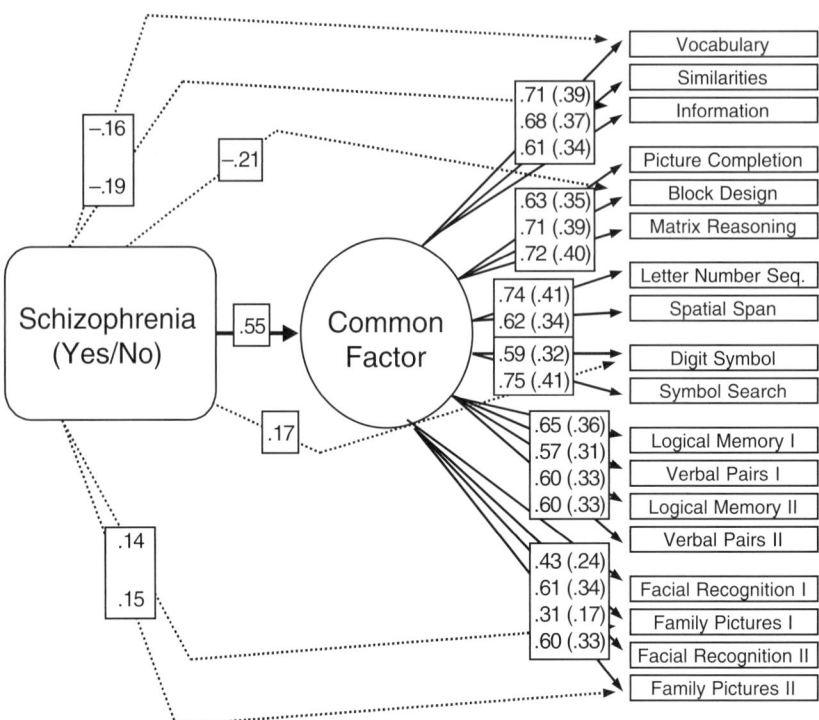

Figure 6.1 Path diagram showing values for two types of pathways from diagnostic grouping to individual Wechsler subtests: (1) two-part pathways from diagnosis through a common factor and on to each of the individual subtests (the solid lines), and (2) direct pathways from diagnosis to the individual subtests that are independent of the common factor (the broken lines). Path coefficients are superimposed on each pathway. Consistent with general practice (Kline, 1998), individual path coefficients that satisfied a *t*-test criterion of $t = 2.0$ were retained in the final model. On the right side of the figure, two coefficients are presented for each subtest. The first coefficient indicates the strength of the association of each subtest with the common factor. The second coefficient (in parentheses) is the product of the first coefficient with the diagnosis group common factor coefficient (i.e., .55) and indicates the overall strength of the association of each subtest with diagnostic grouping, *insofar as that relationship is mediated through the common factor*. For example, the parenthesized value of .32 for the DSST, is the product of the unadjusted common factor Digit Symbol coefficient (.59) and the diagnosis group common factor coefficient (.55). The adjusted coefficients (in parentheses) are thus scaled to be directly comparable to the coefficients for the independent diagnosis group subtest pathways. Comparison of the common factor mediated path coefficients (on the right, in parentheses) with the independent path coefficients (on the left) demonstrates that the independent effects of this illness were selective and small relative to the effects associated with the common factor. Reprinted from Dickinson, Iannone, Wilk, and Gold (2004) with permission from Society of Biological Psychiatry.

be impaired on many others. Thus schizophrenia's greatest effect on cognitive performance seems to occur at a very general level, or through some fundamental process that underlies multiple complex cognitive functions to a similar degree. Second, consistent with findings of the meta-analysis, the schizophrenia deficits on the DSST and in processing speed more generally, while intertwined with other deficits, also tend to be differentially greater in magnitude. As a result, a portion of the association of diagnosis with DSST appears to be independent of other cognitive deficits in this illness, although this is likely to reflect the DSST's differential sensitivity and generality in relation to other measures, rather than some fundamentally distinct process.

Hypotheses about information processing speed impairment in schizophrenia

Examining causal hypotheses

Different hypotheses have been advanced to account for the processing speed deficit in schizophrenia. For example, one familiar proposition is that processing speed is degraded by chronic illness and medication exposure. The current meta-analysis provides a direct way to evaluate the relationship of processing speed to chronicity and medication status. As shown in Table 6.1, three of the meta-analysis studies evaluated *first episode* patients, without a chronic psychiatric or medication history (Bilder et al., 2000; Hill et al., 2004; Mohamed et al., 1999). Across these studies 233 schizophrenia patients with an average age of 26 years were compared with 374 healthy controls with an average age of 24.7 years. The 45 patients from the Hill study were all never-medicated at the time of the evaluation. Seventy-three of the 94 patients from the Mohamed study were never-medicated and the rest had had brief medication exposure. All of the patients from the Bilder study had fewer than 12 weeks of cumulative medication exposure. In contrast, the remaining studies compared more chronic and chronically medicated patients, with an average age of 39 years, to controls aged 35.6 years. The average DSST effect size across the three first episode studies was 1.45 (range 1.22 to 1.58), only trivially different from the overall combined effect size of 1.50 (see Table 6.3). The meta-analysis results are consistent with evidence from longitudinal studies (Censits, Ragland, Gur, & Gur, 1997; Hill et al., 2004; Hoff, Sakuma, Wieneke, Horon, Kushner, & DeLisi, 1999) showing stable DSST and processing speed composite performance from initial first episode evaluations through the early course of schizophrenia treatment. Thus it does not appear that medication exposure or chronicity of illness explains differences between patients and healthy controls on the DSST.

Another hypothesis about processing speed deficits in schizophrenia might be termed the "peripheral motor speed" hypothesis, following the work of Salthouse and colleagues on cognitive changes in normal aging (Salthouse, 1992). The suggestion is that individual performance differences on the DSST result principally from illness-related differences in the speed of executing manual or other movements, as in writing symbol responses, rather than from differences in preceding or intervening cognitive operations. However, the results of the meta-analysis in the present study contradict a "motor speed" explanation. There are substantial and significant differences (i.e., non-overlapping confidence intervals) between the combined DSST effect and the motor speed effects for the Finger Tapping and Grooved Pegboard tasks. Specifically, the DSST effect size of 1.50 (95% CI 1.32–1.67) is more than three times the Finger Tapping effect of 0.44 for simple motor speed (95% CI 0.15–0.73) and half again as large as the Grooved Pegboard effect of 0.99 for more complex motor manipulation (95% CI 0.85–1.13). Further, several studies have examined this issue directly and each has found evidence of cognitive slowing over and above slowing that could be attributed to motor processes (Jogems-Kosterman, Zitman, van Hoof, & Hulstijn, 2001; Nelson, Pantelis, Carruthers, Speller, Baxendale, & Barnes, 1990; van Hoof et al., 1998). For example, van Hoof and colleagues used a digitizing tablet to present an electronic version of the DSST to controls, patients with schizophrenia, and patients with depression. This presentation format allowed precise timing of writing movements and intervals between writing (termed "matching time"). The two psychiatric groups presented an interesting contrast. On the writing time variable, depressed patients were significantly slower than controls and schizophrenia patients. People with schizophrenia did not differ statistically from controls. On the matching time variable, the pattern was reversed, with the schizophrenia patients significantly slower than both depressed patients and controls. The schizophrenia and control findings were subsequently replicated (Jogems-Kosterman et al., 2001). Thus, by a number of accounts, schizophrenia-related motor speed impairment is not sufficient by itself to account for the information processing speed deficits seen in this illness.

Learning and memory deficits in schizophrenia are also well documented (Aleman et al., 1999; Heinrichs & Zakzanis, 1998) and could be another source of performance difficulties on measures of processing speed such as the DSST. Specifically, the DSST may depend in part on the ability to learn and remember digit–symbol pairings (i.e., episodic memory), and also on the active maintenance and updating of information about the pairings (working memory). Deficits in these performance domains might lead schizophrenia patients to spend more time than healthy subjects reinspecting the coding key during performance. However, in the current meta-analysis results, the DSST effect was significantly larger than the effect for working memory variables and for verbal list learning and visual memory (compare the DSST effect of 1.50, 95% CI 1.32–1.67, with the effect for Digit Span 0.72, 95% CI 0.57–0.88, Arithmetic 0.97, 95% CI 0.63–1.31, List Learning 1.13, 95% CI 0.95–1.31, and Visual Reproduction, 0.99, 95% CI 0.80–1.19; see Table 6.3). The DSST effect size estimate was larger in absolute terms than a story memory measure as well, although this difference was not statistically significant (Logical Memory effect 1.24, 95% CI 1.03–1.45). These findings are not consistent with a memory-based explanation of the processing speed deficit captured by DSST performance.

Speeded processing as a foundation for higher functions

A number of other investigations have turned these hypotheses around, speculating that slowed processing speed may actually underlie deficits in higher order processes. For example, Brebion and colleagues suggested that processing speed deficits might actually cause schizophrenia memory difficulties (rather than being *caused by* memory problems) by limiting the possible number of rehearsals during encoding (Brebion, Amador, Smith, & Gorman, 1998; see also Salthouse, 1996). Other studies have investigated whether frequently observed deficits in working memory and executive control processes in schizophrenia could be traced to processing speed impairment. Stratta et al. (1997) found that various WCST variables were associated with DSST, but not with Digit Span and a visual working memory test. Hartman and colleagues also studied processing speed in relation to both working memory and WCST performance (Hartman, Steketee, Silva, Lanning, & Andersson, 2003a; Hartman, Steketee, Silva, Lanning, & McCann, 2003b). Although they did find strong relationships among working memory and WCST variables, controlling for a measure of speed of encoding (i.e., the presentation times necessary to allow an individual to encode information at an 80% accuracy rate) eliminated differences between people with schizophrenia and healthy controls on the WCST (Hartman et al., 2003a). In a further study, these investigators manipulated the speed of stimulus presentation to equate schizophrenia and healthy subjects on initial encoding accuracy in a delayed-match-to-sample task. They found no group differences in delay conditions, suggesting that the oft-cited working memory deficit in the illness may result from slowed processing speed (Hartman et al., 2003b). Again, the results of the current meta-analysis are generally supportive. The DSST deficit was significantly larger in the studies reviewed than the deficits on working memory measures (i.e., Digit Span and Arithmetic; see parenthetical in prior paragraph and Table 6.3). The DSST deficit was also significantly larger than deficits on classic executive functioning variables, including WCST Perseverative Errors (0.98, 95% CI 0.83–1.13) and the Stroop Color–Word test (0.99, 95% CI 0.68–1.30), while the difference in effect sizes approached significance for WCST Categories (1.13, 95% CI 0.87–1.39) and Trails B (1.17, 95% CI 0.96–1.37). Taken together, this work suggests that processing speed impairment in schizophrenia is strongly associated with impairment in higher order cognitive processes, including episodic memory, working memory, and executive functions.

Different task conditions in the Trail Making Test and Stroop Color–Word Test are also informative about the contribution of simple speeded processing to more complex executive control functions. For example, the contrast of Trails B with Trails A is thought to separate flexible set shifting from simpler speeded visual scanning and sequencing (Lezak, 1995). Results from the current meta-analysis (see Table 6.3) are in close agreement with those reported by Heinrichs and Zakzanis (1998). The magnitude of the effect size increment for Trails B over Trails A was non-significant in both reviews (e.g., in the current analysis Trails A effect 1.03, 95% CI 0.84–1.21, compared with Trails B effect 1.17, 95% CI 0.96–1.37), indicating that the simpler, more speed-dependent requirements of the task may account adequately for the observed group differences. Similar results follow from comparisons of the "interference" condition from the Stroop Color–Word Test with the word reading and color naming conditions. These comparisons are purported to distinguish the contribution of inhibitory control from simpler speeded reading or naming (Lezak, 1995). Although results from the word reading and color naming conditions were not reported for most of the studies included in the meta-analysis, we have those data for our vocational outcomes study (Gold et al., in preparation). As noted in Table 6.3, the effect size for the interference condition across the studies was 0.99. The interference condition effect for the Gold study alone was consistent at 1.03. Gold study effect sizes for the word reading and color naming conditions, which require speeded processing but no inhibitory control, were 0.95 and 1.03 respectively, suggesting again that the simple, speed-dependent processes drive performance on this task in schizophrenia more so than executive processes (see also Goldberg, Ragland, Torrey, Gold, Bigelow, & Weinberger, 1990; Purdon, 1998). Computerized, single trial versions of this task have been employed in an effort to increase the precision of Stroop measurements (Barch, Carter, & Cohen, 2004; Carter, Robertson, & Nordahl, 1992; Taylor, Kornblum, & Tandon, 1996). Although schizophrenia patients are slower across neutral and incongruent conditions, and although there are other indications of abnormalities in processing of Stroop stimuli (e.g., increased facilitation in congruent conditions), patients do not show abnormally large interference effects on the computerized Stroop. Across studies, then, it appears that the simpler processing requirements of the non-executive conditions account fully for performance differences between the groups in the executive control condition.

Mechanisms of processing speed impairment in schizophrenia

To review then, information processing speed is conceptualized as a general constraint on cognitive processing: simply, the speed with which many different cognitive operations can be completed. It is a fairly basic capacity that can be adequately measured by simple tasks, such as the DSST, that nearly everyone would complete without error given enough time. It is also a very general capacity, evident in tasks involving a wide variety of stimulus and response modalities. Results of the meta-analysis confirm that processing speed is reliably impaired in schizophrenia. Further, it appears that the schizophrenia impairment in this domain, at least as represented by the

DSST, is selectively somewhat more severe than deficits in other domains that have received greater attention in the schizophrenia literature (e.g., verbal memory, executive functioning). The significance of the deficit is not limited to the schizophrenia/healthy control comparison but, rather, shows an interesting gradation related to disease risk, actual illness, and illness-related disability. Processing speed performance in first degree relatives of people with schizophrenia is intermediate between patients and non-psychiatric comparison groups. Among patients, poorer processing speed performance is associated with greater disability in vocational, independent living and other everyday roles. The cognitive deficit in schizophrenia is quite generalized and the processing speed deficit is best understood as a marker of a very generalized cognitive dysfunction. Although an earlier analysis revealed a degree of independence in the association of diagnosis with DSST, this does not necessarily suggest a separate cognitive or neurobiological mechanism. Rather, the DSST may simply be an especially sensitive, broad, and reliable indicator of the generalized deficit. The processing speed deficit cannot be explained by the experience of chronic illness or long-term medication exposure. It also is not explained by impairment in basic motor processing or memory impairment in this illness. Indeed, some evidence supports the view that processing speed deficits may underlie impairments in higher order processing, for example in working memory and executive control functions.

The question then arises as to the mechanisms through which this basic capacity has such a broad relationship to cognitive task performance. Several cognitive models have been proposed. Versions of a "limited time" mechanism (e.g., Salthouse & Kail, 1983) address situations in which the time available for processing is determined by external constraints. Under this view, an information processing speed deficiency is revealed when relevant cognitive operations cannot be completed in the time allotted. This model might be illustrated by a backward masking paradigm, or a comparison task with a limited inspection time. It is apparent, however, that the speed deficiency in schizophrenia is not limited to situations with externally imposed time constraints. Time constraints and bottlenecks are also created by internal, temporal information processing dynamics (Salthouse, 1996). Plainly, the smooth unfolding of an assembly of cognitive operations involves coordination of various concurrent and successive processing operations. Because information decays, is displaced, or becomes obsolete over time, slow processing at any point reduces or degrades the information simultaneously available for integrative, higher order processing. Note that this model is not inconsistent with findings suggesting a normal pace of information decay in schizophrenia (Javitt, Shelley, Silipo, & Lieberman, 2000; Javitt, Strous, Grochowski, Ritter, & Cowan, 1997; Rabinowicz, Silipo, Goldman, & Javitt, 2000). Rather, slowed processing means less useful information is passed on from one processing stage to the next simply because relevant operations are not completed in the available time. A model incorporating such processing speed constraints would predict that impairments should be manifest in simple cognitive operations (e.g., DSST "matching"), but also in higher order integrated cognitive operations, as in the Letter Number Sequencing task referenced earlier, and other executive working memory tasks that have been a focus of so much schizophrenia research.

A number of very different neurobiological models have emerged that might be consistent with this cognitive model. For example, different lines of evidence point to abnormalities in anatomically segregated, dopamine-mediated frontal-striatal loops in schizophrenia (Pantelis, Barnes, & Nelson, 1992; Robbins, 1990). This research illustrates the idea of a specific deficit with potentially very widespread effects. Although confined to a discrete brain system, defective interactions between the frontal cortex and striatum could cause a response processing bottleneck that might slow performance of almost any task involving effortful response, across the range of stimulus and response modalities. Other models move away from this sort of regionally focused approach. Andreasen and colleagues have posited a more generalized pattern of cortical, subcortical and cerebellar disconnection that they term "cognitive dysmetria" (Andreasen, Paradiso, & O'Leary, 1998). This suggestion of a broad disruption in the temporal dynamics of cognitive operations also appears quite consistent with a broad information processing speed deficit. Still other models posit general neurotransmitter system abnormalities. One prominent example focuses on altered glutamatergic functioning in schizophrenia and, in particular, on disturbances in NMDA receptor-mediated glutamate neurotransmission (Coyle, 1996; Javitt, Liederman, Cienfuegos, & Shelley, 1999; Javitt & Zukin, 1991). Glutamate is distributed throughout the cortex and NMDA receptors have properties that allow them to play a critical role in the fast integration of information from multiple pathways (Javitt, Steinschneider, Schroeder, & Arezzo, 1996). Slowed and inefficient processing across a wide range of cognitive operations could be a manifestation of dysfunction in such a fundamental neurotransmission system (Javitt et al., 1999). Similar arguments could be advanced regarding nicotinic acetylcholine receptors (Leonard et al., 1996) and certain catecholamine neurotransmitter systems. A different neurobiological focus, with intuitive appeal from a processing speed standpoint, is the study of white matter integrity in schizophrenia. White matter defects are well known to cause processing speed deficits in multiple sclerosis (De Sonneville, Boringa, Reuling, Lazeron, Ader, & Polman, 2002; Denney et al., 2004) and normal aging (Garde, Lykke Mortensen, Rostrup, & Paulson, 2005; Longstreth et al., 2005). Recent studies of schizophrenia patients using diffusion tensor imaging techniques have found abnormalities in major fiber tracts, including decreased coherence and density of fibers within tracts, as well as changes in myelination (Kubicki et al., 2005). Interestingly, white matter function and glutamate neurotransmission are closely associated (Davis et al., 2003), providing a possible link between neurobiological models. However, it remains to be tested whether these white matter abnormalities are associated with the schizophrenia processing speed deficit. At an even wider focus are various findings, such as abnormalities in lipid metabolism (Horrobin, 1998; Mahadik & Evans, 2003) and in inflammatory processes associated with vascular functioning (Hanson & Gottesman, 2005). Such processes are not only essential for brain cell development and integrity, but they impact systems throughout the body, helping to support the view of schizophrenia as a general metabolic disorder, rather than simply a brain disease. Again, a specific relationship with processing speed variables seems plausible but remains to be explored.

Conclusions

The goal of this review has been to highlight the evidence that processing speed is reliably impaired in schizophrenia, more so than many of the cognitive functions that have captured the imaginations of researchers in the field. The relative neglect of this dimension of cognitive performance is easily understood given the recent scientific *zeitgeist*, in which neuropsychological research has been largely directed at efforts to locate specific brain regions or systems involved in the pathophysiology of schizophrenia. Given the cognitive complexity and multi-component nature of the DSST, the test does not easily lend itself to such an enterprise. However, current analyses and other work reviewed in this chapter sharpen the hypothesis that slowed information processing is at the core of the cognitive impairment seen in this illness. This hypothesis may lead, in turn, to a focus on emerging neurobiological models that could account for the probably very generalized effects of illness on brain systems.

At the same time, it is important to acknowledge that the biological substrate of the information processing speed construct is unknown. Processing speed impairment may depend on the physiology of neurons and synapses, or dysfunction in large neuronal assemblies or regional brain interactions. It may be associated with imprecision in the formation of initial incoming sensory percepts, faulty coordination among different cognitive processes, or inefficiencies in programming cognitive and motor responses. Indeed, there are likely to be many interacting influences on processing speed in schizophrenia. Thus, while the construct is useful heuristically, in the face of this enormous biological and cognitive complexity it is still not possible to suggest that memory impairments, to take one example, are *caused by* slowed information processing. With recent advances in cognitive neuroscience, however, relevant questions may now be more tractable than in previous decades. For example, it is possible now to integrate millisecond resolution, event-related brain potential techniques with familiar behavioral measures to examine the time course and precision of basic neural processes. New functional and diffusion tensor imaging techniques are other examples of techniques that can be combined with appropriate behavioral measures to test hypotheses about exactly what it is that is slowed in schizophrenia information processing.

References

(Note: Studies included in the meta-analysis are marked with an asterisk.)

Aleman, A., Hijman, R., de Haan, E. H., & Kahn, R. S. (1999). Memory impairment in schizophrenia: A meta-analysis. *American Journal of Psychiatry, 156* (9), 1358–1366.
Andreasen, N. C. (1985). Negative syndrome in schizophrenia: Strategies for long-term management. *Advances in Biochemistry and Psychopharmacology, 40*, 1–7.
Andreasen, N. C., & Olsen, S. (1982). Negative v positive schizophrenia. Definition and validation. *Archives of General Psychiatry, 39* (7), 789–794.
Andreasen, N. C., Paradiso, S., & O'Leary, D. S. (1998). "Cognitive dysmetria" as an integrative theory of schizophrenia: A dysfunction in cortical–subcortical–cerebellar circuitry? *Schizophrenia Bulletin, 24* (2), 203–218.
Barch, D. M., Carter, C. S., & Cohen, J. D. (2004). Factors influencing Stroop performance in schizophrenia. *Neuropsychology, 18* (3), 477–484.
Bellack, A. S., Gold, J. M., & Buchanan, R. W. (1999). Cognitive rehabilitation for schizophrenia: Problems, prospects, and strategies. *Schizophrenia Bulletin, 25* (2), 257–274.
*Bilder, R. M., Goldman, R. S., Robinson, D., Reiter, G., Bell, L., Bates, J. A., et al. (2000). Neuropsychology of first-episode schizophrenia: Initial characterization and clinical correlates. *American Journal of Psychiatry, 157* (4), 549–559.
Bilder, R. M., Volavka, J., Czobor, P., Malhotra, A. K., Kennedy, J. L., Ni, X., et al. (2002). Neurocognitive correlates of the COMT Val(158)Met polymorphism in chronic schizophrenia. *Biological Psychiatry, 52* (7), 701–707.
Birren, J. E., & Fisher, L. M. (1995). Aging and speed of behavior: Possible consequences for psychological functioning. *Annual Review of Psychology, 46*, 329–353.
Brebion, G., Amador, X., Smith, M. J., & Gorman, J. M. (1998). Memory impairment and schizophrenia: The role of processing speed. *Schizophrenia Research, 30* (1), 31–39.
Brekke, J. S., Raine, A., Ansel, M., Lencz, T., & Bird, L. (1997). Neuropsychological and psychophysiological correlates of psychosocial functioning in schizophrenia. *Schizophrenia Bulletin, 23* (1), 19–28.
Buchanan, R. W., Summerfelt, A., Tek, C., & Gold, J. (2003). An open-labeled trial of adjunctive donepezil for cognitive impairments in patients with schizophrenia. *Schizophrenia Research, 59* (1), 29–33.
Cannon, T. D., Zorrilla, L. E., Shtasel, D., Gur, R. E., Gur, R. C., Marco, E. J., et al. (1994). Neuropsychological functioning in siblings discordant for schizophrenia and healthy volunteers. *Archives in General Psychiatry, 51* (8), 651–661.
Carey, C. L., Woods, S. P., Rippeth, J. D., Gonzalez, R., Moore, D. J., Marcotte, T. D., et al. (2004). Initial validation of a screening battery for the detection of HIV-associated cognitive impairment. *Clinical Neuropsychology, 18* (2), 234–248.
Carroll, J. B. (1993). *Human cognitive abilities: A survey of factor-analytic studies*. New York: Cambridge University Press.
Carter, C. S., Robertson, L. C., & Nordahl, T. E. (1992). Abnormal processing of irrelevant information in chronic schizophrenia: Selective enhancement of Stroop facilitation. *Psychiatry Research, 41* (2), 137–146.
Censits, D. M., Ragland, J. D., Gur, R. C., & Gur, R. E. (1997). Neuropsychological

evidence supporting a neurodevelopmental model of schizophrenia: A longitudinal study. *Schizophrenia Research*, *24* (3), 289–298.

Cohen, J. D. (1988). *Statistical power for the behavioral sciences*. Hillsdale, NJ: Lawrence Erlbaum Associates, Inc.

Colbert, J., & Harrow, M. (1967). Psychomotor retardation in depressive syndromes. *Journal of Nervous and Mental Disorders*, *145* (5), 405–419.

Cosway, R., Byrne, M., Clafferty, R., Hodges, A., Grant, E., Abukmeil, S. S., et al. (2000). Neuropsychological change in young people at high risk for schizophrenia: Results from the first two neuropsychological assessments of the Edinburgh High Risk Study. *Psychological Medicine*, *30* (5), 1111–1121.

Coyle, J. T. (1996). The glutamatergic dysfunction hypothesis for schizophrenia. *Harvard Review of Psychiatry*, *3* (5), 241–253.

Crow, T. J. (1980a). Molecular pathology of schizophrenia: More than one disease process? *British Medical Journal*, *280* (6207), 66–68.

Crow, T. J. (1980b). Positive and negative schizophrenic symptoms and the role of dopamine. *British Journal of Psychiatry*, *137*, 383–386.

Cumming, G., & Finch, S. (2005). Inference by eye: Confidence intervals and how to read pictures of data. *American Psychologist*, *60* (2), 170–180.

Davis, K. L., Stewart, D. G., Friedman, J. I., Buchsbaum, M., Harvey, P. D., Hof, P. R., et al. (2003). White matter changes in schizophrenia: Evidence for myelin-related dysfunction. *Archives of General Psychiatry*, *60* (5), 443–456.

De Sonneville, L. M., Boringa, J. B., Reuling, I. E., Lazeron, R. H., Ader, H. J., & Polman, C. H. (2002). Information processing characteristics in subtypes of multiple sclerosis. *Neuropsychologia*, *40* (11), 1751–1765.

Deary, I. J. (2001). Human intelligence differences: A recent history. *Trends in Cognitive Science*, *5* (3), 127–130.

Denney, D. R., Lynch, S. G., Parmenter, B. A., & Horne, N. (2004). Cognitive impairment in relapsing and primary progressive multiple sclerosis: Mostly a matter of speed. *Journal of the International Neuropsychological Society*, *10* (7), 948–956.

Dickerson, F., Boronow, J. J., Ringel, N., & Parente, F. (1996). Neurocognitive deficits and social functioning in outpatients with schizophrenia. *Schizophrenia Research*, *21* (2), 75–83.

Dickinson, D., & Coursey, R. D. (2002). Independence and overlap among neurocognitive correlates of community functioning in schizophrenia. *Schizophrenia Research*, *56* (1–2), 161–170.

Dickinson, D., Iannone, V. N., & Gold, J. M. (2002). Factor structure of the Wechsler Adult Intelligence Scale-III in schizophrenia. *Assessment*, *9* (2), 171–180.

Dickinson, D., Iannone, V. N., Wilk, C. M., & Gold, J. M. (2004). General and specific cognitive deficits in schizophrenia. *Biological Psychiatry*, *55* (8), 826–833.

Dickinson, D., Ragland, J. D., Caulkins, M. E., Gold, J. M., & Gur, R. C. (2006). A comparison of cognitive structure in schizophrenia patients and healthy controls using confirmatory factor analysis. *Schizophrenia Research*, *85*, 20–29.

*Egan, M. F., Goldberg, T. E., Gscheidle, T., Weirich, M., Rawlings, R., Hyde, T. M., et al. (2001). Relative risk for cognitive impairments in siblings of patients with schizophrenia. *Biological Psychiatry*, *50* (2), 98–107.

Frazier, T. W., Demaree, H. A., & Youngstrom, E. A. (2004). Meta-analysis of intellectual and neuropsychological test performance in attention deficit/hyperactivity disorder. *Neuropsychology*, *18* (3), 543–555.

Galletly, C. A., Clark, C. R., McFarlane, A. C., & Weber, D. L. (2000). The effect of clozapine on the speed and accuracy of information processing in schizophrenia. *Progress in Neuropsychopharmacology and Biological Psychiatry*, *24* (8), 1329–1338.

Garde, E., Lykke Mortensen, E., Rostrup, E., & Paulson, O. B. (2005). Decline in intelligence is associated with progression in white matter hyperintensity volume. *Journal of Neurology, Neurosurgery, and Psychiatry*, *76* (9), 1289–1291.

Gladsjo, J. A., McAdams, L. A., Palmer, B. W., Moore, D. J., Jeste, D. V., & Heaton, R. (2004). A six-factor model of cognition in schizophrenia and related psychotic disorders: Relationships with clinical symptoms and functional capacity. *Schizophrenia Bulletin*, *30* (4), 739–754.

Gold, J., Iannone, V. N., McMahon, R. P., & Buchanan, R. W. (2001). Cognitive correlates of competitive employment among patients with schizophrenia (abstract). *Schizophrenia Research*, *49*, 134.

Gold, J. M., Goldberg, R. W., McNary, S. W., Dixon, L. B., & Lehman, A. F. (2002). Cognitive correlates of job tenure among patients with severe mental illness. *American Journal of Psychiatry*, *159* (8), 1395–1402.

*Gold, J. M., McMahon, R. P., Wilk, C., Thaker, G., Bellack, A. S., & Buchanan, R. W. (in preparation). Cognitive correlates of successful vocational outcome in schizophrenia.

Goldberg, T. E., Ragland, J. D., Torrey, E. F., Gold, J. M., Bigelow, L. B., & Weinberger, D. R. (1990). Neuropsychological assessment of monozygotic twins discordant for schizophrenia. *Archives of General Psychiatry*, *47* (11), 1066–1072.

Goodwin, F. K., & Jamison, K. R. (1990). *Manic-depressive illness*. New York: Oxford University Press.

Hanson, D. R., & Gottesman, I. I. (2005). Theories of schizophrenia: a genetic–inflammatory–vascular synthesis. *BMC Medical Genetics*, *6* (1), 7.

Hartman, M., Steketee, M. C., Silva, S., Lanning, K., & Andersson, C. (2003a). Wisconsin Card Sorting Test performance in schizophrenia: The role of working memory. *Schizophrenia Research*, *63* (3), 201–217.

Hartman, M., Steketee, M. C., Silva, S., Lanning, K., & McCann, H. (2003b). Working memory and schizophrenia: Evidence for slowed encoding. *Schizophrenia Research*, *59* (2–3), 99–113.

Hedges, L. V., & Olkin, I. (1985). *Statistical methods for meta-analysis*. Orlando, FL: Academic Press.

Heinrichs, R. W. (2005). The primacy of cognition in schizophrenia. *American Psychologist*, *60* (3), 229–242.

Heinrichs, R. W., & Zakzanis, K. K. (1998). Neurocognitive deficit in schizophrenia: A quantitative review of the evidence. *Neuropsychology*, *12* (3), 426–445.

*Hill, S. K., Schuepbach, D., Herbener, E. S., Keshavan, M. S., & Sweeney, J. A. (2004). Pretreatment and longitudinal studies of neuropsychological deficits in antipsychotic-naive patients with schizophrenia. *Schizophrenia Research*, *68* (1), 49–63.

Hoff, A. L., Sakuma, M., Wieneke, M., Horon, R., Kushner, M., & DeLisi, L. E. (1999). Longitudinal neuropsychological follow-up study of patients with first-episode schizophrenia. *American Journal of Psychiatry*, *156* (9), 1336–1341.

*Hoff, A. L., Svetina, C., Maurizio, A. M., Crow, T. J., Spokes, K., & DeLisi, L. E. (2005). Familial cognitive deficits in schizophrenia. *American Journal of Medical Genetics B. Neuropsychiatric Genetics*, *133* (1), 43–49.

Horrobin, D. F. (1998). The membrane phospholipid hypothesis as a biochemical

basis for the neurodevelopmental concept of schizophrenia. *Schizophrenia Research*, *30* (3), 193–208.
Hoyer, W. J., Stawski, R. S., Wasylyshyn, C., & Verhaeghen, P. (2004). Adult age and digit symbol substitution performance: A meta-analysis. *Psychology and Aging*, *19* (1), 211–214.
*Hughes, C., Kumari, V., Soni, W., Das, M., Binneman, B., Drozd, S., et al. (2003). Longitudinal study of symptoms and cognitive function in chronic schizophrenia. *Schizophrenia Research*, *59* (2–3), 137–146.
Jaeger, J., Czobor, P., Berns, S. M., Donovan-Lepore, A. M., Creech, B., Basile-Sculz, R., et al. (2005). Neurocognitive determinants of functional recovery: A longitudinal examination in 250 recently discharged patients with schizophrenia (abstract). *Schizophrenia Bulletin*, *31* (2), 327.
Javitt, D. C., Liederman, E., Cienfuegos, A., & Shelley, A. M. (1999). Panmodal processing imprecision as a basis for dysfunction of transient memory storage systems in schizophrenia. *Schizophrenia Bulletin*, *25* (4), 763–775.
Javitt, D. C., Shelley, A. M., Silipo, G., & Lieberman, J. A. (2000). Deficits in auditory and visual context-dependent processing in schizophrenia: Defining the pattern. *Archives of General Psychiatry*, *57* (12), 1131–1137.
Javitt, D. C., Steinschneider, M., Schroeder, C. E., & Arezzo, J. C. (1996). Role of cortical N-methyl-D-aspartate receptors in auditory sensory memory and mismatch negativity generation: Implications for schizophrenia. *Proceedings of the National Academy of Science, USA*, *93* (21), 11962–11967.
Javitt, D. C., Strous, R. D., Grochowski, S., Ritter, W., & Cowan, N. (1997). Impaired precision, but normal retention, of auditory sensory ("echoic") memory information in schizophrenia. *Journal of Abnormal Psychology*, *106* (2), 315–324.
Javitt, D. C., & Zukin, S. R. (1991). Recent advances in the phencyclidine model of schizophrenia. *American Journal of Psychiatry*, *148* (10), 1301–1308.
Jensen, A. R. (1998). *The g factor: The science of mental ability*. Westport, CT: Praeger.
Jogems-Kosterman, B. J., Zitman, F. G., van Hoof, J. J., & Hulstijn, W. (2001). Psychomotor slowing and planning deficits in schizophrenia. *Schizophrenia Research*, *48* (2–3), 317–333.
Keefe, R. S., Seidman, L. J., Christensen, B. K., Hamer, R. M., Sharma, T., Sitskoorn, M. M., et al. (2004). Comparative effect of atypical and conventional antipsychotic drugs on neurocognition in first-episode psychosis: A randomized, double-blind trial of olanzapine versus low doses of haloperidol. *American Journal of Psychiatry*, *161* (6), 985–995.
Kirkpatrick, B., & Buchanan, R. W. (1990). The neural basis of the deficit syndrome of schizophrenia. *Journal of Nervous and Mental Disorders*, *178* (9), 545–555.
Kirkpatrick, B., Buchanan, R. W., McKenney, P. D., Alphs, L. D., & Carpenter, W. T., Jr. (1989). The schedule for the deficit syndrome: An instrument for research in schizophrenia. *Psychiatry Research*, *30* (2), 119–123.
Kline, R. B. (1998). *Principles and practice of structural equation modeling*. New York: Guilford Press.
Kubicki, M., Park, H., Westin, C. F., Nestor, P. G., Mulkern, R. V., Maier, S. E., et al. (2005). DTI and MTR abnormalities in schizophrenia: Analysis of white matter integrity. *Neuroimage*, *26*, 1109–1118.
Laurent, A., Biloa-Tang, M., Bougerol, T., Duly, D., Anchisi, A. M., Bosson, J. L., et al. (2000). Executive/attentional performance and measures of schizotypy in

patients with schizophrenia and in their nonpsychotic first-degree relatives. *Schizophrenia Research, 46* (2–3), 269–283.

Laux, L. F., & Lane, D. M. (1985). Information processing components of substitution test performance. *Intelligence, 9,* 111–136.

Leonard, S., Adams, C., Breese, C. R., Adler, L. E., Bickford, P., Byerley, W., et al. (1996). Nicotinic receptor function in schizophrenia. *Schizophrenia Bulletin, 22* (3), 431–445.

Lezak, M. D. (1995). *Neuropsychological assessment* (3rd ed.). New York: Oxford University Press.

Liddle, P. F. (1987). Schizophrenic syndromes, cognitive performance and neurological dysfunction. *Psychological Medicine, 17* (1), 49–57.

Longstreth, W. T., Jr., Arnold, A. M., Beauchamp, N. J., Jr., Manolio, T. A., Lefkowitz, D., Jungreis, C., et al. (2005). Incidence, manifestations, and predictors of worsening white matter on serial cranial magnetic resonance imaging in the elderly: The Cardiovascular Health Study. *Stroke, 36* (1), 56–61.

Mahadik, S. P., & Evans, D. R. (2003). Is schizophrenia a metabolic brain disorder? Membrane phospholipid dysregulation and its therapeutic implications. *Psychiatric Clinics of North America, 26* (1), 85–102.

Miller, W. R. (1975). Psychological deficit in depression. *Psychological Bulletin, 82* (2), 238–260.

Mirsky, A. F., Yardley, S. L., Jones, B. P., Walsh, D., & Kendler, K. S. (1995). Analysis of the attention deficit in schizophrenia: A study of patients and their relatives in Ireland. *Journal of Psychiatric Research, 29* (1), 23–42.

Mishara, A. L., & Goldberg, T. E. (2004). A meta-analysis and critical review of the effects of conventional neuroleptic treatment on cognition in schizophrenia: Opening a closed book. *Biological Psychiatry, 55* (10), 1013–1022.

*Mohamed, S., Paulsen, J. S., O'Leary, D., Arndt, S., & Andreasen, N. (1999). Generalized cognitive deficits in schizophrenia: A study of first-episode patients. *Archives of General Psychiatry, 56* (8), 749–754.

Moher, D., Cook, D. J., Jadad, A. R., Tugwell, P., Moher, M., Jones, A., et al. (1999). Assessing the quality of reports of randomised trials: Implications for the conduct of meta-analyses. *Health Technology Assessment, 3* (12), i–iv, 1–98.

Nelson, H. E., Pantelis, C., Carruthers, K., Speller, J., Baxendale, S., & Barnes, T. R. (1990). Cognitive functioning and symptomatology in chronic schizophrenia. *Psychological Medicine, 20* (2), 357–365.

Niendam, T. A., Bearden, C. E., Rosso, I. M., Sanchez, L. E., Hadley, T., Nuechterlein, K. H., et al. (2003). A prospective study of childhood neurocognitive functioning in schizophrenic patients and their siblings. *American Journal of Psychiatry, 160* (11), 2060–2062.

Pantelis, C., Barnes, T. R., & Nelson, H. E. (1992). Is the concept of frontal-subcortical dementia relevant to schizophrenia? *British Journal of Psychiatry, 160,* 442–460.

Pier, M. P., Hulstijn, W., & Sabbe, B. G. (2004). Differential patterns of psychomotor functioning in unmedicated melancholic and nonmelancholic depressed patients. *Journal of Psychiatric Research, 38* (4), 425–435.

The Psychological Corporation. (1997). *The WAIS-III/WMS-III technical manual.* San Antonio, TX: The Psychological Corporation.

Purdon, S. E. (1998). Olfactory identification and Stroop interference converge in schizophrenia. *Journal of Psychiatry and Neuroscience, 23* (3), 163–171.

Rabinowicz, E. F., Silipo, G., Goldman, R., & Javitt, D. C. (2000). Auditory sensory dysfunction in schizophrenia: Imprecision or distractibility? *Archives of General Psychiatry, 57* (12), 1149–1155.

Ratti, M. T., Bo, P., Giardini, A., & Soragna, D. (2002). Chronic alcoholism and the frontal lobe: Which executive functions are impaired? *Acta Neurological Scandinavica, 105* (4), 276–281.

Richardson, J. T. (2003). Howard Andrew Knox and the origins of performance testing on Ellis Island, 1912–1916. *History of Psychology, 6* (2), 143–170.

Robbins, T. W. (1990). The case of frontostriatal dysfunction in schizophrenia. *Schizophrenia Bulletin, 16* (3), 391–402.

Sackheim, H. A., & Steif, B. L. (1988). Neuropsychology of depression and mania. In A. Georgotas & R. Cancro (Eds.), *Depression and mania* (pp. 265–289). New York: Elsevier.

Salthouse, T. A. (1992). What do adult age differences in the Digit Symbol Substitution Test reflect? *Journal of Gerontology, 47* (3), P121–P128.

Salthouse, T. A. (1996). The processing-speed theory of adult age differences in cognition. *Psychological Review, 103* (3), 403–428.

Salthouse, T. A. (1998). Independence of age-related influences on cognitive abilities across the life span. *Developmental Psychology, 34* (5), 851–864.

Salthouse, T. A., & Becker, J. T. (1998). Independent effects of Alzheimer's disease on neuropsychological functioning. *Neuropsychology, 12* (2), 242–252.

Salthouse, T. A., & Kail, R. (1983). Memory development throughout the lifespan: The role of processing rate. In P. B. Baltes & O. G. Brim (Eds.), *Life span development and behavior* (Vol. 5, pp. 89–116). New York: Academic Press.

*Seidman, L. J., Kremen, W. S., Koren, D., Faraone, S. V., Goldstein, J. M., & Tsuang, M. T. (2002). A comparative profile analysis of neuropsychological functioning in patients with schizophrenia and bipolar psychoses. *Schizophrenia Research, 53* (1–2), 31–44.

Shaddish, W. R., & Haddock, C. K. (1994). Combining estimates of effect size. In H. Cooper & L. V. Hedges (Eds.), *The handbook of research synthesis* (pp. 261–285). New York: Sage.

Stratta, P., Daneluzzo, E., Prosperini, P., Bustini, M., Mattei, P., & Rossi, A. (1997). Is Wisconsin Card Sorting Test performance related to "working memory" capacity? *Schizophrenia Research, 27* (1), 11–19.

Taylor, S. F., Kornblum, S., & Tandon, R. (1996). Facilitation and interference of selective attention in schizophrenia. *Journal of Psychiatric Research, 30* (4), 251–259.

van Hoof, J. J., Jogems-Kosterman, B. J., Sabbe, B. G., Zitman, F. G., & Hulstijn, W. (1998). Differentiation of cognitive and motor slowing in the Digit Symbol Test (DST): Differences between depression and schizophrenia. *Journal of Psychiatric Research, 32*, 99–103.

Wechsler, D. (1955). *Manual for the Wechsler Adult Intelligence Scale*. New York: The Psychological Corporation.

Wechsler, D. (1981). *Manual for the Wechsler Adult Intelligence Scale—Revised*. New York: The Psychological Corporation.

Wechsler, D. (1997). *Wechsler Adult Intelligence Scale—Third Edition*. San Antonio, TX: The Psychological Corporation.

Widlocher, D. J. (1983). Psychomotor retardation: Clinical, theoretical, and psychometric aspects. *Psychiatric Clinics of North America, 6* (1), 27–40.

7 Information processing speed in multiple sclerosis: A primary deficit?

Jessica H. Kalmar and Nancy D. Chiaravalloti

> It is possible that the quality of intelligence may depend upon the number of connections, but also upon the *speed* with which those connections are formed.
>
> (Lemmon, 1927, p. 405)

Multiple sclerosis disease characteristics

Multiple sclerosis (MS) is the most common nontraumatic neurological illness in young and middle-aged adults, with disease onset typically between ages 20 and 40 (Rao, Leo, Bernardin, & Unverzagt, 1991). Current epidemiological studies indicate that women are approximately twice as likely to suffer from MS as men (Kraft, 1981), and MS is more prevalent in certain geographic regions (Rumrill, Kaleta, & Battersby, 1996). It is primarily a white matter disease that particularly affects periventricular areas of the brain bilaterally. MS causes destruction of neuronal myelin sheaths, which are integral to the normal transmission of nerve impulses (Herndon, 2003), and has also recently been associated with axonal damage (Davie, Barker, Thompson, Tofts, McDonald, & Miller, 1997; Trapp, Peterson, Ransohoff, Rudick, Mork, & Bo, 1998). The resulting widespread lesions in the central nervous system (CNS), also known as sclerotic plaques, can cause motor, cognitive, and psychiatric problems (Brassington & Marsh, 1998), with high variability in symptom presentation between individuals (Gordon, Lewis, & Wong, 1994). Currently, the disease course is classified as relapsing remitting (RRMS), secondary progressive (SPMS) or primary progressive multiple sclerosis (PPMS). Previously, individuals with either SPMS or PPMS were classified as chronic progressive (CPMS), but this classification system was eliminated after increasing reports of differences in pathology (Lublin & Reingold, 1996). The wide range in symptoms and disease course creates a significant obstacle in understanding the disease process and identifying effective treatments. While the etiology remains elusive, MS is currently thought to be the result of a combination of immunologic, genetic, and viral factors (Rumrill et al., 1996).

Cognition in MS

Recognition of cognitive impairment as a common consequence of MS is a relatively recent phenomenon. Historically, cognitive deficits were thought to be present in only 3% of individuals with MS (Kurtzke, Beebe, Nagler, Auth, Kurland, & Nefzger, 1972). More recently, prevalence estimates of cognitive dysfunction in MS range as high as 70% (Peyser, Rao, LaRocca, & Kaplan, 1990; Rao, 1997). Cognitive impairments in MS have been documented in specific domains, including attention (Paul, Beatty, Schneider, Blanco, & Hames, 1998), new learning and memory (DeLuca, Barbieri-Berger, & Johnson, 1994; DeLuca, Gaudino, Diamond, Christodoulou, & Engel, 1998), working memory (Lengenfelder, Chiaravalloti, Ricker, & DeLuca, 2003), and executive functions (Arnett et al., 1997). The two most frequently reported cognitive difficulties in MS are impaired long-term episodic memory and compromised information processing efficiency (defined as both working memory "accuracy" and "speed" of processing).

Information processing speed

Processing speed (PS) can be defined as either the amount of time it takes to process a set amount of information, or the amount of information that can be processed within a certain unit of time. PS has been shown to be highly vulnerable to brain damage. For instance, diminished PS has been demonstrated in traumatic brain injury, aging, Parkinson's disease, and schizophrenia, as reviewed in other chapters in this volume. This chapter presents the accumulated evidence for significant difficulties in information PS in persons with MS.

Several investigators have highlighted the similarities between MS and the "subcortical dementias" including widespread white matter pathology with sparing of the cortical mantle and the pattern of cognitive deficits, with slowed PS being one of the cardinal cognitive problems (e.g., Denney, Lynch, Parmenter, & Horne, 2004; Denney, Sworowski, & Lynch, 2005; Litvan, Grafman, Vendrell, & Martinez, 1988; Rao, St Aubin-Faubert, & Leo, 1989). Based on administration of several measures of PS to a sample of individuals with MS and healthy controls (HC), De Sonneville reported that on average participants with MS were 40% slower than HCs (De Sonneville, Boringa, Reuling, Lazeron, Ader, & Polman, 2002). Disease duration and severity were associated with PS, such that those with PPMS were 51% slower, those with SPMS were 50% slower, and those with RRMS were 24% slower, than HCs (De Sonneville et al., 2002). Denney et al. (2004) reported that slowing in MS was evident in automatic and controlled processes, and irrespective of whether speed was an explicit or implicit feature of performance.

Researchers have used various standardized neuropsychological tests and laboratory paradigms to investigate information PS in MS. Perhaps one of the most widely used measures of PS in MS is the Paced Auditory Serial

Addition Test (PASAT; Gronwall, 1977). Several reports indicate that PASAT performance differentiates between individuals with MS and HCs (DeLuca et al., 1994; DeLuca, Johnson, Beldowicz, & Natelson, 1995; DeLuca, Johnson, & Natelson, 1993; Litvan et al., 1988), and between those individuals with RRMS and progressive MS disease courses (Huijbregts, Kalkers, de Sonneville, de Groot, Reuling, & Polman, 2004; Snyder, Cappelleri, Archibald, & Fisk, 2001). Achiron et al. (2005) reported that PASAT performance was correlated with MS disease duration, and was among the indices of cognitive impairment that were evident relatively early in the course of the disease. Researchers have compared two alternate scoring systems for the PASAT—the standard and dyad scoring methods—and found that the dyad scoring system discriminated between individuals with MS and HCs at all presentation rates, while the standard scoring system did not differentiate between the groups at the faster presentation rates (Fisk & Archibald, 2001). Snyder et al. (2001) found that dyad scoring distinguished best between those individuals with RRMS and those with SPMS. A practice effect has been observed with repeat administrations of the PASAT across different subject groups. Barker-Collo (2005) demonstrated that the improvement seen with repeat PASAT performance in individuals with MS is similar to that seen in neurological samples and not HCs. Furthermore, persons with RRMS exhibited greater benefit of repeat PASAT administration than those with CPMS. Thus, considerable data suggest that the PASAT is highly sensitive to the degree of PS impairment in individuals with MS.

Rather than focusing on a single test, some investigators have provided support for the PS deficit in MS based on administration of a battery of tests. Maurelli et al. (1992) administered the Wechsler Adult Intelligence Scale (WAIS) and reported deficits in Performance IQ (PIQ) but not Verbal IQ (VIQ) in individuals with MS relative to HCs. The authors theorized that the observed decrease in PIQ in MS may have been related to the timed nature of the PIQ subtests, and represented a deficit in PS. Kail (1997) posited that if slowing in MS is a result of neural demyelination, the slowing should be global and not restricted to individual tasks. In order to test his theory, Kail conducted a meta-analysis of studies on PS in MS and found that reaction time for MS participants increased systematically as a function of reaction times for comparison participants, irrespective of the PS measures. The slope of the linear increase in individuals with MS was greatest in those with the most severe symptoms (Kail, 1997). In 1998, Kail provided further support for his theory by administering several clinical neuropsychological and laboratory measures of PS to an independent sample of individuals with MS (Kail, 1998). He obtained similar results to those of the meta-analysis, except that reaction time increased by a power function, not linearly.

In addition to the clinical neuropsychological tests used to measure PS, a laboratory paradigm frequently used for the study of PS in MS is the Sternberg Memory Scanning Test. Two groups reported slowing in individuals with MS on the Sternberg paradigm (Archibald & Fisk, 2000; Rao,

St Aubin-Faubert, et al., 1989). Rao and colleagues found that individuals with MS required additional scanning time on the Sternberg paradigm to achieve the same accuracy rate as HCs. Additionally, length of illness correlated with the index of PS obtained from the Sternberg paradigm, while physical disability correlated with a measure of motor speed. It is noteworthy that performance on other measures of PS is also associated with disease course (e.g., Achiron et al., 2005; De Sonneville et al., 2002; Schulz, Kopp, Kunkel, & Faiss, 2006).

Accumulated evidence across studies of the association between length of illness or disease severity and PS ability may be related to the greater probability of cerebral plaque development as the disease advances, and raises the question of whether slowing is related to disease progression in MS. However, direct investigation of the relationship of slowing to disease progression in MS has been limited. Individuals with MS who had longer disease duration showed improvement in PS when treated with amantadine, while those with shorter disease duration did not show the benefit (Sailer, Heinze, Schoenfeld, Hauser, & Smid, 2000). In a longitudinal study of individuals with MS, while the entire sample did not show decline in performance on the neuropsychological battery over a 1-year time period, those participants who did exhibit decline showed it primarily on tests of PS, suggesting that PS may be especially sensitive to cognitive decline in individuals with MS (Hohol et al., 1997).

Information processing efficiency: PS and working memory

Working memory (WM) refers to the ability to maintain and manipulate a limited amount of information over a brief period of time (Baddeley, 1992). In Baddeley's model WM is theorized to be composed of a central executive system (CES) and two "slave" systems, the phonological loop (PL) and the visuospatial sketchpad. The CES is thought to be responsible for the selection, initiation, and termination of processing routines within WM. In contrast, the slave systems are responsible for the temporary maintenance and rehearsal of information. Numerous studies have documented WM impairment in persons with MS. For example, Grigsby and colleagues found that MS subjects performed significantly worse than HCs on tasks requiring the manipulation of stored information, including the Brown-Peterson task, Digit Span Backwards, Symbol Digit Modalities Test, and the PASAT (Grigsby, Ayarbe, Kravcisin, & Busenbark, 1994; Grigsby, Busenbark, Kravcisin, Kennedy, & Taylor, 1994). DeLuca and colleagues have observed this WM deficit in both behavioral (Demaree, DeLuca, Gaudino, & Diamond, 1999) and neuroimaging studies (Chiaravalloti et al., 2005; Hillary et al., 2003).

While deficits in both PS and WM have been clearly shown in persons with MS, the relative contribution of these two elements of information processing is unclear. However, data accumulated by DeLuca and colleagues show that the major contributor to deficits in information processing ability in MS is PS and not WM. Kalmar and colleagues (Kalmar, Bryant, Tulsky, & DeLuca, 2004) examined the relative role of WM versus PS in MS. These researchers compared performance of individuals with MS on the Letter–Number Sequencing (LNS) subtest of the WAIS-III (Wechsler, 1997) to performance on the PASAT. While both tests have a significant WM load, only the PASAT also has a significant speeded component. Thus if the WM load of both tasks is comparable, then any differences in performance between the two tasks could be attributed to the added speed component required of the PASAT. Results indicated that 2% of the MS subjects were impaired on LNS, while a significantly greater proportion of the participants, 39%, were impaired on the PASAT. These data suggest that PS, not WM, is the major determinant in identifying impaired information processing ability in persons with MS (Kalmar et al., 2004).

To further examine this question with larger sample sizes, a follow-up retrospective examination of 215 clinically definite MS subjects, 162 with RRMS and 53 with SPMS, was conducted. Replicating findings from the initial study, the researchers noted that significantly more MS subjects were impaired on the PASAT (30.4%) than on LNS (12.8%). In addition, the authors examined two other common measures of PS and WM: the PS Index score and the WM Index score from the WAIS-III, to examine the *constructs* of PS and WM. These scores were corrected for age, education, gender, and race. Significantly more MS subjects were impaired on the PS Index than on the WM Index. The frequency of impairment was significantly higher among the SPMS than the RRMS subjects. The authors also examined Odd's Ratios (OR) to evaluate the relative risk of a person with MS having a deficit in PS or WM as compared with a healthy individual. In the total MS sample, an OR of 10.4 was observed for the PS Index score, indicating that the risk of MS subjects exhibiting a difficulty in PS is 10.4 times higher that that observed in the general population. In contrast, the WM Index OR for the total MS sample was 2.7. That is, the OR for the PS Index score was almost 4 times greater than that observed for the WM Index score, indicating that PS deficits are a major difficulty in individuals with MS. The SPMS group showed marked impairment on the PS Index, where they obtained an OR of 65.2, indicating a more than 65-fold increased relative risk of exhibiting significant problems in PS compared to what is expected in the general population (Figure 7.1). The RRMS subjects showed an OR of 5.3 for PS, but the OR of 1.3 for WM did not differ from healthy controls. The results of this study provide further evidence that PS is the primary information processing deficit in persons with MS. The data suggest that early during the course of the disease (i.e., RRMS), measures of PS are particularly sensitive to cognitive impairment, while measures of WM are not. Impairment in PS increases dramatically as the disease progresses. Interestingly, with disease progression, there is also increased sensitivity on tests of WM, but substantially less than PS (DeLuca, Chelune, Tulsky, Lengenfelder, & Chiaravalloti, 2004).

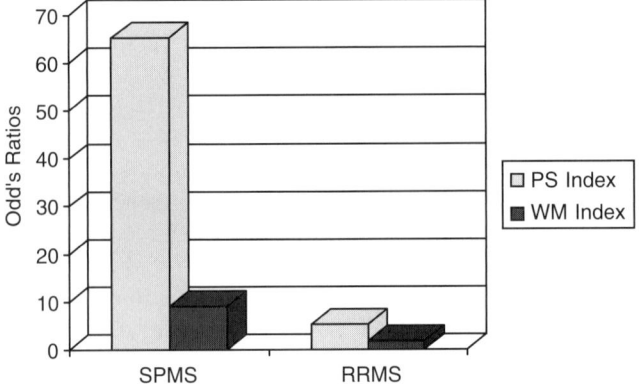

Figure 7.1 Odd's Ratios for Processing Speed versus Working Memory Indices for RRMS and SPMS.

Source: DeLuca, Chelune, Tulsky, Lengenfelder, and Chiaravalloti, 2004. Reprinted with permission.

The next question addressed by Dr. DeLuca's laboratory was whether increasing the difficulty level of a WM task affected PS performance. The Visual Threshold Serial Addition Test (VT-SAT), a visual analogue to the PASAT, was used to address this question. This test is designed to measure PS directly by controlling for accuracy of performance using a Method of Limits procedure. The inter-stimulus interval (ISI, or threshold speed) is adjusted to hold accuracy constant at 50% correct across subjects in both the MS and HC groups. As such, the threshold speed is a direct measure of PS, uncontaminated by accuracy. The VT-SAT is essentially identical to the original PASAT, except for the ISI modulation. To modulate difficulty level, we also employed a more difficult derivative of the original VT-SAT or VT-SAT 1-back, known as the VT-SAT 2-back. Task difficulty was elevated by increasing the amount required to be held in WM (i.e., by increasing the "N" of this "N-back" task). It has been well established that sequential increases of "N" make for a more difficult WM task, and is also known to produce *greater* activation of dorsolateral and left inferior regions of the prefrontal cortex in humans (Braver, Cohen, Nystrom, Jonides, Smith, & Noll, 1997). This design allowed us to examine the influence of WM difficulty on PS. While both the MS and HC groups were equated for accuracy of performance, the MS subjects required significantly longer threshold speed scores (reflecting slower PS) to achieve the same level of accuracy as controls (Demaree et al., 1999; Lengenfelder, Bryant, Diamond, Kalmar, Moore, & DeLuca, 2006). When subjects were then evaluated on the more difficult 2-back condition, it was observed that 70% of the MS subjects performed at or above the 5th percentile of the HCs' scores on the 2-back trial, while 30% performed below the 5th percentile. As such, the MS group was divided into two groups: achievers—those who performed at or above 5th percentile on the 2-back; and non-achievers—those who performed below the 5th percentile on the 2-back task (see Figure 7.2). MS achievers took significantly more time than HCs on the 2-back VT-SAT. Importantly, the MS non-achievers had threshold speeds more than twice as high as the threshold speeds of the MS achievers (Lengenfelder et al., 2006).

To further examine the relationship between PS and WM, DeLuca and colleagues then equated individuals on PS to see what would happen to accuracy of performance. In this part of the study, each subject performed the 2-back version of the VT-SAT a second time, at the optimum threshold speed they each achieved for the 1-back condition; that is, the speed required to achieve 50% correct on the 1-back condition. This method allowed evaluation of performance on the 2-back condition after subjects were equated for PS. If PS is the only problem in information processing in individuals with MS, equating for PS should result in the absence of significant group differences on 2-back accuracy. However, if WM accuracy plays a significant role in, or interacts with, PS, we would expect to see group differences on 2-back accuracy. When accuracy of performance was observed on the 2-back with PS held constant, the MS non-achievers had significantly lower accuracy relative to MS achievers and HCs. These results suggest that with increasing task difficulty and demand on the CES there is an interaction between PS and WM, such that a deficit in WM emerges in a subset of individuals with MS. MS is associated with a slowing of basic information PS and this decrement in PS results in a greater cognitive performance deficit in individuals with MS

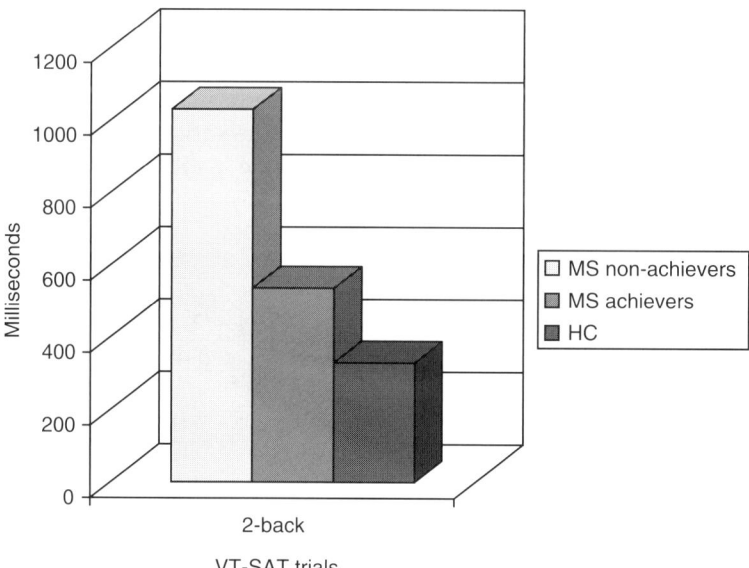

Figure 7.2 Threshold speed on VT-SAT 2-back.

Source: Lengenfelder et al., 2006. Reprinted with permission.

than in healthy individuals in situations that maximize central executive load (Lengenfelder et al., 2006).

The relationship between PS and WM in MS has also been examined using unique measures of these constructs. In preliminary work, DeLuca and colleagues administered the Keeping Track Task (KTT) to individuals with MS and HCs (Lengenfelder, Moore, Bryant, & DeLuca, 2005). The KTT is a computerized task designed to compare performance accuracy under increasing demands on the slave systems (structural load) and the CES of WM (operational load). There were two levels used for both the structural (one or three elements of information) and operational (one or three arithmetic operations) loads. The easiest trial was when structural and operational loads were both low (i.e., one element of information each), while structural and operational loads of three (i.e., three elements for each condition) represented the most difficult. Linear regression analyses were conducted to examine the contributions of PS and WM to performance on the "hard" (three elements) condition of the KTT in individuals with MS. When PS was entered before WM in the model, PS accounted for a significant amount of the variance in "hard" KTT performance, and WM did not make a significant contribution to this model. In the model where WM was entered before speed, WM still did not make a significant contribution to the model. When PS was then entered in step 2, the additional variance accounted for by PS was again significant (Lengenfelder et al., 2005).

Taken together, these data suggest that the variance associated with KTT performance was primarily a result of factors associated with PS and not WM. To replicate these results with different measures of PS and WM, DeLuca and colleagues conducted linear regression analyses similar to those above and examined the relative contribution of PS and WM to PASAT performance. Results for these analyses were virtually identical to the KTT analyses. PS accounted for a larger amount of the variance in PASAT performance than WM did, even when PS was entered in the regression analysis *after* WM (Lengenfelder et al., 2005). These regression analyses provide further support that PS is the major contributing factor associated with performing a complex information processing task in MS. While WM may have an additional independent contribution as well, this remains in a secondary capacity.

Research from other laboratories has also supported the primacy of the PS deficit in MS. Others have shown that PS and WM capacity are separable functions in individuals with MS. For example, performance on the KTT and memory scanning speed on the Sternberg paradigm were not found to be correlated (Archibald et al., 2004). De Sonneville et al. (2002) administered tests that tapped a variety of cognitive functions to HCs and individuals with MS at various disease stages and found widespread deficits in PS and more limited difficulties in accuracy. While the data of De Sonneville and colleagues support the primacy of the PS deficit in MS, they also speak of some interaction between PS and WM abilities, as differences in speed between persons with MS and HCs increased with load and with heightened distraction. This interaction was also observed in our group from the 1-back versus 2-back VT-SAT data of Lengenfelder et al. (2006). Several researchers point out that slowed PS may be one of the earliest cognitive manifestations of MS and impairments are present in the early phase of RRMS (e.g., Nocentini et al., 2006; Olivares, Nieto, Sanchez, Wollmann, Hernandez, & Barroso, 2005; Schulz et al., 2006). Conversely, Archibald and Fisk (2000) and DeLuca et al. (2004) both found that WM deficits were limited to individuals with SPMS, suggesting that WM deficits may only arise with progression of MS.

PS impairment and other cognitive abilities in MS

In addition to examining PS as a cognitive construct in and of itself, it is also important to examine the relative effect that a PS deficit has on other areas of cognition. Despite the general acceptance of the impact of PS on higher cognitive processes (see other chapters in this volume), this relationship has not been extensively evaluated in persons with MS. Some authors hypothesize that impaired PS is a primary consequence of MS, which in turn decreases the ability to acquire new information and to process higher level cognitive functions (Gaudino, Chiaravalloti, DeLuca, & Diamond, 2001; Kail, 1998; Litvan et al., 1988). At early stages of the disease, there is some evidence that there is more impairment in PS than in episodic memory (Achiron & Barak, 2003; Nocentini et al., 2006; Randolph et al., 2005), which supports the idea that slowed PS may arise early in the disease process and contribute to the development of episodic memory disturbance. There is now a substantial amount of literature demonstrating that the episodic memory disturbance observed in MS is primarily a result of difficulty in the acquisition (or learning) of information rather than in retrieval failure (DeLuca et al., 1994; DeLuca et al., 1998; Demaree, Gaudino, DeLuca, & Ricker, 2000; Gaudino et al., 2001). In attempting to elucidate the source of this deficit in the acquisition of new information, DeLuca and colleagues examined the relationship between PS and new learning abilities in a sample of MS participants. These researchers noted a significant relationship between an index of information PS and an index of new learning abilities (Gaudino et al., 2001). Similarly, other research groups have reported correlations between PASAT performance and measures of verbal learning and episodic memory (Fisk & Archibald, 2001; Litvan et al., 1988). Finally, recent preliminary work from the DeLuca laboratory examined a sample of 60 MS participants utilizing multiple regression analysis. Information PS was noted to be a significant predictor of new learning abilities in the visual domain, while tests of WM were not. This relationship was noted after controlling for age and education (Kalmar, Chiaravalloti, & DeLuca, 2005). Taken together, these studies indicate that PS is an important factor underlying episodic memory disturbance in MS.

An important consideration when evaluating cognition in individuals with MS is the contribution of depressive symptomatology to cognitive performance. Findings across studies are inconsistent with regard to the impact of depression on cognition in MS, as well as its specific relationship to information PS. Arnett, Higginson, and Randolph (2001) reported that indices of PS and executive functions each made independent contributions towards predicting the degree of depression in individuals with MS, with PS accounting for a larger share of the variance. Associations between depression and PS were also reported by Landro, Celius, and Sletvold (2004). There is some evidence that even when researchers carefully consider depressive symptomatology in their work, the predominance of impairment in PS is borne out. For instance, Denney et al. (2004) reported deficits in executive function, verbal learning and memory, and PS in RRMS and PPMS, relative to HCs. However, after controlling for degree of fatigue and depression in the MS sample, the only performance deficit that was unexplained was impaired PS, providing further support for the primacy of the PS deficit in MS.

Impact of PS deficit in MS on everyday life

After recognizing the role of PS as an important cognitive deficit in individuals with MS, the relationship between slowed PS and functioning in everyday life requires examination. An association between PS and employment status in individuals with MS has been reported (Schulz et al., 2006). One line of investigation focuses on health-related quality of life (HRQL), or the impact of the disease as perceived by the person suffering from MS. Deloire et al. (2005) reported impairment on measures of PS and other cognitive domains in individuals with RRMS, but found that HRQL was only correlated with indices of PS and not with measures of other cognitive functions. Barker-Collo (2006) investigated the relative contributions of physical and cognitive disability to HRQL in individuals with RRMS or PPMS. Degree of physical disability accounted for a significant portion of the variance in both physical and mental components of HRQL. Measures of PS did not add a significant contribution to the variance explained by physical disability. While the variance explained by PS was not significant (27% of the physical component of HRQL and 23% of the mental component of HRQL), large effect sizes were present. Further research with a larger sample size and using additional measures of PS, as well as HRQL, is required to determine the role of PS in HRQL.

Kalmar and colleagues (Kalmar, Gaudino, Moore, Halper, & DeLuca, submitted) examined the relationship between cognitive functioning and performance on tasks of everyday life, using an objective, structured and standardized assessment battery designed by occupational therapists, the Executive Functional Performance Test (EFPT; Baum & Edwards, 1993; Baum, Morrison, Hahn, & Edwards, 2003). The EFPT includes tasks that vary in their degree of cognitive complexity, ranging from simple and routinized (e.g., hand washing) to complex (e.g., paying two bills when there are insufficient funds in the checking account). Pearson product moment correlations were used to examine the relationship between the Symbol Digit Modalities Test (SDMT, an index of PS) and EFPT performance (see Table 7.1). As anticipated, the SDMT correlated significantly with those EFPT tasks that included a relatively higher level of cognitive complexity. These data suggest that the SDMT is significantly correlated with functional activities performed in everyday life. Despite the fact that the EFPT is not dependent on speed for execution (i.e., subjects are allowed to take their time), a significant relationship with a measure of PS was still observed. A similar relationship between PS and actual performance of everyday life activities was observed by Goverover, Genova, Hillary, and DeLuca (in press). Thus the information processing deficit in MS affects both other higher order cognitive processes and everyday life activities.

Neural substrates of PS deficits in MS

A number of theories attempt to explain the neural mechanism underlying PS deficits in MS. Slowed conduction speed as a result of demyelination in MS has long been known (Filley, 2001), and has been documented in the form of delays in and loss of evoked potentials (Herndon, 2003). Neural conduction speed is not only affected by demyelination, but also by slow axonal transport and nerve fiber fatigue, resulting from loss of the axon's membrane potential (Herndon, 2003). These mechanisms become more apparent with advanced stages of the disease such as in SPMS, where deficits in information PS also increase dramatically (DeLuca et al., 2004).

In an effort to investigate the underlying neural substrates of PS deficits in MS, researchers have employed several techniques to extract morphometric measures from magnetic resonance imaging (MRI) scans. One method used repeatedly is to study the relationship between the extent of brain lesions, or lesion burden, and performance on measures of cognition. Early studies had human operators rate lesions and obtained variable results. Two groups (Franklin, Heaton, Nelson, Filley, & Seibert, 1988; Huber et al., 1987) reported modest correlations between rating scale measures of lesion size and performance on measures of cognition. Conversely, Maurelli et al. (1992) did not find an association between neuroradiologists' ratings of lesion size and

Table 7.1. Correlations between PS and EFPT measures of functional performance

EFPT Test	SDMT
Handwashing	.19
Cooking oatmeal	−.21
Telephone usage	−.18
Medication management	−.50**
Bill payment	−.36*
Cooking casserole	−.43**

Note: Correlations are statistically significant at $*p < .05$ or $**p < .01$.

performance on a battery of neuropsychological tests. However, those participants with most extensive periventricular demyelination exhibited the poorest memory performance.

In order to improve on the subjective nature of the measures extracted from MR images in previous studies, researchers began to use semiautomated methods to quantify lesion area. Using such methodology to measure lesion area and the size of the corpus callosum, Rao and colleagues (Rao, Leo, Haughton, St Aubin-Faubert, & Bernadin, 1989) administered a comprehensive battery of neuropsychological tests to individuals with varied MS disease course. The authors found that while total lesion area predicted cognitive dysfunction in a range of domains, callosal size predicted performance specifically on measures of PS. The authors theorized that speed of information processing may depend on interhemispheric communication that would be disrupted by the demyelination of callosal fiber tracts (Rao, Leo, et al., 1989). While Rao and colleagues employed a battery of cognitive tests, Snyder and Cappelleri (2001) focused their study of total lesion area on its relationship to one measure of PS—the PASAT—and found that total lesion area was correlated with PASAT performance when standard and dyad scoring methods were used. After controlling for age, sex, and education, the correlation only remained statistically significant when using the dyad scoring method. PS deficits were more severe in the participants with greater total lesion area. The authors suggested that deficits in PS in MS may result from disruption of the white matter pathways between subcortical nuclei and the cortical mantle as a result of formation of sclerotic plaques. Swirsky-Sacchetti et al. (1992) also used a semiautomated quantitation system of lesion area in an MS sample that was composed of an equal number of participants with RR and CP disease courses. An index of PS, as well as indices of memory, abstract reasoning, verbal fluency, and visuospatial processing, were correlated with total lesion area with Pearson correlations ranging from .38 to .65.

Advances in MRI processing technologies enabled investigators to begin to study lesion volume, an improvement on previous measurements that were limited to the surface area of the lesions. While Swirksy-Saccheti et al. found that total lesion *area* was related to a range of cognitive functions, Fulton et al. (1999) reported that in individuals with RRMS, total lesion *volume* was only significantly correlated with indices of PS and verbal learning. The neuropsychological battery administered in Fulton's study included measures of PS, WM, verbal fluency, attention, verbal learning, and short-term memory. Further refinement of studies of the relationship between lesion burden and cognition in MS was the practice of employing regional measures of lesion volume. Archibald et al. (2004) reported that while total and frontal lesion volume were not related to PS in MS, a correlation was found between posterior fossa volume and PS as measured by the Sternberg Memory Scan. Performance on an index of WM, the Salthouse KTT, was not related to any of the morphometric measures obtained. The authors theorized that the relationship between posterior fossa volume and PS could be driven by damage to the reciprocal cerebello-cortical pathways that provide the anatomical basis for cerebellar involvement in cognition. Another enhancement of morphometric study in MS was the implementation of an MRI method known to be sensitive to cortical and juxtacortical lesions in MS, and to detecting lesions in neuroanatomical areas associated with multiple cognitive functions, fluid-attenuated inversion recovery (FLAIR). Using semiautomated methods to quantify total lesion volume from these images Randolph et al. (2005) found correlations between total lesion volume and indices of PS ($r = -.57$ to $-.62$) that remained significant after accounting for physical disability.

While the aforementioned studies were all cross-sectional in nature, one group conducted a longitudinal investigation of the relationship between lesion burden and cognitive functioning in individuals with varied MS disease course. Hohol et al. (1997) revealed significant correlations between baseline measures of cognition and total lesion volume obtained on repeated MRI scans over 1 year. The associations between total lesion volume and cognitive performance were most evident on indices of PS and in individuals with a CPMS disease course. In the entire MS sample, the only test that showed a relationship between change in cognitive performance over the 1-year period and change in total lesion volume was an index of PS. A subset of these participants (RRMS and CPMS disease course) was followed for an additional 3 years, and lesion volumes were obtained using automated processes in right and left frontal, temporal, parietal, and posterior regions (Sperling et al., 2001). Participants with MS differed from HCs on indices of PS and verbal memory. Performance on these measures was correlated with frontal and parietal lesion volumes at all time points, with Spearman rank correlations ranging from .55 to .73. The authors suggest that disruption of frontoparietal subcortical networks may underlie impairments in PS and verbal memory in MS.

A second approach to studying the neural substrate of cognitive impairment in MS is to focus on brain atrophy, rather than lesion burden. Benedict et al. (2005) measured regional, whole brain, and central atrophy in patients with RRMS and SPMS and found that regional atrophy in the temporal lobe was the primary predictor of memory performance, while central and general atrophy measures were the primary predictors of PS ability. These findings suggest that while PS may be mediated by widely dispersed cortical regions connected by long white matter tracts, memory may be more cortically mediated in a distinct area. On the other hand, another group found that volume measurements of brain atrophy did not correlate with any measures in their battery of cognitive tests, while lesion load quantified from FLAIR images was associated with indices of PS performance (Deloire et al., 2005). A third group that studied the relationship between brain atrophy and cognitive performance employed voxel-based morphometry. They reported that PASAT performance was correlated with gray matter volume, and not white matter volume or white matter lesion burden. Their findings of a relationship between PASAT performance and gray matter volume were localized to bilateral PFC, precentral gyrus, superior parietal cortex, and right cerebellum (Morgen et al., 2006).

A variety of reasons exist for the variability in findings across these morphometric imaging studies. Comparisons across studies are complicated by differences in group composition, such as sample size and MS disease course of the participants. The variability in presentation across individuals with MS further confounds the study of group differences. Methodological disparities include choice of neuropsychological tests, MRI scanning parameters, and morphometric measures. Findings of no relationship between cognition and morphometric measures may relate to the insensitivity of the neuropsychological tests or the nonspecificity of lesion burden. Future research employing other MR methods, such as diffusion tensor imaging, may shed further light on the parameters of the disease process that are more precisely related to cognitive dysfunction.

Conclusions and future directions

While it is evident that persons with MS have a significant impairment in information processing abilities, the precise mechanism underlying this dysfunction remains unclear. Reduced speed of information processing was viewed by some as representing the fundamental cognitive deficit associated with MS, and was thought to reflect the diffusely distributed changes in neural efficiency secondary to demyelination and axonal damage. Cumulative evidence from studies conducted in Dr. DeLuca's laboratory and by others has clearly shown that deficient PS accounts for the vast majority of the variance on tasks of information processing ability, which affects everyday life activities. On the other hand, accuracy of WM performance is minimally related to the information processing deficit characteristic of individuals with MS. This suggests that persons with MS may perform complex WM tasks as well as HCs, but simply need more time to do so.

Review of extant literature on PS in MS highlights several factors that should be weighed in future research. It is important to keep in mind when conducting research into PS in individuals with MS that test performance may be affected by motor/sensory dysfunction and therefore motor, primary sensory, and cognitive speed should be teased apart. An additional challenge to this line of research is the fact that neuropsychological tests often engage multiple cognitive mechanisms and, more specifically, that several tests which target PS also place significant demands on WM. As such, the same neuropsychological measures can be interpreted as tapping either PS or WM (or both). Attempts should be made to develop paradigms that target and manipulate PS while holding other cognitive abilities constant, such as that employed by the DeLuca group and described above. Another complicated issue is the intrinsic heterogeneity of persons with the disease. Ideally, research efforts would group individuals with MS based on clinical and demographic variables and not disease course alone (e.g., Olivares et al.,

2005), enabling minimization of the heterogeneity of individuals studied. Finally, the impact of medications that affect CNS functioning should be systematically considered when studying cognition in MS. One group reported that individuals with MS on CNS-active medications showed greater impairment on measures of PS and other areas of cognition than those not on CNS-active medications (Oken et al., 2006). These confounding factors should be carefully addressed before inferences about PS in MS are made.

Despite the aforementioned limitations, accumulated data demonstrate that deficits in information PS may lie at the root of cognitive problems in persons with MS, and that this deficiency in PS itself influences higher order cognitive processes and everyday life activities. Future research examining the contribution of impaired PS to higher cognitive functioning, as well as everyday life functional activity, in individuals with MS, is necessary. With regard to remediation, the presence of a PS deficit in MS argues for giving people with MS increased time to complete tasks to avoid the tradeoff of accuracy for speed. If PS lies at the core of cognitive deficits and everyday life activities that rely on cognition, cognitive rehabilitation interventions geared toward improving PS may substantially improve the social, occupational, and everyday functional status of persons with MS.

References

Achiron, A., & Barak, Y. (2003). Cognitive impairment in probable multiple sclerosis. *Journal of Neurology, Neurosurgery and Psychiatry*, 74 (4), 443–446.

Achiron, A., Polliack, M., Rao, S. M., Barak, Y., Lavie, M., Appelboim, N., et al. (2005). Cognitive patterns and progression in multiple sclerosis: Construction and validation of percentile curves. *Journal of Neurology, Neurosurgery and Psychiatry*, 76 (5), 744–749.

Archibald, C. J., & Fisk, J. D. (2000). Information processing efficiency in patients with multiple sclerosis. *Journal of Clinical and Experimental Neuropsychology*, 22 (5), 686–701.

Archibald, C. J., Wei, X., Scott, J. N., Wallace, C. J., Zhang, Y., Metz, L. M., et al. (2004). Posterior fossa lesion volume and slowed information processing in multiple sclerosis. *Brain*, 127 (Pt. 7), 1526–1534.

Arnett, P. A., Higginson, C. I., & Randolph, J. J. (2001). Depression in multiple sclerosis: Relationship to planning ability. *Journal of the International Neuropsychological Society*, 7 (6), 665–674.

Arnett, P. A., Rao, S. M., Grafman, J., Bernardin, L., Luchetta, T., Binder, J. R., et al. (1997). Executive functions in multiple sclerosis: An analysis of temporal ordering, semantic encoding, and planning abilities. *Neuropsychology*, 11 (4), 535–544.

Baddeley, A. (1992). Working memory. *Science*, 255 (5044), 556–559.

Barker-Collo, S. L. (2005). Within session practice effects on the PASAT in clients with multiple sclerosis. *Archives of Clinical Neuropsychology*, 20 (2), 145–152.

Barker-Collo, S. L. (2006). Quality of life in multiple sclerosis: Does information-processing speed have an independent effect? *Archives of Clinical Neuropsychology*, 21 (2), 167–174.

Baum, C. M., & Edwards, D. F. (1993). Cognitive performance in senile dementia of the Alzheimer's type: The Kitchen Task Assessment. *American Journal of Occupational Therapy, 47* (5), 431–436.

Baum, C. M., Morrison, T., Hahn, M., & Edwards, D. F. (2003). *Test manual for the executive function performance test*. St. Louis, MO: Washington University.

Benedict, R. H., Zivadinov, R., Carone, D. A., Weinstock-Guttman, B., Gaines, J., Maggiore, C., et al. (2005). Regional lobar atrophy predicts memory impairment in multiple sclerosis. *AJNR American Journal of Neuroradiology, 26* (7), 1824–1831.

Brassington, J. C., & Marsh, N. V. (1998). Neuropsychological aspects of multiple sclerosis. *Neuropsychology Review, 8* (2), 43–77.

Braver, T. S., Cohen, J. D., Nystrom, L. E., Jonides, J., Smith, E. E., & Noll, D. C. (1997). A parametric study of prefrontal cortex involvement in human working memory. *Neuroimage, 5* (1), 49–62.

Chiaravalloti, N., Hillary, F., Ricker, J., Christodoulou, C., Kalnin, A., Liu, W. C., et al. (2005). Cerebral activation patterns during working memory performance in multiple sclerosis using FMRI. *Journal of Clinical and Experimental Neuropsychology, 27* (1), 33–54.

Davie, C. A., Barker, G. J., Thompson, A. J., Tofts, P. S., McDonald, W. I., & Miller, D. H. (1997). 1H magnetic resonance spectroscopy of chronic cerebral white matter lesions and normal appearing white matter in multiple sclerosis. *Journal of Neurology, Neurosurgery and Psychiatry, 63* (6), 736–742.

De Sonneville, L. M., Boringa, J. B., Reuling, I. E., Lazeron, R. H., Ader, H. J., & Polman, C. H. (2002). Information processing characteristics in subtypes of multiple sclerosis. *Neuropsychologia, 40* (11), 1751–1765.

Deloire, M. S., Salort, E., Bonnet, M., Arimone, Y., Boudineau, M., Amieva, H., et al. (2005). Cognitive impairment as marker of diffuse brain abnormalities in early relapsing remitting multiple sclerosis. *Journal of Neurology, Neurosurgery and Psychiatry, 76* (4), 519–526.

DeLuca, J., Barbieri-Berger, S., & Johnson, S. K. (1994). The nature of memory impairments in multiple sclerosis: Acquisition versus retrieval. *Journal of Clinical and Experimental Neuropsychology, 16* (2), 183–189.

DeLuca, J., Chelune, G. J., Tulsky, D. S., Lengenfelder, J., & Chiaravalloti, N. D. (2004). Is speed of processing or working memory the primary information processing deficit in multiple sclerosis? *Journal of Clinical Experimental Neuropsychology, 26* (4), 550–562.

DeLuca, J., Gaudino, E. A., Diamond, B. J., Christodoulou, C., & Engel, R. A. (1998). Acquisition and storage deficits in multiple sclerosis. *Journal of Clinical and Experimental Neuropsychology, 20* (3), 376–390.

DeLuca, J., Johnson, S. K., Beldowicz, D., & Natelson, B. H. (1995). Neuropsychological impairments in chronic fatigue syndrome, multiple sclerosis, and depression. *Journal of Neurology, Neurosurgery and Psychiatry, 58* (1), 38–43.

DeLuca, J., Johnson, S. K., & Natelson, B. H. (1993). Information processing efficiency in chronic fatigue syndrome and multiple sclerosis. *Archives of Neurology, 50* (3), 301–304.

Demaree, H. A., DeLuca, J., Gaudino, E. A., & Diamond, B. J. (1999). Speed of information processing as a key deficit in multiple sclerosis: Implications for rehabilitation. *Journal of Neurology, Neurosurgery and Psychiatry, 67* (5), 661–663.

Demaree, H. A., Gaudino, E. A., DeLuca, J., & Ricker, J. H. (2000). Learning impairment is associated with recall ability in multiple sclerosis. *Journal of Clinical and Experimental Neuropsychology*, *22* (6), 865–873.

Denney, D. R., Lynch, S. G., Parmenter, B. A., & Horne, N. (2004). Cognitive impairment in relapsing and primary progressive multiple sclerosis: Mostly a matter of speed. *Journal of the International Neuropsychological Society*, *10* (7), 948–956.

Denney, D. R., Sworowski, L. A., & Lynch, S. G. (2005). Cognitive impairment in three subtypes of multiple sclerosis. *Archives of Clinical Neuropsychology*, *20* (8), 967–981.

Filley, C. M. (2001). *The behavioral neurology of white matter*. New York: Oxford University Press.

Fisk, J. D., & Archibald, C. J. (2001). Limitations of the Paced Auditory Serial Addition Test as a measure of working memory in patients with multiple sclerosis. *Journal of the International Neuropsychological Society*, *7* (3), 363–372.

Franklin, G. M., Heaton, R. K., Nelson, L. M., Filley, C. M., & Seibert, C. (1988). Correlation of neuropsychological and MRI findings in chronic/progressive multiple sclerosis. *Neurology*, *38* (12), 1826–1829.

Fulton, J. C., Grossman, R. I., Udupa, J., Mannon, L. J., Grossman, M., Wei, L., et al. (1999). MR lesion load and cognitive function in patients with relapsing–remitting multiple sclerosis. *AJNR American Journal of Neuroradiology*, *20* (10), 1951–1955.

Gaudino, E. A., Chiaravalloti, N. D., DeLuca, J., & Diamond, B. J. (2001). A comparison of memory performance in relapsing–remitting, primary progressive and secondary progressive, multiple sclerosis. *Neuropsychiatry, Neuropsychology and Behavioral Neurology*, *14* (1), 32–44.

Gordon, P. A., Lewis, M. D., & Wong, D. (1994). Multiple sclerosis: Strategies for rehabilitation counselors. *Journal of Rehabilitation*, *60*, 34–38.

Goverover, Y., Genova, H. M., Hillary, F. G., & DeLuca, J. (in press). The relationship between neuropsychological measures and the timed instrumental activities of daily living task in multiple sclerosis. *Multiple Sclerosis*.

Grigsby, J., Ayarbe, S. D., Kravcisin, N., & Busenbark, D. (1994). Working memory impairment among persons with chronic progressive multiple sclerosis. *Journal of Neurology*, *241* (3), 125–131.

Grigsby, J., Busenbark, D., Kravcisin, N., Kennedy, P. M., & Taylor, D. (1994). Impairment of the working memory system in relapsing–remitting multiple sclerosis. *Archives of Clinical Neuropsychology*, *9*, 134–135.

Gronwall, D. M. (1977). Paced auditory serial-addition task: a measure of recovery from concussion. *Perceptual Motor Skills*, *44* (2), 367–373.

Herndon, R. M. (2003). *Multiple sclerosis: Immunology, pathology and pathophysiology*. New York: Demos Medical Publishing.

Hillary, F. G., Chiaravalloti, N. D., Ricker, J. H., Steffener, J., Bly, B. M., Lange, G., et al. (2003). An investigation of working memory rehearsal in multiple sclerosis using fMRI. *Journal of Clinical and Experimental Neuropsychology*, *25* (7), 965–978.

Hohol, M. J., Guttmann, C. R., Orav, J., Mackin, G. A., Kikinis, R., Khoury, S. J., et al. (1997). Serial neuropsychological assessment and magnetic resonance imaging analysis in multiple sclerosis. *Archives of Neurology*, *54* (8), 1018–1025.

Huber, S. J., Paulson, G. W., Shuttleworth, E. C., Chakeres, D., Clapp, L. E., Pakalnis, A., et al. (1987). Magnetic resonance imaging correlates of dementia in multiple sclerosis. *Archives of Neurology*, *44* (7), 732–736.

Huijbregts, S. C., Kalkers, N. F., de Sonneville, L. M., de Groot, V., Reuling, I. E., &

Polman, C. H. (2004). Differences in cognitive impairment of relapsing remitting, secondary, and primary progressive MS. *Neurology, 63* (2), 335–339.

Kail, R. (1997). The neural noise hypothesis: Evidence from processing speed in adults with multiple sclerosis. *Aging, Neuropsychology, and Cognition, 4* , 157–165.

Kail, R. (1998). Speed of information processing in patients with multiple sclerosis. *Journal of Clinical and Experimental Neuropsychology, 20* (1), 98–106.

Kalmar, J. H., Bryant, D., Tulsky, D., & DeLuca, J. (2004). Information processing deficits in multiple sclerosis: Does choice of screening instrument make a difference? *Rehabilitation Psychology, 49* (3), 213–218.

Kalmar, J. H., Chiaravalloti, N. D., & DeLuca, J. (2005). Information processing deficits impact new learning in multiple sclerosis. *Journal of the International Neuropsychological Society, 11* (S1), 42 (Published online April 6, 2005).

Kalmar, J. H., Gaudino, E. A., Moore, N. B., Halper, J., & DeLuca, J. (submitted). The relationship between cognitive deficits and everyday functional activities in multiple sclerosis.

Kraft, G. I. (1981). Multiple sclerosis. In W. C. Stolov & M. R. Cloers (Eds.), *Handbook of severe disability* (pp. 111–118). Washington, DC: United States Department of Education and Rehabilitation Services Administration.

Kurtzke, J. F., Beebe, G. W., Nagler, B., Auth, T. L., Kurland, L. T., & Nefzger, M. D. (1972). Studies on the natural history of multiple sclerosis. 6. Clinical and laboratory findings at first diagnosis. *Acta Neurologica Scandinavica, 48* (1), 19–46.

Landro, N. I., Celius, E. G., & Sletvold, H. (2004). Depressive symptoms account for deficient information processing speed but not for impaired working memory in early phase multiple sclerosis (MS). *Journal of the Neurological Sciences, 217* (2), 211–216.

Lemmon, V. W. (1927). The relation of reaction time to measures of intelligence, memory, and learning. *Archives of Psychology, 94,* entire issue.

Lengenfelder, J., Bryant, D., Diamond, B. J., Kalmar, J. H., Moore, N. B., & DeLuca, J. (2006). Processing speed interacts with working memory efficiency in multiple sclerosis. *Archives of Clinical Neuropsychology, 21* (3), 229–238.

Lengenfelder, J., Chiaravalloti, N. D., Ricker, J. H., & DeLuca, J. (2003). Deciphering components of impaired working memory in multiple sclerosis. *Cognitive and Behavioral Neurology, 16* (1), 28–39.

Lengenfelder, J., Moore, N. B., Bryant, D., & DeLuca, J. (2005). Does increasing information processing time improve working memory accuracy in MS? *Journal of the International Neuropsychological Society, 10 (S1),* 73 (Published online January 31, 2005).

Litvan, I., Grafman, J., Vendrell, P., & Martinez, J. M. (1988). Slowed information processing in multiple sclerosis. *Archives of Neurology, 45* (3), 281–285.

Lublin, F. D., & Reingold, S. C. (1996). Defining the clinical course of multiple sclerosis: Results of an international survey. National Multiple Sclerosis Society (USA) Advisory Committee on Clinical Trials of New Agents in Multiple Sclerosis. *Neurology, 46* (4), 907–911.

Maurelli, M., Marchioni, E., Cerretano, R., Bosone, D., Bergamaschi, R., Citterio, A., et al. (1992). Neuropsychological assessment in MS: Clinical, neurophysiological and neuroradiological relationships. *Acta Neurologica Scandinavica, 86* (2), 124–128.

Morgen, K., Sammer, G., Courtney, S. M., Wolters, T., Melchior, H., Blecker, C. R., et al. (2006). Evidence for a direct association between cortical atrophy and cognitive impairment in relapsing-remitting MS. *Neuroimage, 30* (3), 891–898.

Nocentini, U., Pasqualetti, P., Bonavita, S., Buccafusca, M., De Caro, M. F., Farina, D., et al. (2006). Cognitive dysfunction in patients with relapsing–remitting multiple sclerosis. *Multiple Sclerosis, 12* (1), 77–87.

Oken, B. S., Flegal, K., Zajdel, D., Kishiyama, S. S., Lovera, J., Bagert, B., et al. (2006). Cognition and fatigue in multiple sclerosis: Potential effects of medications with central nervous system activity. *Journal of Rehabilitation Research Development, 43* (1), 83–90.

Olivares, T., Nieto, A., Sanchez, M. P., Wollmann, T., Hernandez, M. A., & Barroso, J. (2005). Pattern of neuropsychological impairment in the early phase of relapsing–remitting multiple sclerosis. *Multiple Sclerosis, 11* (2), 191–197.

Paul, R. H., Beatty, W. W., Schneider, R., Blanco, C., & Hames, K. (1998). Impairments of attention in individuals with multiple sclerosis. *Multiple Sclerosis, 4* (5), 433–439.

Peyser, J. M., Rao, S. M., LaRocca, N. G., & Kaplan, E. (1990). Guidelines for neuropsychological research in multiple sclerosis. *Archives of Neurology, 47* (1), 94–97.

Randolph, J. J., Wishart, H. A., Saykin, A. J., McDonald, B. C., Schuschu, K. R., MacDonald, J. W., et al. (2005). FLAIR lesion volume in multiple sclerosis: Relation to processing speed and verbal memory. *Journal of the International Neuropsychological Society, 11* (2), 205–209.

Rao, S. M. (1997). Neuropsychological aspects of multiple sclerosis. In C. S. Raine, H. F. McFarland, & W. W. Tourtellotte (Eds.), *Multiple sclerosis: Clinical and pathogenic basis* (pp. 357–362). London: Chapman & Hall.

Rao, S. M., Leo, G. J., Bernardin, L., & Unverzagt, F. (1991). Cognitive dysfunction in multiple sclerosis. I. Frequency, patterns, and prediction. *Neurology, 41* (5), 685–691.

Rao, S. M., Leo, G. J., Haughton, V. M., St Aubin-Faubert, P., & Bernardin, L. (1989). Correlation of magnetic resonance imaging with neuropsychological testing in multiple sclerosis. *Neurology, 39* (2, Pt 1), 161–166.

Rao, S. M., St Aubin-Faubert, P., & Leo, G. J. (1989). Information processing speed in patients with multiple sclerosis. *Journal of Clinical and Experimental Neuropsychology, 11* (4), 471–477.

Rumrill, P. D., Kaleta, D. A., & Battersby, J. C. (1996). Etiology, incidence, and prevalence. In P. D. Rumrill (Ed.), *Employment issues and multiple sclerosis*. New York: Demos Vermande.

Sailer, M., Heinze, H. J., Schoenfeld, M. A., Hauser, U., & Smid, H. G. (2000). Amantadine influences cognitive processing in patients with multiple sclerosis. *Pharmacopsychiatry, 33* (1), 28–37.

Schulz, D., Kopp, B., Kunkel, A., & Faiss, J. H. (2006). Cognition in the early stage of multiple sclerosis. *Journal of Neurology, 253* (8), 1002–1010.

Snyder, P. J., & Cappelleri, J. C. (2001). Information processing speed deficits may be better correlated with the extent of white matter sclerotic lesions in multiple sclerosis than previously suspected. *Brain and Cognition, 46* (1–2), 279–284.

Snyder, P. J., Cappelleri, J. C., Archibald, C. J., & Fisk, J. D. (2001). Improved detection of differential information-processing speed deficits between two disease-course types of multiple sclerosis. *Neuropsychology, 15* (4), 617–625.

Sperling, R. A., Guttmann, C. R., Hohol, M. J., Warfield, S. K., Jakab, M., Parente, M., et al. (2001). Regional magnetic resonance imaging lesion burden and cognitive function in multiple sclerosis: A longitudinal study. *Archives of Neurology, 58* (1), 115–121.

Swirsky-Sacchetti, T., Field, H. L., Mitchell, D. R., Seward, J., Lublin, F. D., Knobler, R. L., et al. (1992). The sensitivity of the Mini-Mental State Exam in the white matter dementia of multiple sclerosis. *Journal of Clinical Psychology, 48* (6), 779–786.

Trapp, B. D., Peterson, J., Ransohoff, R. M., Rudick, R., Mork, S., & Bo, L. (1998). Axonal transection in the lesions of multiple sclerosis. *New England Journal of Medicine, 338* (5), 278–285.

Wechsler, D. (1997). *Wechsler Adult Intelligence Scale—Third Edition*. San Antonio, TX: The Psychological Corporation.

8 Traumatic brain injury and processing speed

Glynda J. Kinsella

Although prevalence rates vary across countries, traumatic brain injury (TBI) is the most common cause of death and morbidity in young people (Baguley, Slewa-Younan, Lazarus, & Green, 2000; Gharjar, 2000; Kraus & McArthur, 1996), and cognitive disability is a common outcome (Satz et al., 1998). The significance of this point is that TBI represents a major community health-risk in our society, and persisting cognitive deficit reduces quality of life and goal-attainment for many young adults surviving trauma (Cifu et al., 1997; Mazaux, Masson, Levin, Alaoui, Maurette, & Barat, 1997; Prigatano, 1987). Isolating the nature of trauma-related cognitive impairment is critical in directing effective approaches in rehabilitation and supporting ongoing management of residual sequelae of trauma.

Slowing in processing speed has been identified as one of the most pervasive of cognitive changes post-TBI and impacts on performance of everyday tasks and activities (Ponsford & Kinsella, 1991; Stuss, Stethem, Picton, Leech, & Pelchat, 1989). In this chapter, I first introduce issues within TBI that are relevant to an appraisal of processing speed within this clinical population; I then review the research relating to processing speed and TBI; and finally, I consider the impact of slowing in processing speed in relation to performance of everyday activities following TBI.

Traumatic brain injury

Heterogeneity of injury within a clinical sample

Severity of traumatic injury may range from simple concussion and rapid recovery to lengthy periods of unconsciousness and post-traumatic amnesia (PTA), which can persist for days or months and is associated with major ongoing psychosocial deficits. A simple estimation of severity of injury is notoriously difficult to determine but a common guiding method is by use of the Glasgow Coma Scale (GCS), which provides an internationally accepted method for documenting the presence, degree, and duration of coma (Jennett & Bond, 1975; Lezak, Howieson, & Loring, 2004). Using the GCS, severity of injury can be classified into three general categories: severe injury (a score of 8 or less), moderate injury (a score of 9–12), and mild injury (a score of 13–15). By no means perfect, the GCS has been found to offer some prediction of outcome (Asikainen, Kaste, & Sarna, 1998; Felmingham, Baguley, & Crooks, 2001; Levin et al., 1990; Ponsford, Olver, Curran, & Ng, 1995b). In clinical practice, the GCS is frequently combined with clinical signs of neurological abnormality and duration of post-traumatic amnesia to provide more information about severity of injury (Lezak et al., 2004).

Although most cases of mild injuries have been considered to produce transient cognitive impairment (Binder, Rohling, & Larrabee, 1997; Dikmen, McClean, & Temkin, 1986; Schretlen & Shapiro, 2003), a minority will continue to demonstrate troubling cognitive outcomes at long-term follow-up (Vanderploeg, Curtiss, & Belanger, 2005). In contrast, moderate to severe injuries are consistently associated with a range of cognitive problems that tend to persist over time (Levin et al., 1990; Olver, Ponsford, & Curran, 1996; Ponsford, Olver, & Curran, 1995a; Tate & Broe, 1999; Teasdale & Engberg, 2005). By implication, the severity of the injury and the timing of the assessment post-injury will demand different interpretations of obtained data from test performance (Sherer, Sander, Nick, High, Malec, Rosenthal, 2002; Shum, McFarland, Bain, & Humphreys, 1990). The variation in severity of TBI and factors moderating neuropsychological outcomes makes comparisons across studies of outcome a complex process (Belanger, Curtiss, Demery, Lebowitz, & Vanderploeg, 2005; Tate & Broe, 1999). Nevertheless, a majority of the research suggests a dose–response relationship between severity of injury and neuropsychological outcome (Kesler, Adams, & Bigler, 2000).

Underlying neuropathology

In most countries, road traffic accidents continue to be the leading cause of TBI (Baguley et al., 2000), accounting for approximately 60% of presenting cases (Hillier, Hiller, & Metzer, 1997). Consequently, as extreme, rapid, acceleration–deceleration forces contribute to the majority of TBI, the nature of TBI pathology is not only reflective of localized damage (contusions, haemorrhages, etc.) but also of significant diffuse lesions throughout the brain leading to complex pathology (Adams, Graham, & Jennett, 2001; Blumbergs, Scott, Manavis, Wainwright, Simpson, & McLean, 1994; Fork, Bartels, Ebert, Grubich, Synowitz, & Wallesch, 2005; Strich, 1969). Furthermore, physiological changes are frequently disruptive (Bigler, 2001a); and although the relationship between neurochemical change and neuropsychological deficit is still evolving, involvement of the cholinergic system is identified as contributory to cognitive sequelae (Salmond, Chatfield, Menon, Pickard, & Sahakian, 2005).

Bigler (2001a) reviews the neuropathology of TBI by first separating the acute and chronic effects. Acute effects revolve around contusions, haemorrhages, oedema, and shearing of nerve fibres, predominantly in the inferior frontal and antero-temporal lobes (Walsh, 1985). An outcome of these acute changes is the development of non-specific abnormality affecting the fronto-temporal poles (Fork et al., 2005; Gentry, Godersky, & Thompson, 1988; Gurdijan & Gurdijan, 1976; Kesler et al., 2000). Diffuse axonal injury occurs in the white matter of the brain as a consequence of the mechanical shaking and rotational forces projected on the brainstem and brain within the skull at the time of the injury, thereby producing shearing injuries. Diffuse axonal injury was initially considered a key characteristic of more severe injuries, however recent investigations (Fork et al., 2005; Mittl et al., 1994) have demonstrated evidence of the presence of diffuse axonal injury in milder cases of injury (GCS > 13, loss of consciousness < 20 minutes), supporting the view of a broad dose–response relationship between the severity of the injury and the extent of diffuse axonal injury (Fork et al., 2005; Gentry et al., 1988). Diffuse axonal injury is disruptive of subcortical white matter, providing the neural substrate for aspects of the neuropsychological changes associated with TBI (Felmingham, Baguley, & Green, 2004: Fork et al., 2005).

Common cognitive outcomes

Considering the diffuse nature of injury, a range of presenting deficits post-TBI are expected, however impairments in episodic memory, working memory, executive attention, and cognitive slowing tend to dominate neuropsychological outcome. Working memory is most easily articulated in the model provided by Baddeley and colleagues (Baddeley, 2001; Baddeley & Hitch, 2000; Baddeley & Logie, 1999), and describes a system consisting of multiple specialized components of cognition that allow humans to formulate and act on current goals through both an executive attentional control system (central executive) and specialized temporary memory storage systems (slave systems). Executive attention (in this chapter the term is used to represent the central executive of working memory) is closely associated with prefrontal regions (D'Esposito & Postle, 2002) and output is determined by a combination of skills including focusing attention and inhibiting distraction, switching attention, dividing attention, and activating representations within long-term memory (Baddeley, 2001). Some degree of deficit in episodic memory (Curtiss, Vanderploeg, Spencer, & Salazar, 2001; DeLuca, Schultheis, Madigan, Christodoulou, & Averill, 2000, Levin et al., 1990), working memory and attention (Leclercq et al., 2000; McDowell, Whyte, & D'Esposito, 1997; Perlstein et al., 2004), including dual-task performance (McDowell et al., 1997; Park, Moscovitch, & Robertson, 1999; Perlstein et al., 2004), and slowing in processing speed (Ponsford & Kinsella, 1992; Spikman, van der Naalt, van Weerden, & van Zomeren, 2004; van Zomeren & Brouwer, 1994) have been commonly reported cognitive outcomes from TBI, irrespective of severity of injury (Robertson, Manly, Andrade, Baddlely, & Yiend, 1997; van Zomeren & van den Berg, 1985; Whyte, Polansky, Fleming, Coslett, & Cavallucci, 1995); however, residual deficits in the post-acute phase of recovery are generally only associated with at least moderate to severe injury, and measures of pre-injury sociodemographic variables are also important predictors of long-term outcome (Hoofien, Vakils, Gilboa, Donovick, & Barak, 2002; Tate & Broe, 1999).

Given the common underlying neuropathology of frontotemporal dysfunction and diffuse axonal injury, the presence of memory and executive attention deficits is intuitively understandable. Nevertheless, the nature of the memory and attention deficit is disputed, and for many the presence of difficulties in tasks assessing executive attention (controlled processing) or complex memory and new learning has been explainable by a generic model of slowing in processing speed (Chiaravalloti, Christodoulou, Demaree, & DeLuca, 2003; Madigan, DeLuca, Diamond, Tramontano, & Averill, 2000; Ponsford & Kinsella, 1992; van Zomeren & Brouwer, 1994).

Within this approach there is an assumption that more difficult tasks require more processing, and therefore will be more likely to show TBI effects as a result of slowing in the speed of processing. This provides a test of the processing speed hypothesis of injury effects. If processing speed is operative in TBI deficits, as a task becomes more complex and demands more processing it would be expected that the more complex tasks will be performed more slowly than simpler tasks. If there is no interaction found between groups and task difficulty this would be consistent with a generalized slowing effect affecting TBI participants. Alternatively, if an interaction is found across groups and task difficulty this would suggest that, in addition to processing speed issues, a separate component of cognition is operative.

Traumatic brain injury and slowing in processing speed

Slowness in processing information has been identified as one of the most disruptive cognitive consequence of TBI by several research groups (Azouvi, Jovik, Van der Linden, Marlier, & Bussel, 1996; Madigan et al., 2000; Mathias, Beall, & Bigler, 2004; Ponsford & Kinsella, 1992; Spikman et al., 2004; Stuss et al., 1989; van Zomeren & Brouwer, 1994). Slowing in processing speed has been proposed to be reflected in the invariant presence of diffuse axonal injury in significant TBI, either by diffuse cell loss demanding indirect neural transmission, or from reduced dendritic branching or loss of myelination resulting in slower transmission (Bigler, 2001b; Felmingham et al., 2004; van Zomeren & Brouwer, 1994). Speed of processing information is not a unidimensional concept. Within the field of cognitive ageing, Salthouse and colleagues (1996, 2000) provide an influential model to interpret processing speed and its impact on cognitive tasks (see also chapter 10 in this volume). Salthouse (1996) proposed that there are at least two ways in which processing speed impacts on cognition: *a limited time mechanism* or *a simultaneity mechanism*. Limited time in performing the operations of complex cognitive tasks suggests that the time to perform later operations will be impacted or restricted when a significant proportion of the time available for task completion is devoted to completion of the preliminary steps of the process. The *simultaneity process* suggests that the outcomes of early processing will be lost by the time the later processing of task demands is completed. Applying these concepts to performance on many neuropsychological tests could explain poor performance by TBI patients who are often slow in performing early stages of a complex task, and this can result in later stages never being reached because earlier operations or stages are no longer accessible. The impact of slowing in processing speed is assumed to be global, and will impact on tasks even if they are not overtly timed.

However, researchers have proposed that variation in the tests or approaches used to assess processing speed contributes to ongoing ambiguity in interpretation of results across studies. Via factor analysis of commonly used tests of information processing speed, Chiaravalloti et al. (2003) contrasted reaction time measures and a complex measure of information processing speed requiring divided attention (the Paced Serial Addition Test, PASAT; Gronwall & Wrightson, 1981), and reported that these processing speed measures did not load on a single factor. They interpreted this by arguing that reaction time measures require recognition of a stimulus and a simple motor response, whereas measures such as the PASAT need more complex mental manipulation requiring greater cognitive resources, including both speed and working memory. Chiaravalloti et al. (2003) propose that the demands in complex information processing speed tasks such as PASAT include the additional coordinating functions of executive attention of working memory, although this is either not required or minimally required for simple reaction time measures. This conceptualization of processing speed as multifactorial provides the basis for the expectation that persons with TBI may cope effectively with the demands in measures of *simple* processing speed, whereas they may show impairments on *complex* tasks of information processing.

Speed–accuracy trade-off

An important methodological aspect of assessing processing speed in any demanding cognitive task is that varying the speed of response required in the task can impact on the accuracy of the response, and vice versa. For example, impairment in speed of processing can lead to errors as there is less time for efficient encoding of information and slower retrieval of accurate information. A trade-off between these two components of task response can occur such that accuracy on the task can be maintained if speed of processing is sacrificed, or alternatively efficient speed in task performance can be maintained if task performance is less regulated, leading to an increase in errors.

In an early study (Ponsford & Kinsella, 1992) we addressed this issue by comparing a series of 47 participants with severe TBI and an orthopaedically injured control group on a range of neuropsychological tasks to index processing speed in reaction time measures and executive attention tasks. As expected, we found that there was a large and significant effect of group status so that the TBI group were identifiably slower than the healthy controls across all the tasks. However, when error scores across the tasks were compared for groups, the only significant effect was in the PASAT, which was the most cognitively demanding task, requiring executive attention skills of working memory. From these results of slower but no less accurate performance for the TBI participants, we suggested that a trade-off in performance may be occurring for the TBI groups, and they were sacrificing speed for accuracy in performance. A problem with this research was that in the single task in which errors occurred in accuracy as well as speed, the PASAT, the speed of the task was controlled externally so that participants were unable to sacrifice speed of performance to achieve grater accuracy; which may have been the strategy used on the less cognitively demanding tasks.

Using a more controlled paradigm to carefully manipulate speed and accuracy task demands, Madigan et al. (2000) compared response to task demands by 22 participants with moderate to severe TBI and 20 healthy adult controls. Their approach was to control for accuracy of response in the first instance so that speed of response could be directly measured. They designed a task to measure processing speed by adjusting the presentation rate on a serial addition task, similar to the procedure used in the PASAT (Brittain, La Marche, Reeder, Roth, & Boll, 1991) to achieve a performance criterion for accuracy. This criterion was indexed by varying the duration of the interstimulus interval to identify the optimal interval at which each participant could correctly respond to at least 50% of the trials. This was referred to as threshold speed and was argued to index processing speed while controlling for accuracy of performance (Madigan et al., 2000). Using this approach, the authors were able to confirm that even after accounting for response accuracy, TBI participants were substantially slower than healthy adults on the serial addition task.

Furthermore, in order to directly evaluate whether performance at an individual's optimum threshold speed would improve accuracy, the researchers administered an additional task condition in which they assessed performance using the participant's threshold speed, so that the serial-addition task was performed at each participant's optimal processing speed. As a consequence they found that performance did not differ between the two groups, indicating that if given sufficient time to respond, participants with TBI were generally able to respond accurately. As the researchers suggested, these results provide encouragement for focusing rehabilitation effort post-TBI towards modifying environmental or task demand so that the processing speed demand is self-paced, thereby allowing sufficient time for accuracy of response.

Slowing and stages in information processing

Research has provided conflicting results in relation to attempts to characterize the stage at which slowing in information processing post-TBI is considered to be maximal. There are various models of information processing but Shum et al. (1990) based their investigation of post-TBI information processing on Sternberg's (1969) additive structural model (see Figure 8.1). In this model there is an assumption of four discrete stages in information processing: stimulus encoding and memory comparisons (these are input stages concerning the identification and selection of relevant stimuli), decision-making and response selection (these are output stages concerning the selection of the response). This type of model assumes that stages can be manipulated independently and Shum et al. (1990) found in their study of cognitive consequences following severe TBI, that patients in the acute phase of recovery (less than 1 year after injury) were impaired (slower reaction time) in both the identification and output response-selection phase of tasks, whereas chronic patients (more than 1 year after injury) were impaired only in the output response-selection phase; thereby suggesting a recovery in speed of information processing of attentional tasks over time post-injury.

However, there has been some dissonance in reports of the stages in information processing in which slowing of processing speed is apparent post-TBI (Schmitter-Edgecombe, Marks, Fahy, & Long, 1992). Slowness in processing speed post-TBI has been reported to affect each stage of information processing, but is especially evident in tasks in which the demands are complex and time pressure is increased (Ponsford & Kinsella, 1992; Stuss et al., 1989). Gron (1996) concluded that although slowing may be apparent across information processing stages post-TBI, it can generally be found that with increasing task complexity the impairment post-TBI becomes greater, and therefore the output stages of decision making and response selection appear to contribute more to the slowing in the final task response. In reality, this is another example of the interaction between processing speed and accuracy of performance (i.e., decreased accuracy with increased task demands).

Spikman et al. (2004) investigated this issue further by evaluating the performance of 44 participants with moderate to severe TBI and 36 healthy adults on a range of neuropsychological tests of simple and complex attention tasks, which provided speed of information processing indices, and also

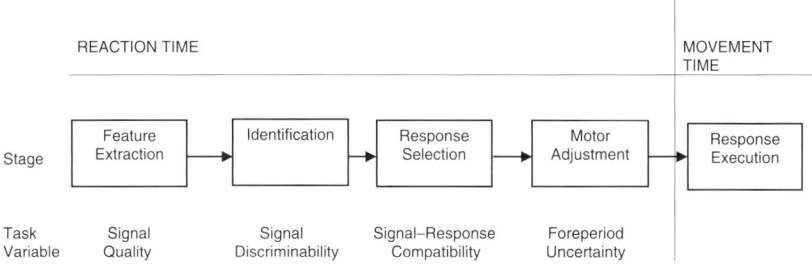

Figure 8.1 Diagram of the four stages of information processing and task variables (reprinted from Shum, McFarland, Bain, & Humphreys, 1990).

recorded event-related potentials during an auditory task using an oddball paradigm. All the neuropsychological tests were described as being performed under time pressure, and the TBI group were found to be generally slower across tasks than the healthy adults. However, by comparing the event-related potentials during task performance, and relating these to indices of severity of injury and neuropsychological test performance, the results were interpreted to suggest that TBI does affect the input stage of information processing through slowing in the identification and evaluation of a stimulus; that is, feature analysis. However, this was only apparent on neuropsychological tests that the researchers argued emphasized the stimulus evaluation processes or encoding stage of information processing, and did not require significant attention to output-related processes; for example, the colour trial of the Stroop test in which study participants were simply required to name ink patches of colour as quickly as possible. In contrast, the researchers argued that most neuropsychological tests, for example, the colour–word interference trial of the Stroop in which the participant is required to name the colour of the ink in which incongruent colour words are printed, emphasize the output-related processes in information processing, and consequently slowness in these stages disguises the slowing in earlier input-related stages, and appears to be the major determinant of performance. However, it should be noted that many of the clinical tests used within the study have not been originally designed to isolate discrete aspects of information processing; therefore, interpretation of the precise localization of dysfunction in information processing through analysis of performance on clinical measures can be problematic (Stuss et al., 2005). Nevertheless, Spikman et al. (2004) concluded that their results confirm the argument of Gron (1996) that persons in the chronic phase post-TBI as compared to healthy controls are slower in both the input- and the output-related stages of information processing. It would be expected that this would also be apparent in the acute phase post-injury.

Variability in severity of injury and slowing in processing speed

Slowing in processing speed has been predominantly demonstrated following moderate to severe TBI, and it has been questioned whether such deficits will be apparent following less severe injuries (Madigan et al., 2000). Van Zomeren & Brouwer (1994) have suggested that slowing following TBI results from shearing of long, white matter nerve fibres. If this is the case, it may be argued that the extent of shearing in mild cases of TBI is insufficient to significantly impact on processing speed. However, a recent case study (Bigler, 2004) of a 47-year-old male who, 7 months prior to an unexpected death, had sustained a mild TBI, provides support for slowed processing speed following mild TBI. Microscopic analysis at autopsy was able to demonstrate observable shearing and disruption of white matter, thereby suggesting a neuronal basis for the reported complaint of insidious cognitive change in everyday tasks, as well as slowness on neuropsychological tests and lowered performance on the initial encoding trial of list-learning on a verbal learning task (Bigler, 2004). These data would suggest that it is the extent of the "shearing" and not the initial level of TBI severity as defined by measures such as loss of consciousness or post-traumatic amnesia that is important in determining processing speed impairment (van Zomeren & Brouwer, 1994; Felmingham et al., 2004).

Relationship between processing speed and executive attention of working memory in TBI

An interesting question is whether cognitive impairments following TBI can be explained by slowing in processing speed, or whether additional deficits in cognition, specifically executive attentional control of working memory, can be observed. To a certain extent the answer to this question is yet to be determined through large-scale modelling of post-TBI cognition, although preliminary research is providing some direction. Attention post-TBI has been described as relatively preserved at the more automatic level (Schmitter-Edgecombe & Beglinger, 2001; van Zomeren & Brouwer, 1994), whereas deficits have been reported in tasks that require attentional allocation or executive attention of working memory (McDowell et al., 1997; Park et al., 1999; Perlstein et al., 2004; Rios, Perianez, & Munoz-Cespedes, 2004; Zoccolotti et al., 2000). Executive attention can be fractionated into different roles or sub-processes that include focusing attention and inhibition, dividing attention (dual-tasking), and set-shifting (Baddeley, 2001); but although performance on various attention-demanding tasks that require different sub-processes of executive attention have been demonstrated post-TBI, researchers have frequently been unable to demonstrate a significant attention allocation deficit once accounting for slowing in processing speed (Madigan et al., 2000; Spikman, van Zomeren, & Deelman, 1996; Spikman, Deelman, & van Zomeren, 2000). This raises the question as to whether the decline in performance on executive attention-demanding tasks simply reflects task difficulty.

Support for the centrality of processing speed deficits post-TBI in comparison to an index of general working memory deficits (including executive attention), is provided by Martin, Donders, and Thompson (2000) who found in a sample of 60 participants with TBI that although WAIS-III Full Scale IQ was not able to distinguish between participants with mild versus moderate to severe injuries, the WAIS-III Processing Speed index was the only one of the WAIS-III indices, including the Working Memory index, to be able to detect a significant effect of injury severity. However, in a recent study, Rios et al. (2004) reported on the performance of 29 patients with severe TBI and 30 healthy controls on three neuropsychological tests commonly used clinically to index different roles of executive attention (Wisconsin Card Sorting Test, Trail Making Test, and the Stroop Test). Covariance analysis was used to interpret the importance of slowness in the TBI patients' difficulties on these measures of executive attention. The researchers found that although slowing in processing speed partially explained impaired performance on these tests, their results also suggested that additional aspects of impaired cognition were being assessed within the executive attention tasks. Specifically, they found that some patients following TBI were impaired on a task that assessed set-shifting ability in attention (Trail Making Test); that is, the capacity for shifting between one schema of action to another. In contrast, slowing in processing speed was sufficient to explain group differences on a measure of focused attention and capacity to resist interference (the Stroop Test). This study provides preliminary evidence to suggest that in addition to slowing in processing speed, executive attention dysfunction may be present after TBI; and yet these impairments in executive attention may be specific rather than general—a potential difficulty in attention set-shifting rather than focused attention and capacity to resist interference. This suggestion waits to be reliably supported.

Further argument for selective deficits in executive attention in addition to slowness in processing speed has been provided by the dual-task methodology to investigate capacity for divided attention. Using this approach a number of researchers have reported poorer performances in TBI populations as compared to control participants (Azouvi et al., 1996; Leclerq et al., 2000; McDowell et al., 1997; Park et al., 1999; van Zomeren & Brouwer, 1994; Zoccolotti et al., 2000). However, as noted by Perlstein et al. (2004), many of the dual-task paradigms have also obtained group differences on the individual tasks when performed singly (baseline), thereby creating ambiguity in the interpretation of dual-task performance when the tasks are performed simultaneously. Furthermore, Park et al. (1999) also note that the effects of dual-task performance are only reliably demonstrated when both tasks place demand on executive attention or controlled processing, whereas deficits in dual-task performance are not observed post-TBI when the individual tasks can be achieved relatively automatically.

In conclusion, it is indisputable that processing speed is a pervasive impairment invariably impacting on cognitive performance post-TBI, and as tasks become more cognitively complex and the number of cognitive operations to be completed increases, processing speed is further slowed. Nevertheless, a body of research is arguing that although significant TBI-related variance in neuropsychological test performance is mediated by processing speed, speed also operates through executive attention of working memory and this can provide an additional contribution to performance. In addition to the number of cognitive operations to be completed, the nature or type of cognitive operation is also critical to successful task performance (Park et al., 1999; Rios et al., 2004).

Recovery

Schretlen and Shapiro (2003) reported from a meta-analysis of 39 studies of the cognitive effects of mild to severe TBI from the acute phase to long-term follow-up, that findings generally suggest that cognitive functioning recovers most rapidly during the first few weeks following mild TBI and broadly returns to baseline within 1–3 months; cognitive functioning also improves during the first 2 years after moderate to severe TBI, but remains significantly impaired among patients even assessed > 2 years post-injury. Although long-term follow-up studies of TBI have generally reported persisting problems in terms of neuropsychological deficit and psychosocial impairment (Olver et al., 1996; Teasdale & Engberg, 2005), there is limited information available about the specific recovery patterns of speed of processing. However, Millis et al. (2001), in a study reporting on neuropsychological outcome up to 5 years after injury in persons with TBI who received inpatient rehabilitation, found that although neuropsychological recovery is highly variable across individuals and neuropsychological domains, improvement from 1–5 years post-injury was most apparent on measures of cognitive speed (Trail Making Test), visuoconstruction, and verbal memory. Furthermore, Haslam, Batchelor, Fearnside, Haslam, Hawkins, and Kenway (1994) reported that length of initial PTA predicted processing speed 1 year post-injury; that is, the severity of injury was the most useful predictor of performance status in slowing of processing speed at follow-up.

Within a study that demonstrated the relationship between slowed processing speed in TBI and the presence of diffuse axonal injury, Felmingham et al. (2004) reported that patients with diffuse axonal injury showed proportionally greater recovery in processing speed between 1 and 5 months post-injury than patients with predominantly focal lesions (mixed TBI) or controls. By 5 months post-injury, the patients with axonal injury had reached equivalent levels of performance to the mixed TBI group on tasks of basic processing speed (Stroop reading task and the Symbol Digit Modalities test), although impaired speed of processing on more complex tasks was still evident (Trail Making Test-B, Stroop colour–word task, Complex RT tasks). Felmingham et al. suggested that although initial cognitive presentation of patients with diffuse axonal injury may be low, they can recover basic processing speed over the sub-acute period and by 5 months post-injury can reach a level of performance at which they may benefit from interventions as prescribed for less severely injured patients.

Although early improvement in test performance has been reported, persisting impairments in processing speed are still apparent at the post-acute phase. Spikman et al. (2000) reported that patients with TBI in a chronic stage (2–5 years) post-injury are still impaired on reaction time measures. However, importantly, differences were only apparent on those reaction time tasks in which time pressure could not be compensated for by using efficient response procedures or strategies. In tasks in which time-pressure demands were still evident but there was an opportunity to manage this time pressure by using specific strategies, the patients were not impaired compared to controls. Spikman et al. suggested that although the patients with TBI are still slower in processing information, in tasks that allow them to manage the speed demand by developing strategies or procedures, the patients will perform at an equivalent level to controls. As the researchers note, their findings are important in relation to prediction of performance in everyday activities. For example, certain everyday tasks such as cleaning the house can be complex but can also be self-paced.

These studies provide some support for the view that processing speed can improve over time post-TBI, at least by the development of strategies of compensation in tasks in which opportunity for such strategies is created. This provides the foundation for considering interventions for improving processing speed.

Processing speed and implications for management

Intervention

As slowness in processing speed is such a common problem post-TBI, and the impact on everyday activities is clear to observe, attempts at remediation strategies have been targeted. Direct treatment of processing speed can be both cognitive-behavioural and pharmacological. In an early cognitive-behavioural study (Ponsford & Kinsella, 1988) we evaluated a computer-mediated cognitive training programme to improve speed of information processing for 10 patients following severe TBI. Once spontaneous recovery and practice effects were accounted for, significant treatment effects were not found. Nevertheless, we did observe considerable individual differences in response to aspects of the programme. Similarly, individual variation in neuropsychological recovery (including information processing speed) has been noted by many researchers (e.g., Hetherington, Stuss, & Finlayson, 1996; Millis et al., 2001), and this needs to be considered when evaluating response to treatment.

A more recent study by Fasotti, Kovacs, Eling, and Brouwer (2001) evaluated a time-pressure management strategy that was based on a set of cognitive strategies that could be used to compensate for the consequences of slow information processing in daily activities, for example in preparing a meal. Twenty-two participants with severe to very severe TBI were assigned to either the experimental group (time-pressure management) or the control group (concentration training) in a randomized pre-, post- and follow-up group study. In the time-pressure management intervention, using a framework of hierarchical task analysis, participants learned strategies to give themselves enough time to deal with the required task, and this approach was compared with concentration training. Both training conditions were found to improve performance on a task that involved listening to a videotaped story with instructions to remember as much information as possible. However, time-pressure management was found to lead to greater gains than concentration training, and also generalized to measures of speed of processing and memory function. As processing speed deficits post-TBI have been consistently reported in tasks under time pressure, the utility of this approach is noteworthy. A similar view was reported by Cicerone (2002), who found that an intervention for attention deficits in participants with mild TBI was effective as measured by the ability to temporally maintain and manipulate information during task performance, but in this study had no direct effect on processing speed. Cicerone suggested that the benefit of the training is in relation to improved ability to compensate for residual slowing by consciously adopting strategies for more effective allocation of remaining attention resources, thereby reducing time-pressure demands in task performance. The importance of a speed–accuracy trade-off has been argued by Madigan et al. (2000) in a study reported earlier in this chapter. Madigan et al. found that when participants with TBI performed a task at their optimal processing speed, their accuracy on task performance did not differ from that of healthy controls.

One of the few controlled medication studies is reported by Whyte et al. (2004), who investigated the effects of methylphenidate on attention deficits and processing speed after TBI. Thirty-four adults with moderate to severe TBI in the post-acute phase of recovery were enrolled in a 6-week, double-blind study of methylphenidate. A range of attention and processing speed measures were administered weekly, as well as behavioural observations during the programme and caregiver (family) and research staff ratings of attention in everyday life. Out of 13 test factors, the three factors that showed an intervention effect were speed of information processing, attentiveness during individual work tasks, and family ratings of attention, with effect sizes in the small to medium range. In relation to a speed–accuracy trade-off, improved processing speed was not associated with a significant lowering in accuracy. No intervention effect was noted in divided attention, sustained attention, or susceptibility to distraction. Whyte et al. conclude that methylphenidate can produce clinically significant positive effects on speed of processing following moderate to severe TBI. Importantly, they comment that this effect impacts not only on laboratory-based tasks but also on ability to attend to naturalistic tasks and everyday behaviour as assessed by families on attention rating scales. From this encouraging result, the researchers advocate further clinical trials on larger samples.

Driving

Loss of capacity to drive has a significant impact on ability to maintain independence within society and represents a critical functional skill that can be jeopardized by the cognitive consequences of TBI (Brouwer, Withaar, Tant, & van Zomeren, 2002; Olver et al., 1996). For example, Kreutzer et al. (2003) reported from a 4-year follow-up of 186 TBI survivors (aged

18–26 years at injury) that driving independence was highly influential and significantly related to post-injury employment stability.

Neuropsychological test performances are frequently reviewed in order to assist in the process of determining fitness to drive post-TBI. Processing speed, as indicated by reaction time measures, provides a modest ability to predict specific driving skills and yet, as Brouwer & Withaar (1997) aptly commented, it is not whether we can predict how fast a driver someone may be but the safety of the driving behaviour. It may not be the operational level of driving (elementary driving skills) that is critical in evaluating competence in driving post-TBI, but the tactical skills of driving (judgement of traffic situations and anticipatory risk avoidance). Van Zomeren & Brouwer (1994) argue that judgement of fitness to drive requires caution as there are many opportunities to compensate during driving for noted deficits in processing speed, for example deciding to drive only outside the rush hour, and only in low density streets. They argue that driving is an expert skill and highly practised throughout our lives, therefore level of pre-injury driving skills will necessarily exert a moderating influence between presenting cognitive impairment and driving performance post-TBI, and many studies have demonstrated that poor test performance is not necessarily related to poor driving. However, this argument may be lessened by the consideration that the TBI population tends to be dominated by young inexperienced drivers, therefore maintaining driving skill is particularly at risk in a TBI population because driving has not necessarily become a skilled behaviour.

The Useful Field of View is a measure of visual information processing that has been found to be a good predictor of vehicle crash risk in older adults. Fisk, Novack, Mennemeier, and Roenker (2002) evaluated the Useful Field of View within a sample of survivors of TBI as compared to healthy young adults, and found that, as predicted, survivors of TBI have a more constrained Useful Field of View. They argued that the Useful Field of View may be used as a predictor for assessing driving readiness following TBI. Nevertheless, as with so many other clinical measures, this test is multifaceted and requires at least three cognitive processes: ability to divide attention, ability to avoid distracters, and processing speed (Park & Gutchess, 2000). Clinically, it will be important to disentangle which component aspect of cognition is the most potent in test performance. For example, Lengenfelder, Schultheis, Al-Schihabi, Mourant, and DeLuca (2002) have provided some preliminary information about the use of virtual reality technology in investigating the relationship between specific features of driving performance (divided attention) and performance on neuropsychological tests. They found that through analysing performance on a virtual reality driving task by three individuals with TBI as compared to three healthy controls, there were no differences in driving speed between the groups; however, TBI participants made more errors on secondary tasks (divided attention tasks) while driving. This development in analysis of component skills in driving is important if driving training is to be considered.

Brouwer and Withaar (1997) argue that neuropsychological testing, including indexing processing speed, for fitness to drive post-TBI should not only be used as a hurdle requirement for regaining a licence, but should also be used more productively for providing direction for driving education. Brouwer et al. (2002) report on training in time-pressure management using a hierarchical task analysis that separates driving skill into different levels of response. They argue that on the operational level there is insufficient opportunity for compensation, and even though this is the level of driving in which processing speed deficits post-TBI will emerge, it doesn't necessarily lead to unsafe driving practices if the tactical level allows for compensation. Brouwer et al. and other researchers are arguing that in relation to driving post-TBI, speed of processing is necessarily an important cognitive resource to consider, but additional skills, including dividing attention and maintaining focused attention against distractions, are critical features of determining ongoing cognitive competence to drive.

Employment

Sherer et al. (2002) reviewed 23 studies of the relationship between neuropsychological test results and employment outcome after TBI, and concluded that there is strong support for the use of early (but not late) neuropsychological assessment to predict late employment outcome. However, as there was a wide range of neuropsychological measures used in the various studies, the investigators were unable to determine which neuropsychological tests may be most predictive, demanding a larger sample to address the question. Preliminary information about the role of speed of processing was provided in an early study by van Zomeren & van den Berg (1985), who found significant correlations between work outcome and the injured person's complaints of slowness and inability to do two things at once. In a later study, Ruff et al. (1993) investigated the occupational outcome of 53 adults who had experienced severe TBI. From the range of neuropsychological predictors to determine return to work at 1-year post-TBI, age, verbal IQ, and speed of processing information were the strongest predictors of outcome. The contribution of speed of processing to prediction of later employability was confirmed in a later study reported by Asikainen, Nybo, Muller, Sarna, and Kaste (1999), who investigated the clinical usefulness of neuropsychological tests in evaluating long-term (at least 5 years post-TBI) functional and vocational outcome of patients with moderate to severe TBI. They found that measures of speed of information processing (Stroop and Purdue Pegboard) were predictive of capacity for later employment. Understandably it would be expected that slowness in processing information would be highly disruptive in the workplace where, for example, meeting externally imposed deadlines is often critical. Whether provision of time-management training to compensate for processing speed deficits, as advocated in other core areas of disability post-TBI, is a realistic option in the workplace is a socioeconomic challenge and is yet to be substantially addressed.

Summary

Slowing in speed of processing is a pervasive and disruptive legacy of TBI, especially following moderate to severe injury. Typically, slowed processing speed has been found to mediate performance post-TBI on a range of cognitive tasks, including those tests that index executive attention of working memory. Slowing in speed of information processing appears persistent, and impairment can still be identified at 5 years post-injury follow-up. There is some support for response to treatment, but this is mainly through the use of compensatory techniques or environmental modulation. Speed has been identified as an important predictor of various components of psychosocial functioning post-TBI, including driving and return to employment. The TBI population is heterogenous in pre-existing status, severity and nature of injury, so large populations for investigation are necessary to allow further theoretical and practical development in the field. With the emergence of larger data bases, more extended follow-up, and more routine neuropsychological assessment and use of standardized tests, we will have the opportunity to evaluate emergent neuropsychological changes on larger clinical populations than have been readily available to date. An important question still to be addressed is the relationship post-TBI between speed and working memory, and how they interrelate in complex cognitive tasks. On a more immediate practical level, there is a need to further evaluate the efficacy of cognitive-behavioural and psychopharmacological approaches to intervention.

References

Adams, J. H., Graham, D. I., & Jennett, B. (2001). The structural basis of moderate disability after traumatic brain damage. *Journal of Neurology, Neurosurgery, and Psychiatry*, *71*, 521–524.

Asikainen, I., Kaste, M., & Sarna, S. (1998). Predicting late outcome for patients with traumatic brain injury referred to a rehabilitation programme: A study of 508 Finnish patients 5 years or more after injury. *Brain Injury*, *12*, 95–107.

Asikainen, I., Nybo, T., Muller, K., Sarna, S., & Kaste, M. (1999). Speed performance and long-term functional and vocational outcome in a group of young patients with moderate or severe traumatic brain injury. *European Journal of Neurology*, *6*, 179–185.

Azouvi, P., Jovik, C., Van der Linden, M., Marlier, N., & Bussel, B. (1996). Working memory and supervisory control after severe closed head injury. A study of dual task performance and random generation. *Journal of Clinical and Experimental Neuropsychology*, *18*, 317–337.

Baddeley, A. D. (2001). Is working memory still working? *American Psychologist*, *56*, 851–864.

Baddeley, A. D., & Hitch, G. J. (2000). Development of working memory: Should the Pascual-Leone and the Baddeley and Hitch models be merged? *Journal of Experimental Child Psychology, 77,* 128–137.

Baddeley, A. D., & Logie, R. H. (1999). Working memory: The multiple-component model. In A. Miyake and P. Shah (Eds.), *Models of working memory: Mechanisms of active maintenance and executive control* (pp. 28–61) Cambridge: Cambridge University Press.

Baguley, I., Slewa-Younan, S., Lazarus, R., & Green, A. (2000). Long-term mortality trends in patients with traumatic brain injury. *Brain Injury, 14,* 505–512.

Belanger, H. G., Curtiss, G., Demery, J. A., Lebowitz, B. K., & Vanderploeg, R. D. (2005). Factors moderating neuropsychological outcomes following mild traumatic brain injury: A meta-analysis. *Journal of the International Neuropsychological Society, 11,* 215–227.

Bigler, E. D. (2001a). Quantitative magnetic resonance imaging in traumatic brain injury. *The Journal of Head Trauma Rehabilitation, 16,* 117–134.

Bigler, E. D. (2001b). The lesion(s) in traumatic brain injury: Implications for clinical neuropsychology. *Archives of Clinical Neuropsychology, 16,* 95–131.

Bigler, E. D. (2004). Case study. Neuropsychological results and neuropathological findings at autopsy in a case of mild traumatic brain injury. *Journal of the International Neuropsychological Society, 10,* 794–806.

Binder, L. M., Rohling, M. L., & Larrabee, G. J. (1997). A review of mild head trauma, Part 1: Meta-analytic review of neuropsychological studies. *Journal of Clinical and Experimental Neuropsychology, 19,* 421–431.

Blumbergs, P. C., Scott, G., Manavis, J., Wainwright, H., Simpson, D. A., & McLean, A. J. (1994). Staining of amyloid precursor protein to study axonal damage in mild head injury. *Lancet, 344,* 1055–1066.

Brittain, J. L., La Marche, J. A., Reeder, K. P., Roth, D. L., & Boll, T. J. (1991). Effects of age and IQ in paced serial addition task (PASAT) performance. *The Clinical Neuropsychologist, 5,* 163–175.

Brouwer, W. H., & Withaar, F. K. (1997). Fitness to drive after traumatic brain injury. *Neuropsychological Rehabilitation, 7,* 177–193.

Brouwer, W. H., Withaar, F. K., Tant, M. L. M., & van Zomeren, A. H. (2002). Attention and driving in traumatic brain injury: A question of coping with time-pressure. *Journal of Head Trauma Rehabilitation, 17,* 1–15.

Chiaravalloti, N. D., Christodoulou, C., Demaree, H. A., & DeLuca, J. (2003). Differentiating simple versus complex processing speed: Influence on new learning and memory performance. *Journal of Clinical and Experimental Neuropsychology, 25,* 489–501.

Cicerone, K. D. (2002). Remediation of "working attention" in mild traumatic brain injury. *Brain Injury, 16,* 185–195.

Cifu, D. X., Keyser-Marcus, L., Lopez, E., Wehman, P., Kreutzer, J. S., Englander, J., et al. (1997). Acute predictors of successful return to work 1 year after traumatic brain injury: A multicentre analysis. *Archives of Physical Medicine and Rehabilitation, 78,* 125–131.

Curtiss, G., Vanderploeg, R. D., Spencer, J., & Salazar, A. M. (2001). Patterns of verbal learning and memory in traumatic brain injury. *Journal of the International Neuropsychological Society, 7,* 574–585.

DeLuca, J., Schultheis, M. T., Madigan, N. K., Christodoulou, C., & Averill, A. (2000). Acquisition vs retrieval deficits in traumatic brain injury: Implications for memory rehabilitation. *Archives of Physical Medicine and Rehabilitation, 81,* 1327–1333.

D'Esposito, M., & Postle, B. R. (2002). The neural basis of working memory storage, rehearsal, and control processes: Evidence from patient and functional magnetic resonance imaging studies. In L. Squire & D. Schacter (Eds.), *Neuropsychology of memory.* New York: Guilford.

Dikmen, S., McClean, A., & Temkin, N. (1986). Neuropsychological and psychosocial consequences of minor head injury. *Journal of Neurology, Neurosurgery, and Psychiatry, 49,* 1227–1232.

Fasotti, L., Kovacs, F., Eling, P. A. T. M., & Brouwer, W. H. (2004). Time pressure management as a compensatory strategy training after closed head injury. *Neuropsychological Rehabilitation, 10,* 47–65.

Felmingham, K. L., Baguley, I. J., & Crooks, J. (2001). A comparison of acute and postdischarge predictors of employment 2 years after traumatic brain injury. *Archives of Physical Medicine and Rehabilitation, 82,* 435–439.

Felmingham, K. L., Baguley, I. J., & Green, A. (2004). Effects of diffuse axonal injury on speed of information processing following severe traumatic brain injury. *Neuropsychology, 18,* 564–571.

Fisk, G. D., Novack, T., Mennemeier, M., & Roenker, D. (2002). Useful field of view after traumatic brain injury. *Journal of Head Trauma Rehabilitation, 17,* 16–25.

Fork, M., Bartels, C., Ebert, A. D., Grubich, C., Synowitz, H., & Wallesch, C.-W. (2005). Neuropsychological sequelae of diffuse traumatic brain injury. *Brain Injury, 19,* 101–108.

Gentry, J. R., Godersky, J. C., & Thompson, B. (1988). MR imaging of head trauma: Review of the distribution and radiographic features of traumatic brain lesions. *American Journal of Radiology, 150,* 663–672.

Ghajar, J. (2000). Traumatic brain injury. *Lancet, 356,* 923–929.

Gron, G. (1996). Cognitive slowing in patients with acquired brain damge: An experimental approach. *Journal of Clinical and Experimental Neuropsychology, 18,* 406–415.

Gronwall, D., & Wrightson, P. (1981). Memory and information processing capacity after closed head injury. *Journal of Neurology, Neurosurgery, and Psychiatry, 44,* 889–895.

Gurdijan, E. S., & Gurdijan, E. S. (1976). Cerebral contusions: Re-evaluation of the mechanism of their development. *Journal of Trauma, 16,* 35–51.

Haslam, C., Batchelor, J., Fearnside, M. R., Haslam, S. A., Hawkins, S., & Kenway, E. (1994). Post-coma disturbance and post-traumatic amnesia as nonlinear predictors of cognitive outcome following severe closed head injury: Findings from the Westmead Head Injury project. *Brain Injury, 8,* 519–528.

Hetherington, C. R., Stuss, D. T., & Finlayson, M. A. J. (1996). Reaction time and variability 5 and 10 years after traumatic brain injury. *Brain Injury, 10,* 473–486.

Hillier, S. L., Hiller, J. E., & Metzer, J., (1997). Epidemiology of traumatic brain injury in South Australia. *Brain Injury, 11,* 649–659.

Hoofien, D., Vakils, E., Gilboa, A., Donovick, P. J., & Barak, O. (2002). Comparison of the predictive power of socio-economic variables, severity of injury and age on long-term outcome of traumatic brain injury: Sample-specific variables versus factors as predictors. *Brain Injury, 16,* 9–27.

Jennett, B., & Bond, M. (1975). Assessment of outcome after severe brain damage. *Lancet, 1,* 480–484.

Kesler, S. R., Adams, H. F., & Bigler, E. D. (2000). SPECT, MR and quantitative MR imaging: Correlates with neuropsychological and psychological outcome in traumatic brain injury. *Brain Injury, 14*, 851–857.

Kraus, J. F., & McArthur, D. L. (1996). Epidemiologic aspects of brain injury. *Neurologic Clinics, 14*, 435–450.

Kreutzer, J. S., Marwitz, J. H., Walker, W., Sander, A., Sherer, M., Bogner, J., et al. (2003). Moderating factors in return to work and job stability after traumatic brain injury. *Journal of Head Trauma Rehabilitation, 18*, 128–138.

Leclerq, M., Couillet, J., Azouvi, P., Marlier, N., Martin, Y., Strypstein, E., et al. (2000). Dual task performance after severe diffuse traumatic brain injury or vascular prefrontal damage. *Journal of Clinical and Experimental Neuropsychology, 22*, 339–350.

Lengenfelder, J., Schultheis, M. T., Al-Schihabi, M. T., Mourant, R., & DeLuca, J. (2002). Divided attention and driving: A pilot study using virtual reality technology. *Journal of Head Trauma Rehabilitation, 17*, 26–37.

Levin, H. E., Gary, H., Eisenberg, H., Ruff, R., Barth, J., Kreutzer, J., et al. (1990). Neuro-behavioural outcome 1 year after severe head injury: Experience of the Traumatic Coma Data Bank. *Journal of Neurosurgery, 73*, 699–709.

Lezak, M. D., Howieson, D. B., & Loring, D. W. (2004). *Neuropsychological Assessment* (2nd Ed.). Oxford: Oxford University Press.

Madigan, N. K., DeLuca, J., Diamond, B. J., Tramontano, G., & Averill, A. (2000). Speed of information processing in traumatic brain injury: Modality-specific factors. *The Journal of Head Trauma Rehabilitation, 15*, 943–956.

Martin, T. A., Donders, J., & Thompson, E. (2000). Potential of and problems with new measures of psychometric intelligence after traumatic brain injury. *Rehabilitation Psychology, 45* (4), 402–408.

Mathias, J. L., Beall, J. A. & Bigler, E. D. (2004). Neuropsychological and information processing deficits following mild traumatic brain injury. *Journal of the International Neuropsychological Society, 10*, 286–297.

Mazaux, J. M., Masson, F., Levin, H. S., Alaoui, P., Maurette, P., & Barat, M. (1997). Long-term neuropsychological outcome and loss of social autonomy after traumatic brain injury. *Archives of Physical Medicine and Rehabilitation, 78*, 1316–1320.

McDowell, S., Whyte, J., & D'Esposito, M. (1997). Working memory impairments in traumatic brain injury: Evidence from a dual-task paradigm. *Neuropsychologia, 35*, 1341–1345.

Millis, S. R., Rosenthal, M., Novack, T. A., Sherer, M., Nick, T. G., Kreutzer, J. S., et al. (2001). Long-term neuropsychological outcome after traumatic brain injury. *Journal of Head Trauma Rehabilitation, 16*, 343–355.

Mittl, R. L., Grossman, R. I., Hiehle, J. F., Hurst, R. W., Kander, D. R., Gennarelli, T. A., et al. (1994). Prevalence of MR evidence of diffuse axonal injury in patients with mild head injury and normal head CT findings. *American Journal of Neuroradiology, 15*, 1583–1589.

Olver, J. H., Ponsford, J. I., & Curran, C. A. (1996). Outcome following traumatic brain injury: A comparison between 2 and 5 years after injury. *Brain Injury, 10*, 841–848.

Park, D. C., & Gutchess, A. H. (2000). Cognitive aging and everyday life. In D. Park & N. Schwarz (Eds.), *Cognitive aging. A primer* (pp. 217–232). Philadelphia: Psychology Press.

Park, N. W., Moscovitch, M., & Robertson, I. H. (1999). Divided attention impairments after traumatic brain injury. *Neuropsychologia, 37*, 1119–1133.

Perlstein, W. M., Cole, M. A., Demery, J. A., Seignourel, P. J., Dixit, N. K., Larson, M. J., et al. (2004). Parametric manipulation of working memory load in traumatic brain injury: Behavioral and neural correlates. *Journal of the International Neuropsychological Society, 10*, 724–741.

Ponsford, J. L., & Kinsella, G. (1988). Evaluation of a remedial programme for attentional deficits following closed-head injury. *Journal of Clinical and Experimental Neuropsychology, 10*, 693–708.

Ponsford, J. L., & Kinsella, G. (1991). The use of a rating scale of attentional behaviour. *Neuropsychological Rehabilitation, 1*, 241–257.

Ponsford, J., & Kinsella, G. (1992). Attentional deficits following closed head injury. *Journal of Clinical and Experimental Neuropsychology, 14*, 822–838.

Ponsford, J. L., Olver, J. H., & Curran, C. (1995a). A profile of outcome: 2 years after traumatic brain injury. *Brain Injury, 9*, 1–10.

Ponsford, J. L., Olver, J. H., Curran, C., & Ng, K. (1995b). Prediction of employment status 2 years after traumatic brain injury. *Brain Injury, 9*, 11–20.

Prigatano, G. P. (1987). Personality and psychosocial consequences after brain injury. In M. J. Meier & A. L. Benton (Eds.), *Neuropsychological rehabilitation* (pp. 335–378), New York: Guilford Press.

Rios, M., Perianez, J. A., & Munoz-Cespedes, J. M. (2004). Attentional control and slowness of information processing after severe traumatic brain injury. *Brain Injury, 18*, 257–272.

Robertson, I. H., Manly, T., Andrade, J., Baddlely, B. T., & Yiend, J. (1997). "Oops!": Performance correlates of everyday attentional failures in traumatic brain injured and normal subjects. *Neuropsychologia, 35*, 747–758.

Ruff, R., Marshall, L. F., Crouch, J., Klauber, J., Levin, H. S., Barth, J., et al. (1993). Predictors of outcome following severe head trauma: Follow-up data from the Traumatic Coma Data Bank. *Brain Injury, 7*, 101–111.

Salmond, C. H., Chatfield, D. A., Menon, D. K., Pickard, J. D., & Sahakian, B. J. (2005). Cognitive sequelae of head injury: Involvement of basal forebrain and associated structures. *Brain, 128*, 189–200.

Salthouse, T. A. (1996). The processing-speed theory of adult age differences in cognition. *Psychological Review, 103*, 403–428.

Salthouse, T. A. (2000). Steps towards the explanation of adult age differences in cognition. In T. J. Perfect & E. A. Maylor (Eds.), *Models of cognitive aging* (pp. 19–49). Oxford: Oxford University Press.

Satz, P., Forney, D. L., Zaucha, K., Asarnow, R. R., Light, R., McCleary, C., et al. (1998). Depression, cognition, and functional correlates of recovery outcome after traumatic brain injury. *Brain Injury, 12*, 537–551.

Schmitter-Edgecombe, M. E., & Beglinger, L. (2001). Acquisition of skilled visual search performance following severe closed-head injury. *Journal of the International Neuropsychological Society, 7*, 615–630.

Schmitter-Edgecombe, M. E., Marks, W., Fahy, J. F., & Long, C. J. (1992). Effects of severe closed-head injury on three stages of information processing. *Journal of Clinical and Experimental Neuropsychology, 14*, 717–737.

Schretlen, D. J., & Shapiro, A. M. (2003). A quantitative review of the effects of traumatic brain injury on cognitive functioning. *International Review of Psychiatry, 15*, 341–349.

Sherer, M., Sander, A. M., Nick, T. G., High, W. M., Malec, J. F., & Rosenthal, M. (2002). Early cognitive status and productivity outcome after traumatic brain injury: Findings from the TBI model systems. *Archives of Physical Medicine and Rehabilitation*, 83, 183–192.

Shum, D. H., McFarland, K., Bain, J. D., & Humphreys, M. S. (1990). Effects of closed-head injury on attentional processes: An information processing stage analysis. *Journal of Clinical and Experimental Neuropsychology*, 12, 247–264.

Spikman, J. M., Deelman, B. G., & van Zomeren, A. H. (2000). Executive functioning, attention and frontal lesions in patients with chronic CHI. *Journal of Clinical and Experimental Neuropsychology*, 22, 325–338.

Spikman, J. M., van der Naalt, J., van Weerden, T. W., & van Zomeren, A. (2004). Indices of slowness of information processing in head injury patients: Tests for selective attention related to ERP latencies. *Journal of the International Neuropsychological Society*, 10, 851–861.

Spikman, J. M., van Zomeren, A. H., & Deelman, B. G. (1996). Deficits of attention after closed-head injury: Slowness only? *Journal of Clinical and Experimental Neuropsychology*, 18, 755–767.

Sternberg, S. (1969). On the discovery of processing stage. *Acta Psychologica*, 51, 41–59.

Strich, S. J. (1969). The pathology of brain damage due to blunt head injuries. In A. E. Walker, W. F. Caveness, & M. Critchley (Eds.), *The late effects of head injury*. Springfield, IL: Charles C. Thomas.

Stuss, D. T., Alexander, M. P., Schallice, T., Picton, T. W., Binns, M. A., MacDonald, R., et al. (2005). Multiple frontal systems controlling response speed. *Neuropsychologia*, 43, 396–417.

Stuss, D. T., Stethem, L. L., Picton, T. W., Leech, E. E., & Pelchat, G. (1989). Traumatic brain injury, aging and reaction time. *Canadian Journal of Neurological Science*, 16, 161–167.

Tate, R. L., & Broe, G. A. (1999). Psychosocial adjustment after traumatic brain injury: What are the important variables? *Psychological Medicine*, 29, 713–725.

Teasdale, T. W., & Engberg, A. W. (2005). Subjective well-being and quality of life following traumatic brain injury in adults: A long-term population-based follow-up. *Brain Injury*, 19, 1041–1048.

van Zomeren, A. H., & Brouwer, W. H. (1994). *Clinical neuropsychology of attention*. New York: Oxford University Press.

van Zomeren, A. H., & van den Berg, W. V. (1985). Residual complaints of patients two years after severe head injury. *Journal of Neurology, Neurosurgery, and Psychiatry*, 48, 21–28.

Vanderploeg, R. D., Curtiss, G., & Belanger, H. (2005). Long-term neuropsychological outcomes following mild traumatic brain injury. *Journal of the International Neuropsychological Society*, 11, 228–236.

Walsh, K. W. (1985). *Understanding brain damage. A primer of neuropsychological evaluation*. Edinburgh: Churchill Livingstone.

Whyte, J., Hart, T., Vaccaro, M., Grieb-Neff, P., Risser, A., Polansky, M., et al. (2004). Effects of methylphenidate on attention deficits after traumatic brain injury. A multidimensional, randomized, controlled trial. *American Journal of Physical Medicine and Rehabilitation*, 83, 401–420.

Whyte, J., Polansky, M., Fleming, M., Coslett, H. B., & Cavallucci, C. (1995).

Sustained arousal and attention after traumatic brain injury. *Neuropsychologia*, *33*, 797–813.

Zoccolotti, P., Matano, A., Deloche, G., Cantagello, A., Passadori, A., Leclercq, M., et al. (2000). Patterns of attentional impairment following closed head injury: A collaborative European study. *Cortex*, *36*, 93–107.

9 Frontal-subcortical determinants of processing speed in Parkinson's disease

Roderick K. Mahurin

Cognitive slowing, or bradyphrenia, is a hallmark symptom of subcortical disorders (SCDs), which otherwise are clinically characterized by their pathognomonic motor symptoms and associated neurobehavioral alterations. Although bradyphrenia commonly is defined as a slowing of cognitive processes (Rogers, 1986), more broadly it has been described as "slowness of thought, impaired attention and motivation, lack of spontaneity, inflexibility and forgetfulness" (Lees, 1994, p. 823). SCDs include Parkinson's disease (PD), Huntington's disease (HD), progressive supranuclear palsy (PSP), Wilson's disease, multiple system atrophy (MSA), Tourette's syndrome, spinocerebellar ataxia (SCA), Shy-Drager syndrome, and olivopontocerebellar atrophy (Cummings, 1986; Rinne, 2003). In addition to bradyphrenia, cognitive impairments in SCDs include problems with attention, verbal fluency, executive functions, recall, visuospatial ability, visual learning memory, and acquisition of motor skills (Albert, Feldman, & Willis, 1974; Cummings, 1990; Dubois, Defontaines, Deweer, Malapani, & Pillon, 1995). In contrast to many cortical disorders, in SCDs there generally is an absence of "instrumental" deficits of apraxia, aphasia, and agnosia (Cummings, 1986; Pillon, Ertle, Deweer, Sarazin, Agid, & Dubois, 1996). Since cognitive slowing also is evident in many cortical disorders (e.g., stroke, traumatic brain injury and Alzheimer's disease (AD)), it is unclear to what extent bradyphrenia as a presenting symptom has utility for distinguishing subcortical from cortical disorders.

For purposes of this chapter, cognitive speed is used synonymously with information processing speed (IPS), and is defined as the time taken for completion of a single, or series of, mental event(s) independent of motor output. Neurophysiological indices (e.g., nerve conduction velocity, event-related potentials) provide relatively direct measures of IPS. However clinical evaluation of cognitive abilities usually relies on motor output by the patient (e.g., speaking, writing, or manipulating objects). Since SCDs are characterized by motor impairment, assessment of IPS in these disorders depends on dissociating the relative contribution of motor from cognitive influences. As summarized by Rafal and co-authors (Rafal, Posner, Walker, & Friedrich, 1984, p. 1084), the term "bradyphrenia" has been applied to this presumed slowing of thought in PD [and other subcortical disorders] and implies (1) that increased response latencies are not strictly motoric but are due to slowed information processing, and (2) that the mental slowing is analogous to the bradykinesia observed in the motor domain and, hence, attributable to dysfunction of dopaminergic basal ganglia mechanisms.

Only after this dissociation has been achieved can comparisons of IPS between cortical and SCDs be accurately established.

The focus of the chapter is on PD, which is the most prevalent and most studied of the SCDs. The chapter is divided into three parts: (1) a summary of subcortical structures and their connections with the cortex, (2) a review of studies characterizing bradyphrenia in PD, and (3) a report by the author and colleagues comparing bradyphrenia in PD with slowed IPS in AD. It is postulated that: (a) bradyphrenia in PD results from dysfunction of specific frontal-subcortical pathways and their cortical and subcortical target regions, (b) bradyphrenia is related to reduction in dopaminergic activity that affects both motor and higher-order executive control processes, and (c) bradyphrenia in PD is not clearly distinguishable from slowed cognition in AD, but the clinical presentation of bradyphrenia in PD qualitatively differs that seen in AD.

The basal ganglia

SCDs involve the basal ganglia (BG), a network of subcortical processing centers critical to many neurobehavioral functions, ranging from motor control to attention and emotion. The BG include the striatum (caudate, putamen, and ventral striatum), substantia nigra (pars reticularis and pars compacta), internal and external globus pallidus, subthalamic nucleus, and thalamic nuclei. Additional structures, including the amygdala, nucleus accumbens, red nucleus and reticular formation, often are classified as BG components (Young & Penney, 1993).

The BG are connected with cortical regions through functionally organized closed loops, or "circuits." The principal cortical targets are orbital, lateral, and mid-prefrontal regions, with additional connections to inferotemporal and posterior parietal cortex (Alexander & Crutcher, 1990; Lichter & Cummings, 2001). These circuits are of a feedforward re-entrant nature, and maintain consistent topographic mapping throughout the striato-thalamocortical pathways (Strick, Hoover, & Mushiake, 1993). A specific cortical region receives convergent information from other cortical sites, both adjacent and distant, and this information is topographically segregated at smaller target zones within the BG (Hoover & Strick, 1993). It has been postulated that the BG circuits strictly maintain structural and functional segregation, however recent findings have questioned this assumption (Middleton & Strick, 2001).

Initial descriptions of the BG loops included five segregated pathways: skeletomotor, oculomotor, dorsolateral prefrontal cortex (DLPFC), lateral orbitofrontal, and anterior cingulate/medial orbitofrontal (Alexander, DeLong, & Strick, 1986). Two of these pathways are associated with motor control, while the remaining circuits are related to cognitive and affective regulation (Alexander, Crutcher, & DeLong, 1991; Mahurin, 1998) (see Figure 9.1). Subsequent investigations using neurotropic viral tracing techniques have modified the number of cortical–subcortical loops to seven, with formal characterization of anterior cingulate, medial orbitofrontal, and inferotemporal/posterior parietal loops (Hoover & Strick, 1999; Middleton & Strick, 2001).

Frontal-subcortical circuits (FSCs), in particular, play a major role in motor and cognitive processing in SCDs (Cummings, 1990). The skeletomotor loops connect to motor and premotor areas involved with planning and execution of movement (e.g., supplementary motor area and premotor cortex), while oculomotor loops target frontal eye fields and related areas contributing to both saccadic and smooth pursuit eye movements. Lateral orbitofrontal loops are involved in the production of emotional behavior, and

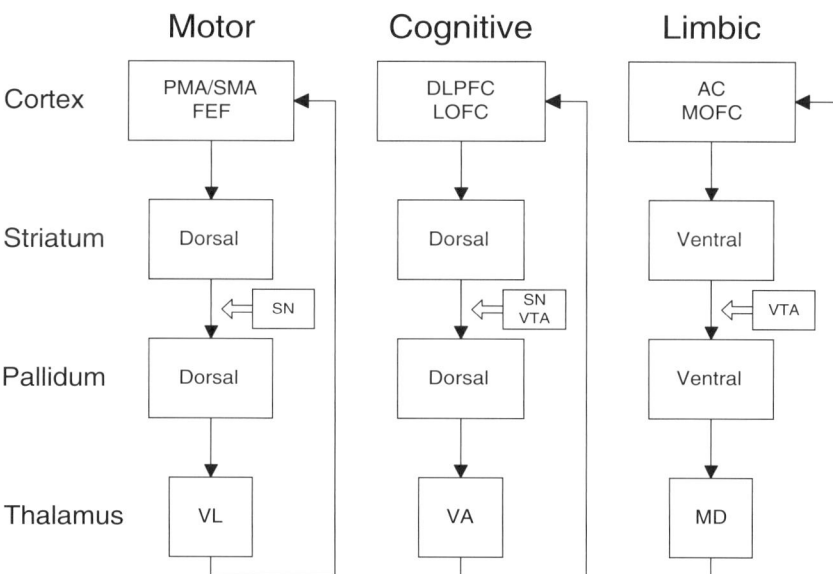

Figure 9.1 Schematic of three types of cortical–subcortical circuits. Note the dorsolateral connectivity of the motor and cognitive circuits, and the ventral connectivity of the limbic circuit. PMA/SMA = primary motor area/supplementary motor area, FEF = frontal eye fields, DLPFC = dorsal lateral prefrontal cortex, LOFC = lateral orbital frontal cortex, MOFC = medial orbital frontal cortex, AC = anterior cingulate, SN = substantia nigra, VTA = ventral tegmental area, VL = ventral lateral, VA = ventral anterior, MD = medial dorsal. Adapted from Mahurin (1998).

medial orbitofrontal circuits integrate visceral and limbic functions. The anterior cingulate circuit is associated with motivation and the modulation of emotional arousal. DLPFC circuits primarily are associated with executive functions involving the planning, monitoring, and regulation of goal-directed cognition and actions. The DLPFC connections with the BG are of particular relevance to SCDs because of their influence on motor programming and executive control functions (Jacobs, Levy, & Marder, 2003; Salmon, Heindel, & Hamilton, 2001).

Cortical input to the BG is via the striatum. The striatum connects to other BG structures through the "direct" and "indirect" pathways. These multisynaptic pathways project to the thalamus, which is the principal source of excitatory output to the cortex. The direct pathway affects BG output by reducing thalamic inhibition, thus facilitating the tonic excitatatory output of thalamic nuclei to their respective cortical targets. The indirect pathway includes an additional synaptic connection from striatum to the internal globus pallidus, which projects to the subthalamic nucleus, thalamus and cortex. In contrast to the direct pathway, a relative increase in excitation of the indirect pathway results in tonic inhibitory influence on the thalamus, effectively reducing output to the cortex. In general, the direct basal ganglia pathway facilitates thalamic output, while the indirect pathway inhibits it (Houk, 2001; Lichter, 2001).

The basal ganglia and processing speed

The balance between activity of direct and indirect pathways largely contributes to the clinical presentation of specific SCDs (Lichter, 2001). Hypokinetic syndromes result from disruption of the direct, facilitatory pathway from the BG to the thalamus, resulting in reduced output to cortical target zones. As a consequence, hypokinetic syndromes are associated with a reduction in the speed, amplitude and frequency of movement (i.e., bradykinesia), as well as limb rigidity, postural instability, gaze restriction, and gait disturbance. Examples of hypokinetic disorders include PD, PSP, MSA and SCA. Hyperkinetic syndromes, in contrast, are marked by increased spontaneous, uncontrolled movements, including motor and speech tics, chorea, and ballismus. These syndromes result from disruption of the indirect (inhibitory) pathway, with a consequent increase in thalamocortical output. The most common examples of hyperkinetic disorders are HD and Tourette's syndrome. Although disorders with hyperkinetic motor disturbance, such as HD, show rapid uncontrolled movements, cognitive speed is not increased but, rather, slowed (Hanes, Andrewes, & Pantelis, 1995). Similar findings in other hyperkinetic disorders suggest that disruption of the BG and connections, regardless of the specific disease considered, results in cognitive slowing.

The importance of the BG to processing speed was shown in a magnetic resonance imaging study examining the impact of subcortical white matter lesions on cognitive function in a large sample of nondemented elderly adults

(O'Brien et al., 2002). Hyperintense lesions (HLs) were found in almost half of the participants. The extent of subcortical lesions in the caudate and thalamus was significantly correlated with impaired performance on tests of processing speed and of executive function. No significant associations were found between HLs and either episodic or working memory, indicating a major role for the BG with regard to processing speed, but a lesser role in memory processes.

Both the prefrontal cortex and the BG, in particular the mediodorsal striatum, play an important role in movement initiation. Several neurotransmitters, including dopamine, glutamate and gamma aminobutyric acid (GABA) appear to be involved at cortical and subcortical levels (Houk, 2001). Processing of temporal information in the seconds-to-minutes range (e.g., duration discrimination and timing sequences) appears linked to dopamine function in the BG. In contrast, memory and attentional mechanisms concerned with temporal processing are associated with acetylcholine activity, primarily in the frontal cortex (Meck, 1996). The FSCs link these two timing systems, underscoring the importance of cortical–subcortical connections to rapid and efficient cognitive processing.

Studies of psychostimulant effects on motor behavior show an interaction between striatal dopamine and glutamate that is postulated to enhance the signal-to-noise ratio of afferent information to the BG (Rebec, 2006). This effect would potentially increase response speed to an external stimulus. Additionally, results from several dopaminergic challenge studies (Rammsayer, 1994, 1997) indicate that automatic temporal processing of brief duration (in the range of milliseconds) is dependent on dopaminergic activity in the mesostriatal system. Many cognitive processes occur in this brief temporal range and thus can be affected in disorders involving the BG. Temporal processing of longer duration is under greater cognitive control, and appears related to mesolimbocortical dopamine influence on higher-order working memory (Rammsayer, 1994).

Processing speed in Parkinson's disease

Clinical features and neuropathology

PD is the second most common neurodegenerative disorder of the elderly, with a prevalence approaching 1% in the population aged 60 years and older (Padovani, Costanzi, Gilberti, & Borroni, 2006). Age of onset is variable, with initial symptoms often appearing in the fifth or sixth decade. The disease course is slowly progressive, but the rate of decline varies among patients. Clinically, PD is defined by bradykinesia, resting tremor and cogwheel-type rigidity. Although not universal, postural instability, shuffling gait, stooped posture, poverty of spontaneous facial and limb movement, micrographia and hypophonia are common.

PD is associated with a variety of etiologies, including viral encephalitis, neuroleptic usage, manganese toxicity, insecticide exposure, carbon monoxide poisoning, and multiple cerebral infarcts (Golbe & Langston, 1993; Gray, Poirier, & Scaravilli, 1991). However, approximately 80% of cases of PD are of undetermined etiology ("sporadic"), with indications that many of these cases are due to interaction between nongenetic factors and susceptibility genes (Benmoyal-Segal & Soreq, 2006; de Lau & Breteler, 2006). Recent findings have implicated a variety of gene–environment interactions in the pathogenesis of PD, with emphasis on mutations of genes involved in protection from oxidative stress (Farrer, 2006; Schapira, 2006). In particular, heterozygous parkin mutations are estimated to account for as much as 50% of familial PD and 18% of sporadic PD (Clark et al., 2006).

Neuropathological features in PD include progressive degeneration of pigmented brainstem nuclei, predominantly the pars compacta of the substantia nigra, with subsequent dopamine reduction in the caudate and putamen. Although dopamine plays a major role in PD, other neurotransmitters are implicated, notably acetylcholine, but also serotonin, glutamate, GABA, and various neuropetides (Agid, 1991; Bronstein, 2001). In addition, pathology of other subcortical structures, including the locus coeruleus, dorsal vagal nucleus, ventral tegmentum and sympathetic ganglia, contributes to deficits seen in PD (Agid, 1991; Young & Penney, 1993). Histopathological appearance of intracellular Lewy bodies confirms the degenerative changes in these areas (Lerner & Whitehouse, 2002).

Brain imaging studies show decreased contralateral striatal dopamine in hemiparkinsonism and bilateral reductions in bilateral parkinsonism, with greatest reductions in the region of the putamen (Garnett, Nahmias, & Firnau, 1984; Leenders et al., 1986). Changes in regional cerebral blood flow (rCBF) are seen in cortical regions as well. For example, reduced rCBF in mesial and dorsolateral prefrontal regions is associated with executive dysfunction in PD, becoming increasingly pronounced as the disorder progresses (Bissessur, Tissingh, Wolters, & Scheltens, 1997; Weder et al., 2000). Frontal-temporal changes have been implicated with regard to working and recent memory (Davidson, Anaki, Saint-Cyr, Chow, & Moscovitch, 2006; Monetta & Pell, 2006), mesiofrontal pathology with apathy (Alexander & Stuss, 2000), and temporoparietal association areas with object discrimination (Weder et al., 2000). It is unclear to what extent these cortical changes reflect remote effects of neuropathology in the BG.

Major depression is common in PD, with a prevalence of between 20–40%, and is associated with increased cognitive impairment relative to non-depressed PD patients (Lieberman, 2006b; Troster, Stalp, Paolo, Fields, & Koller, 1995). Depression often occurs early in the disorder and may precede motor and cognitive symptoms, and appears to involve serotonergic mesolimbic and mesocortical, as well as dopaminergic, cortical–subcortical pathways (Mayberg, 1994). Depression and dementia in PD commonly are accompanied by apathy and fatigue, complicating the clinical picture (Oved, Ziv, Treves, Paleacu, Melamed, & Djaldetti, 2006). Apathy can occur in the absence of depression, and appears to be a core feature of the disorder (Kirsch-Darrow, Fernandez, Marsiske, Okun, & Bowers, 2006). Recognizing the presence of depression and apathy is important in the assessment of bradyphrenia in PD since both can exacerbate existing disease-related cognitive slowing, particularly when dementia is present (Comijs, Jonker, Beekman, & Deeg, 2001; Lieberman, 2006a).

Cognitive changes generally are mild in early stages of PD, but increase with disease progression. In addition to bradyphrenia, impairment is found in areas of executive function (e.g., planning, sequencing, set-shifting), visual-spatial abilities, attention, verbal fluency and memory (Brown & Marsden, 1990; Hannay, Howieson, Loring, Fischer, & Lezak, 2004; Mahurin, Feher, Nance, Levy, & Pirozzolo, 1993; Whittington, Podd, & Stewart-Williams, 2006). PD with dementia (PDD) occurs in later stages of the disorder in approximately 15–40% of patients, with varying estimates depending on how dementia is defined (Cummings, 1988; Padovani et al., 2006). Executive dysfunction, which is evident early in the disease, becomes especially prominent if dementia is present in later stages (Dubois et al., 1995).

Event-related potentials

Event-related potentials (ERPs) measure neuronal electrophysiological response to stimuli, providing a more direct measure of IPS than do tests of behavioral performance. Presentation of stimuli need not be accompanied by the potentially confounding effect of a motor response (e.g., oddball paradigms). Or, if motor responses are used as part of the task, ERPs provide an index of cognitive speed that can be examined in relation to speed and accuracy of the responses (e.g., reaction time (RT) and visual discrimination tasks). ERPs have been used extensively in cognitive research as well as having a long history of clinical use, primarily in assessing the integrity of sensory systems. For PD, as well as other SCDs, ERPs provide a unique means of dissociating the cognitive aspects of bradyphrenia from co-existing motor impairment.

ERPs in PD typically show slowing in mid- and long-latency auditory evoked potentials (N1, N2, and P3) (Starkstein, Esteguy, Berthier, Garcia, & Leiguarda, 1989). When measured in conjunction with RT tasks of increasing complexity, ERPs in PD patients show delayed latencies of N1, N2 and P3 that worsen as task difficulty increases (Kutukcu, Marks, Goodin, & Aminoff, 1998). A report by Wang, Wang, Wang, Cui, Tian, and Zhang (2002) showed delayed N270 component in PD patients for a conflict condition matching task. The same researchers used single photon emission computed tomography (SPECT) in conjunction with ERPs to investigate the P3 response to an oddball paradigm. They found prolonged P3 latency that correlated with rCBF of the bilateral temporal lobes. The corresponding RT was slowed and correlated significantly with rCBF of right prefrontal regions, as well as areas of the temporal, occipital, and parietal lobes (Wang et al., 2000). Tanaka,

Koenig, Pascual-Marqui, Hirata, Kochi, and Lehmann (2000) employed an oddball paradigm in PD patients with no, moderate, or severe dementia and found a positive correlation between P3 latency and severity of dementia. Similarly, a PD study comparing cognitive speed with clinical features found slowed RT and longer latencies for P3 and N2, all of which were significantly correlated with motor disability, intelligence, and rCBF (Li et al., 2005). The effect of medication treatment on ERPs also has been explored, with findings of normal P3 latency and slower response time before levodopa treatment, but prolonged P3 latency and faster response time after treatment, consistent with a dopamine-induced dissociation between cognitive speed and motor performance (Prasher & Findley, 1991) (see studies by Muller et al. presented below).

Movement-related potentials (MRPs) are complementary to sensory-related ERPs in that they record electrophysiological changes associated with the production of motor responses, but without the confound of peripheral motor impairment. In an experimental protocol involving a size discrimination task, PD patients showed delayed onset of MRPs, as well as overall response slowing, that worsened with increased task complexity (Low, Miller, & Vierck, 2002). Onset and peaks of MRPs associated with preparation and execution of internally determined movements also are delayed in PD patients relative to healthy controls, suggesting abnormal activity of the supplementary motor area and its connections to the BG (Cunnington, Iansek, Bradshaw, & Phillips, 1995). Overall, findings of EPR and MRP studies of PD patients are consistent with nonmotoric cognitive slowing. The magnitude of slowing is associated with level of cognitive impairment as well as task complexity.

Reaction time

Speed of voluntary response to an external stimulus (i.e., RT) has been used for over a century in the investigation of human cognition (Donders, 1868; Luce, 1986; Mahurin & Pirozzolo, 1986). The literature on RT is extensive and, like ERPs, the methodology has been widely employed in experimental as well as clinical research. Because the structure of RT tasks allows for dissociation of cognitive and motor processing components, the methods are particularly well suited to studying bradyphrenia.

The majority of studies are consistent with slowed RT in PD, affecting both the preparation and execution of rapid voluntary movements (Cooper, Sagar, Tidswell, & Jordan, 1994; Johnson, Vernon, Almeida, Grantier, Singarayer, & Jog, 2004; Montgomery, Nuessen, Nuessen, & Douglas, 1991). Furthermore, slowed processing speed in PD has been found in various RT studies, even after controlling for potential confounds of age, cognitive status, and depression (Dobbs et al., 1993a; Montgomery, Baker, Lyons, & Koller, 2000). RT was investigated in the ERP study by Kutukcu et al. cited above (1998). RTs of PD patients were longer than those of control subjects in all three of the administered tasks. In addition, RTs of the PD group showed disproportionately greater slowing as task complexity increased, implicating central as well as peripheral response slowing. Pate and Margolin (1994) compared RT performance of PD and AD patients with young and elderly healthy control subjects. Relative to the pattern in AD patients, cognitive slowing in both nondemented and demented PD patients was disproportionate to their general cognitive status. The authors suggest that this disproportionality be used to differentiate the concepts of bradyphrenia and "nonspecific" cognitive slowing such as seen in AD.

Choice RT (i.e., presentation of more than one response alternative) has been employed to investigate the effects of congruent and incongruent response cuing in PD (Hocherman, Moont, & Schwartz, 2004). Although PD patients did not differ from healthy controls in error rate, they were slower to respond except under 100% congruent cuing. These results suggest that slowed choice RT in PD results from cognitive delays in stimulus–response linking, rather than from impaired motor initiation and execution. A study by Bherer and colleagues (Bherer, Belleville, & Gilbert, 2003) also found that PD patients were slower than healthy controls for simple and choice RT tasks. Greater slowing was seen for longer preparatory intervals between a warning signal and presentation of the visual target, suggesting RT slowing in PD may, in part, result from problems with temporal response preparation.

Findings of slowed RT in PD are not universal, however. A review of RT studies concluded that although the data generally support a slowing of simple RT in PD, there is less consistent evidence for a slowing of choice RT. Unlike studies cited above, the authors of this review did not find evidence for a specific motor programming deficit (Gauntlett-Gilbert & Brown, 1998). Other investigators also report simple RT slowing, but no disproportionate slowing in choice RT conditions (Evarts, Teravainen, & Calne, 1981). Smith and colleagues (Smith, Goldman, Janer, Baty, & Morris, 1998) studied early stage nonmedicated PD subjects using timed verbal, quantitative, and spatial information discrimination tasks of differing difficulty levels, a memory scanning paradigm, and a simple manual RT task. The discrimination and scanning tasks required a verbal, but not manual, response. The PD group performed as fast as the control group on all measures except movement time, a finding consistent with motor, but not cognitive, slowing. A study comparing focused attention in patients with PD or HD found that HD patients had disproportionately longer RTs to inconsistent stimuli relative to an age-matched control group, while RTs of patients with PD were comparable to those of the control subjects, regardless of stimulus consistency (Roman et al., 1998). Difference scores between RTs for inconsistent versus consistent stimuli were not correlated with overall level of dementia or disease severity. To summarize the above investigations, although many RT studies support the premise of bradyphrenia in PD, other reports implicate motor, rather than cognitive, slowing.

Timed cognitive tasks

Another approach to investigating bradyphrenia is through use of timed cognitive tasks specifically designed to allow for dissociation of cognitive and motor components. This methodology is exemplified in mental rotation tasks. As stated by Duncombe and co-authors (Duncombe, Bradshaw, Iansek, & Phillips, 1994, p. 1383), "mental rotation provides an internal or cognitive analogue of real movement and enables us to determine the speed of such mental processes independent of any concurrent motor slowing in response initiation and execution." Some studies have found impairment in PD for mental rotation (e.g., Lee, Harris, & Calvert, 1998), although other studies have failed to find slowing, especially in PD patients without dementia or depression (Duncombe et al., 1994). Performance on the Sternberg character classification paradigm also has been used to measure speed of nonmotoric short-term memory scanning. Speed on this task was slowed in elderly PD patients, but scanning accuracy showed only mild impairment, consistent with slowed processing of information in working memory (Wilson, Kaszniak, Klawans, & Garron, 1980). Other investigators also have found slowed scanning speed in PD patients, with greater slowing evident in patients with more advanced disease (e.g., Ransmayr et al., 1990). In the latter study, cognitive slowing correlated significantly with bradykinesia and severity of motor symptoms, and was independent of severity of depression. Another study found that PD patients had slowed inspection time, relative to healthy controls, in judging the temporal sequence of four single letters presented at varying rates, indicating the presence of bradyphrenia in a task without motor demands (Shipley, Deary, Tan, Christie, & Starr, 2002).

Results from a study requiring serial updating of mental representations in response to a series of visual stimuli showed slowing in PD patients compared with healthy control subjects, with increased slowness at higher speeds of stimulus presentation (Sawamoto, Honda, Hanakawa, Fukuyama, & Shibasaki, 2002). Because of the nonmotoric nature of the task the authors interpreted the findings as evidence for bradyphrenia as a "cognitive mental operation." It has been suggested that if PD patients have difficulty shifting mental set because of cognitive slowing, then delayed auditory feedback should disrupt speech output more in PD patients than in healthy control subjects (Dobbs et al., 1993b). This hypothesized result was obtained, which the authors interpreted as indicative of bradyphrenia in the absence of motor output. Speech disruption was significantly associated with cued RT, but was independent of cognitive test scores, antiparkinsonian therapy or depression.

There are discrepant findings, however. For example, a study of nonmotoric inspection time that required judging the order of onset of two rapidly presented lights showed no difference between PD patients and a group of age-matched control subjects, although both were slower than a group of younger control subjects (Phillips, Schiffter, Nicholls, Bradshaw, Iansek, & Saling, 1999). A novel approach to measuring IPS was conducted by Vardy and colleagues (Vardy, Bradshaw, & Iansek, 2003) who used a modification of an "attentional blink" paradigm. In this task, the subject identifies the second target following a previously attended target in rapidly presented series. Although error patterns differed between the PD and healthy control groups, processing and clearance of information were largely preserved, again suggesting an absence of bradyphrenia.

In summary, use of carefully constructed, timed cognitive tasks allows for separation of cognitive from motor components of processing speed. Results overall support the presence of bradyphrenia in PD, but there are contradictory findings as well. More so than for ERP or RT studies, the wide variety of methodologies makes difficult the comparisons of studies such as those presented above.

Executive functions in PD

The role of FSCs in integrating frontal and BG processes suggests that frontal-mediated executive functions may play an important role in the expression of bradyphrenia (Jacobs et al., 2003; Partiot, Verin, Pillon, Teixeira-Ferreira, Agid, & Dubois, 1996; Taylor, Saint-Cyr, & Lang, 1986). Executive dysfunction in PD has been demonstrated in a variety of cognitive processes, including initiation, reasoning and planning (Uekermann et al., 2004), cognitive and motor response-switching (Inzelberg, Plotnik, Flash, Schechtman, Shahar, & Korczyn, 2001), deployment of attentional resources (Woodward, Bub, & Hunter, 2002), memory (Bondi, Kaszniak, Bayles, & Vance, 1993), and category learning (Price, 2006). Meiran and colleagues (Meiran, Friedman, & Yehene, 2004) found goal-setting deficits during task switching for PD subjects, although normal task-rule implementation was indicated by a preparation-related reduction in the RT task-switching cost. The authors suggest that slowed RT in PD reflects a specific deficit in goal setting (an executive task), reflected in a difficulty determining which task is currently relevant. Longer response latencies have been reported in PD for frontally mediated automatic and inhibitory tasks, often with no difference in error rates between groups (e.g., Bouquet, Bonnaud, & Gil, 2003). Slowed response time for voluntary visual saccades also has been demonstrated in PD, with patients showing increased errors relative to healthy control subjects in inhibiting reflexive antisaccades (i.e., eye movement opposite to the direction cue) (Amador, Hood, Schiess, Izor, & Sereno, 2006). Speed and accuracy measures were significantly correlated in this study, suggesting that bradyphrenia interacts with executive control of inhibitory functions in the frontal cortex.

Processing speed also has been examined in PD by use of sentence comprehension tasks (Lee, Grossman, Morris, Stern, & Hurtig, 2003). In this study, PD patients were slowed relative to healthy controls in recognizing specific types of errors, and their performance was correlated with timed executive measures of planning. This pattern of results suggests the influence of both cognitive speed and executive dysfunction on sentence comprehension. Another approach to investigating the relationship between bradyphrenia and executive function is to examine response readiness by manipulating the probability of response in an RT-based task. This method has demonstrated abnormal patterns of response force in PD patients, as well as difficulty in inhibiting responses on no-go trials (an executive function) (Franz & Miller, 2002). The results are consistent with other reports of both motor activation impairment and executive dyscontrol of response modulation in PD. Additional evidence for an interaction between executive function and motor response has been demonstrated in an ERP study (Bokura, Yamaguchi, & Kobayashi, 2005). No differences between PD and healthy control subjects were found for P3 latency and amplitude of the "Go" component of a standard Go/No Go task. However, the corresponding "No Go" latency, requiring inhibitory control, was significantly longer in the PD group. Additionally, P3 latency for the "No Go," but not the "Go," task was significantly correlated with other tests of executive function.

An investigation of "paradoxical kinesis" in PD assessed patients as to whether they responded more quickly to externally generated responses than to responses requiring self-generated, nonroutine decision-making (Siegert, Harper, Cameron, & Abernethy, 2002). Healthy control subjects reacted quickest when they initiated responses themselves (i.e., internal cuing), but PD patients were quicker to respond when responses were externally cued, further suggesting difficulty in executive regulation of response generation. Berry and co-authors (Berry, Nicolson, Foster, Behrmann, & Sagar, 1999) reported on the performance of "frontal" and "nonfrontal" PD patients (based on scores from the Wisconsin Card Sorting Test and the picture arrangement subtest of the Wechsler Adult Intelligence Scale) on visual attention tests designed to dissociate motoric response speed from "central" IPS. Performance of the nonfrontal PD group did not differ from healthy control subjects in either speed or accuracy. In contrast, the frontal group was significantly slower than the other two groups, although error rates did not differ. To summarize, the above studies suggest that executive dysfunction in PD is closely related to cognitive slowing, consistent with the important role FSC integrity plays in both processes.

Bradyphrenia and bradykinesia

Evaluation of subtypes of motor impairment in PD generally shows a significant relationship of cognitive performance and bradykinesia, but not between cognition and tremor (Mortimer, Pirozzolo, Hansch, & Webster, 1982). Zetusky, Jankovic, and Pirozzolo (1985) examined data from a large sample of patients with idiopathic PD and found positive correlations of cognitive deficits with bradykinesia, postural instability, and gait difficulty, but a negative correlation between cognitive decline and tremor. A study focused just on IPS and symptom subtype examined simple and choice RT in

PD patients and found significant slowing compared to healthy control subjects (Mahurin, 1984). Again, bradykinesia, but not tremor, was significantly correlated with response times. Other investigators have reported similar findings (Ebmeier, Calder, Crawford, Stewart, Besson, & Mutch, 1990; Huber, Christy, & Paulson, 1991). A more recent study found that PD patients with postural instability and gait difficulty had a higher incidence of dementia and a faster rate of cognitive decline than patients with predominant tremor (Burn, Rowan, Allan, Molloy, O'Brien, & McKeith, 2006).

The co-expression of cognitive and motor slowing in PD suggests a shared neurochemical substrate related to subcortical dopamine depletion. For example, a study compared neuropsychological test scores with physical symptoms and levels of homovanillic acid (HVA), a dopamine metabolite, in cerebrospinal fluid of patients with PD, AD or major depression (Wolfe et al., 1990). The authors found significant associations between HVA levels, information processing speed, and verbal fluency in all groups. Patients with low HVA had more parkinsonian features, but also were more depressed. Another study examined the relationship between nigrostriatal dopaminergic denervation in PD, as measured by SPECT with (123) Iodine-beta-CIT, and speed of performance in a simultaneous processing task (Duchesne, Soucy, Masson, Chouinard, & Bedard, 2002). Bradyphrenia was found in those PD subjects off dopamine medication, but not those on medication. Further, a significant correlation was found between task performance and dopamine levels, suggesting a role for dopamine in executive function tasks with a high demand for processing resources and speed.

A study examining the effect of uncertainty of rules in determining response speed on a go/no go task found that, unlike healthy control subjects, untreated PD patients showed significant response slowing that increased with the degree of response uncertainty (Pessiglione et al., 2005). The authors interpreted this finding as reflecting an abnormal temporal coupling between deliberation and execution processes in PD. This interference was minimized by dopaminergic treatment, but was unchanged with deep brain stimulation, suggesting a dopaminergic effect on functional segregation of motor response from the pre-response deliberation stages. Another investigation examined cognitive speed in patients with either PD or primary depression, using several computerized digit symbol substitution tests (Rogers, Lees, Smith, Trimble, & Stern, 1987). Both groups showed slowed response time as compared with matched healthy control subjects. Slowing was correlated with structural brain changes and depression in the PD group, and with motor impairment in the depression group. Following six months of levodopa treatment, PD patients showed little change in response time on the digit symbol test. However, treated depressed patients improved on ratings for both affective and motor impairment, as well as digit symbol scores. These results suggest that bradyphrenia and psychomotor retardation are closely related, but that bradyphrenia is less likely to respond to treatment than is depression.

Other studies, however, have failed to demonstrate an association between bradyphrenia and bradykinesia. For example, motor disability in early untreated PD has been shown to strongly correlate with severity of depression, but weakly with cognitive impairment (Cooper, Sagar, Jordan, Harvey, & Sullivan, 1991). In contrast to other reports, the authors of this study suggest that cognitive dysfunction in PD may largely be independent of the frontal-striatal dopamine deficiency postulated to underlie motor disability. An investigation of effects of levodopa treatment in PD employed three experiments designed to separate motor speed from cognitive speed: rate of memory scanning, visual orientation speed, and movement preparation time (Rafal et al., 1984). RT for all tasks was slowed for patients in the untreated state, but this effect appeared related to motor slowing rather than bradyphrenia. The authors suggest that the "slowing of thought" often reported in PD is not necessarily associated with bradykinesia, and thus may not be related to dopaminergic dysfunction.

Several studies by Muller and colleagues (Muller, Benz, & Bornke, 2001; Muller, Eising, Kuhn, Buttner, Coenen, & Przuntek, 1999) further explored the relationship between cognitive speed and dopamine levels in PD. In a SPECT brain imaging study the authors found that for untreated PD patients, rCBF in the striatal region was associated with both cognitive and motor components of an RT task. A treatment study by the same authors found that the cognitive component of RT was significantly slower after levodopa intake, but movement time did not change, indicating a selective slowing effect of dopamine on cognitive speed. A similar slowing of RT, but no change in movement time, was found following injection of apomorphine, a dopamine agonist (Muller, Benz, & Przuntek, 2002). The authors relate this finding to sedative effects of levodopa, or an interaction with dopamine overflow in prefrontal regions, with subsequent cholinergic dysfunction. This slowing is significantly more pronounced in previously untreated PD patients, suggesting development of tolerance to the effect with continued medication treatment (Muller, Benz, & Przuntek, 2000).

In summary, although conceptually appealing, not all studies support a close association between bradyphrenia and bradykinesia in PD. Comprehensive modeling of the interaction between dopamine levels, disease stage, cognitive impairment, and motor slowing continues to be a challenging area of investigation. Findings that levodopa does not consistently improve cognitive speed, and even may adversely affect it, are important considerations in interpretation of PD treatment studies that use IPS as an outcome variable.

A study of processing speed in PD and AD

As described above, PD patients typically show a subcortical pattern of cognitive impairment that may be distinguished from cortical dementia, such as seen in AD. However, both PD and AD are characterized by slowing of IPS and impaired executive functions, consistent with involvement of frontal regions and their connections (Elias & Treland, 1999; Janvin, Larsen, Salmon, Galasko, Hugdahl, & Aarsland, 2006; Royall, Mahurin, & Gray, 1992). Given this overlap in symptom presentation, it is unclear whether bradyphrenia in PD is a distinct finding from cognitive slowing in AD. The following study by the author and colleagues approached this question by use of factor analysis and an information processing model to investigate motor and cognitive processing speed in PD and AD. There are few previous studies comparing processing speed in PD and AD by use of these methods.

Subjects consisted of three age- and education-matched groups, AD, PD, and healthy elderly controls (EC) ($n = 20$ in each group). Physical evaluation of AD patients was negative for primary motor involvement (e.g., weakness, decreased reflexes) or extrapyramidal signs that might overlap with PD (e.g., tremor, rigidity, or bradykinesia). All PD patients were in early to mid-stages of disease course and were receiving standard levodopa treatment. No PD patients showed generalized dementia.

Neuropsychological data from all three groups are presented in Table 9.1. Verbal IQ, a relatively motor free measure of intellectual status (Wechsler, 1981) was significantly lower for AD patients compared to the other groups ($p < .01$), consistent with the diagnosis of dementia. Verbal IQ did not significantly differ between the PD and EC groups, confirming absence of dementia in the PD patients. Subjects were administered a battery of timed motor and cognitive tasks, including Grip Strength, Finger Tapping, Two-Goal Tapping, Purdue Pegboard, Grooved Pegboard, Pursuit Rotor, Name Writing, Letter Cancellation, Symbol Digit Modalities Test, Trail Making Parts A and B, Simple Reaction Time, and Choice Reaction Time (Lezak, Howieson, & Loring, 2004; Strauss, Sherman, & Spreen, 2006). An additional measure, the Timed Card Sorting Task (TCST), was administered and analyzed separately in order to better characterize IPS in the three subject groups.

Data from all 60 subjects were submitted to exploratory principal component analysis (jackknife procedure) to reduce the number of variables under consideration (Johnson & Wichern, 2002). Varimax rotation yielded three principal factors, "simple motor," "psychomotor," and "reaction time," that accounted for 76% of the total variance (see Table 9.2).

Analysis of variance revealed significant between-group effects for the simple motor ($p < .001$), psychomotor ($p < .001$) and reaction time ($p < .01$) factors. The PD group was significantly worse than either the AD or EC group on the simple motor factor ($p < .001$). Although the group mean scores for the AD and PD groups were worse than controls on the psychomotor ($p < .001$) and reaction time factors ($p < .01$), they did not significantly differ from each other ($p > .05$).

Performance on the TCST was measured in the three groups described above, with the addition of a second control group of 20 young healthy adults (YC). The experimental procedure required the rapid sorting of 40 standard playing cards according to four different conditions: (1) all cards into a single

Table 9.1 Between-group comparisons (mean, SD) for simple motor, complex motor and reaction time tasks

Group	Parkinson	Alzheimer	Control
Age (yrs)	65.8 (7.8)	67.7 (7.9)	65.5 (5.8)
Education (yrs)	13.6 (3.3)	13.0 (2.4)	13.8 (3.1)
Female	30%	50%	65%
Verbal IQ	105.9 (16.2)	88.6 (14.2)[a,c]	105.6 (17.0)
Simple motor			
Grip Strength (kg)	17.9 (10.5)[a,b]	27.3 (14.3)	26.5 (13.1)
Finger Tapping (taps/10 s)	35.2 (12.2)[a]	41.9 (11.5)	48.7 (8.5)
Two-Goal Tapping (taps/10 s)	33.4 (7.0)[a,b]	42.8 (8.4)	46.7 (6.7)
Purdue Pegboard (pegs/30 s)	8.3 (3.9)[a,b]	12.1 (1.6)[a]	14.5 (2.0)
Grooved Pegboard (pegs/60 s)	9.1 (4.6)[a,b]	13.2 (5.6)[a]	20.1 (2.8)
Pursuit Rotor (TOT/30 s)	14.1 (6.8)[a]	14.7 (8.1)[a]	22.9 (3.9)
Psychomotor			
Letter Cancellation[d] (time, s)	70.1 (26.9)[a]	62.6 (20.5)[a]	45.0 (12.0)
Trail Making Part A[d] (time, s)	60.4 (25.7)[a]	109.7 (91.8)[a]	37.4 (13.0)
Trail Making Part B[d] (time, s)	156.2 (79.5)[a]	245.5 (80.8)[a,c]	88.1 (31.1)
Name Writing (letters/s)	0.9 (0.4)[a]	1.1 (0.8)	1.8 (0.8)
Symbol Digit (digits/90 s)	28.0 (12.9)[a]	16.6 (14.9)[a]	41.2 (10.4)
Reaction time			
Simple Reaction Time[d] (time, ms)	309.4 (110.8)	288.6 (285.7)	266.5 (51.9)
Choice Reaction Time[d] (time, ms)	752.8 (194.1)[a]	916.1 (516.4)[a]	610.6 (93.0)

Notes: TOT = time on target in seconds. Mean score Significantly worse ($p < .01$) than [a]Control group, [b]Alzheimer group, [c]Parkinson group. [d]Lower value indicates better performances.

Table 9.2 Factor loadings from principal component analysis of PD, AD, and EC groups

	Factor 1 "Simple motor"	Factor 2 "Psychomotor"	Factor 3 "Reaction time"
Grip Strength	.711*	−.160	−.057
Finger Tapping	.848*	−.047	.254
Two-Goal Tapping	.819*	.173	.297
Purdue Pegboard	.798*	.447	−.028
Grooved Pegboard	.637*	(.618)	.126
Pursuit Rotor	.601*	.397	.341
Letter Cancellation	(−.571)	−.629*	.024
Trail Making Part A	.061	−.685*	(−.625)
Trail Making Part B	−.073	−.896*	−.192
Name Writing	(.482)	−.513*	.165
Symbol–Digit Substitution	.248	.864*	.246
Simple Reaction Time	−.221	−.061	−.881*
Choice Reaction Time	−.200	−.459	−.765*
Proportion of total variance accounted for	30.9%	28.4%	16.7%

Notes: *Maximum factor loading for task. Secondary loadings are indicated by parentheses.

pile, (2) two piles, one all black, the other all red, (3) four piles corresponding to the four suits (diamonds, hearts, clubs, and spades), and (4) 10 piles by rank order, from ace (corresponding to 1) to the number 10 (for details, see Mahurin & Pirozzolo, 1993). Significant mean effects were found for group ($p < .0001$) and sorting condition ($p < .0001$). The data for each group followed the log-linear relationship $RT = a + b(\log2(n + 1))$, in which n equals the number of response alternatives. However, the slopes of the regression lines significantly differed among the four subject groups, with AD and PD groups showing steeper slopes than either control group ($p < .0001$) (see Figure 9.2).

The two parts of this study demonstrate slowed processing speed in both PD and AD, but with different patterns of impairment. Specifically, the factor analysis revealed greater motor impairment in PD than AD, in accord with clinical descriptions of the two disorders. Additionally, both groups were impaired on tasks comprising the psychomotor factor. The added executive demands of these more complex tasks, such as selective attention, mental tracking, and symbol decoding, suggest the additional involvement of frontal regions in both disorders. The TCST results are consistent with Hick's law, which states that a subject's response time to equiprobable stimuli increases linearly with the logarithm of the number of alternative targets (Hick, 1952; Hyman, 1953). In terms of information theory, each additional binary decision (i.e., doubling the number of response alternatives) increases the cognitive processing load by one "bit" of information (Shannon, 1948; Teichner & Krebs, 1974). Although slopes of the regression line differed across groups, data from both patient and control subjects were consistent with Hick's law,

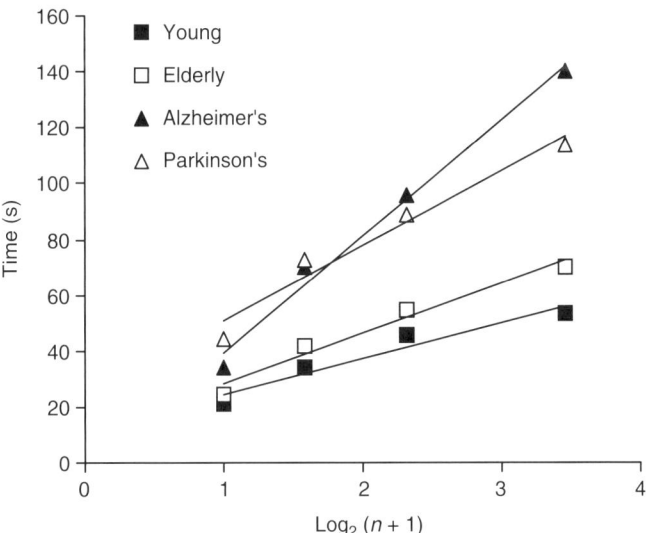

Figure 9.2 Group mean card sorting times as a log-linear function of the number of response alternatives (n). Regression lines represent $RT = a + b(\log2(n + 1))$. Adapted from Mahurin and Pirozzolo (1993).

reflecting a common structure to the organization of IPS, even when slowed by disease processes.

Summary and conclusions

Taken together, the studies in this chapter are consistent with the premise that bradyphrenia in PD is a dissociable cognitive impairment, although motor deficits also contribute to task slowing. There is increased latency of ERPs and MRPs in PD, with greater slowing evident as task complexity increases. RT is slowed in PD, but it is unclear to what extent this slowing is related to bradykinesia rather than bradyphrenia. Slowing of RT is more apparent for internally initiated than for externally cued behaviors. Certain nonmotoric cognitive tasks also are slowed, for example memory scanning. Bradyphrenia is influenced by, and interacts with, frontal-executive dysfunction, which contributes to significantly greater slowing in PDD compared with PD without dementia. Finally, bradyphrenia, a cognitive deficit, appears associated with bradykinesia, a motor deficit, and both types of impairment correlate with dopamine levels. Conflicting results from different studies may result from choice of diagnostic criteria, stage of disease course, presence of dementia, age of subjects, influence of secondary disease characteristics (e.g., apathy, depression, motivation), and treatment status (e.g., medicated or nonmedicated at the time of assessment).

Both PD and AD are associated with prominent executive impairment. Executive dysfunction in PD is consistent with disruption of FSCs connecting the BG and frontal systems (Padovani et al., 2006). When no dementia is present in PD, cognitive slowing appears primarily associated with BG pathology, whereas in AD slowing is associated with pathology of frontal regions. Rapid IPS requires executive control of response initiation, task shifting, working memory, selective attention, and efficient use of behavioral strategies, all of which are influenced by integrity of FSCs and their target regions. As PD progresses, greater involvement of frontal regions contributes to executive deficits that interact with bradyphrenia. Although cognitive slowing in PD and AD differs primarily in degree rather than pattern of impairments, slowing in PD has a distinct clinical quality that differs from cortical dementia, such as AD. Specifically, a PD patient's cognitive processes may give the clinical impression of "stickiness," hesitancy in thought, effortful shifting of attention set, and a "labored" quality to cognition. This pattern of cognitive slowing in PD is similar to observed motor impairment, further supporting the premise of common frontal-subcortical mechanisms underlying both bradyphrenia and bradykinesia.

References

Agid, Y. (1991). Parkinson's disease: Pathophysiology. *Lancet, 337*, 1321.
Albert, M. L., Feldman, R. G., & Willis, A. (1974). The "subcortical dementia" of

progressive supranuclear palsy. *Journal of Neurology, Neurosurgery, and Psychiatry, 37*, 121–130.

Alexander, G. E., & Crutcher, M. D. (1990). Functional architecture of basal ganglia circuits: Neural substrates of parallel processing. *Trends in Neuroscience, 13*, 266–271.

Alexander, G. E., Crutcher, M. D., & DeLong, M. R. (1991). Basal ganglia-thalamocortical circuits: Parallel substrates for motor, oculomotor, "prefrontal" and "limbic" functions. *Progress in Brain Research, 85* (119), 145.

Alexander, G. E., DeLong, M. R., & Strick, P. L. (1986). Parallel organization of functionally segregated circuits linking basal ganglia and cortex. *Annual Review of Neuroscience, 9*, 357–381.

Alexander, M. P., & Stuss, D. T. (2000). Disorders of frontal lobe functioning. *Seminars in Neurology, 20* (4), 427–437.

Amador, S. C., Hood, A. J., Schiess, M. C., Izor, R., & Sereno, A. B. (2006). Dissociating cognitive deficits involved in voluntary eye movement dysfunctions in Parkinson's disease patients. *Neuropsychologia, 44* (8), 1475–1482.

Benmoyal-Segal, L., & Soreq, H. (2006). Gene–environment interactions in sporadic Parkinson's disease. *Journal of Neurochemistry, 97* (6), 1740–1755.

Berry, E. L., Nicolson, R. I., Foster, J. K., Behrmann, M., & Sagar, H. J. (1999). Slowing of reaction time in Parkinson's disease: The involvement of the frontal lobes. *Neuropsychologia, 37* (7), 787–795.

Bherer, L., Belleville, S., & Gilbert, B. (2003). Temporal preparation strategy may inflate RT deficit in patients with Parkinson's disease. *Journal of Clinical and Experimental Neuropsychology, 25* (8), 1079–1089.

Bissessur, S., Tissingh, G., Wolters, E. C., & Scheltens, P. (1997). rCBF SPECT in Parkinson's disease patients with mental dysfunction. *Journal of Neural Transmission Supplement, 50*, 25–30.

Bokura, H., Yamaguchi, S., & Kobayashi, S. (2005). Event-related potentials for response inhibition in Parkinson's disease. *Neuropsychologia, 43* (6), 967–975.

Bondi, M. W., Kaszniak, A. W., Bayles, K. A., & Vance, K. T. (1993). Contributions of frontal system dysfunction to memory and perceptual abilities in Parkinson's disease. *Neuropsychology, 7*, 89–102.

Bouquet, C. A., Bonnaud, V., & Gil, R. (2003). Investigation of supervisory attentional system functions in patients with Parkinson's disease using the Hayling task. *Journal of Clinical and Experimental Neuropsychology, 25* (6), 751–760.

Bronstein, Y. L. (2001). Neurochemistry of frontal-subcortical disorders. In D. G. Lichter & J. L. Cummings (Eds.), *Frontal-subcortical circuits in psychiatric and neurological disorders* (pp. 59–91). New York: Guilford.

Brown, R. G., & Marsden, C. D. (1990). Cognitive function in Parkinson's disease: From description to theory. *Trends in Neurosciences, 13*, 21–29.

Burn, D. J., Rowan, E. N., Allan, L. M., Molloy, S., O'Brien, J. T., & McKeith, I. G. (2006). Motor subtype and cognitive decline in Parkinson's disease, Parkinson's disease with dementia, and dementia with Lewy bodies. *Journal of Neurology, Neurosurgery and Psychiatry, 77* (5), 585–589.

Clark, L. N., Afridi, S., Karlins, E., Wang, Y., Mejia-Santana, H., Harris, J., et al. (2006). Case-control study of the parkin gene in early-onset Parkinson disease. *Archives of Neurology, 63* (4), 548–552.

Comijs, H. C., Jonker, C., Beekman, A. T., & Deeg, D. J. (2001). The association between depressive symptoms and cognitive decline in community-dwelling elderly persons. *International Journal of Geriatric Psychiatry*, *16* (4), 361–367.

Cooper, J. A., Sagar, H. J., Jordan, N., Harvey, N. S., & Sullivan, E. V. (1991). Cognitive impairment in early, untreated Parkinson's disease and its relationship to motor disability. *Brain*, *114*, 2095–2122.

Cooper, J. A., Sagar, H. J., Tidswell, P., & Jordan, N. (1994). Slowed central processing in simple and go/no-go reaction time tasks in Parkinson's disease. *Brain*, *117*, 517–529.

Cummings, J. L. (1986). Subcortical dementia. Neuropsychology, neuropsychiatry, and pathophysiology. *British Journal of Psychiatry*, *149*, 682–697.

Cummings, J. L. (1988). The dementia of Parkinson disease: Prevalence, characteristics, neurobiology, and comparison with dementia of the Alzheimer type. *European Neurology*, *28* (Suppl. 1), 15–23.

Cummings, J. L. (1990). Introduction: Subcortical dementia. In J. L. Cummings (Ed.), *Subcortical dementia* (pp. 3–16). New York: Oxford University Press.

Cunnington, R., Iansek, R., Bradshaw, J. L., & Phillips, J. G. (1995). Movement-related potentials in Parkinson's disease. Presence and predictability of temporal and spatial cues. *Brain*, *118* (Pt 4), 935–950.

Davidson, P. S., Anaki, D., Saint-Cyr, J. A., Chow, T. W., & Moscovitch, M. (2006). Exploring the recognition memory deficit in Parkinson's disease: Estimates of recollection versus familiarity. *Brain*, *129* (Pt 7), 1768–1779.

de Lau, L. M., & Breteler, M. M. (2006). Epidemiology of Parkinson's disease. *Lancet Neurology*, *5* (6), 525–535.

Dobbs, R. J., Bowes, S. G., Charlett, A., Henley, M., Frith, C., Dickins, J., et al. (1993a). Hypothesis: The bradyphrenia of Parkinsonism is a nosological entity. *Acta Neurologica Scandinavica*, *87* (4), 255–261.

Dobbs, R. J., Bowes, S. G., Henley, M., Charlett, A., O'Neill, C. J., Dickins, J., et al. (1993b). Assessment of the bradyphrenia of Parkinsonism: A novel use of delayed auditory feedback. *Acta Neurologica Scandinavica*, *87* (4), 262–267.

Donders, F. C. (1868). On the speed of mental processes. Reprinted in W. G. Koster (Ed.). (1969), *Attention and performance II*. Amsterdam: North Holland.

Dubois, B., Defontaines, B., Deweer, B., Malapani, C., & Pillon, B. (1995). Cognitive and behavioral changes in patients with focal lesions of the basal ganglia. *Advances in Neurology*, *65*, 29–41.

Duchesne, N., Soucy, J. P., Masson, H., Chouinard, S., & Bedard, M. A. (2002). Cognitive deficits and striatal dopaminergic denervation in Parkinson's disease: A single photon emission computed tomography study using 123iodine-beta-CIT in patients on and off levodopa. *Clinical Neuropharmacology*, *25* (4), 216–224.

Duncombe, M. E., Bradshaw, J. L., Iansek, R., & Phillips, J. G. (1994). Parkinsonian patients without dementia or depression do not suffer from bradyphrenia as indexed by performance in mental rotation tasks with and without advance information. *Neuropsychologia*, *32* (11), 1383–1396.

Ebmeier, K. P., Calder, S. A., Crawford, J. R., Stewart, L., Besson, J. A., & Mutch, W. J. (1990). Clinical features predicting dementia in idiopathic Parkinson's disease: A follow-up study. *Neurology*, *40*, 1222–1224.

Elias, J. W., & Treland, J. E. (1999). Executive function in Parkinson's disease and subcortical disorders. *Seminars in Clinical Neuropsychiatry*, *4* (1), 34–40.

Evarts, E. V., Teravainen, H., & Calne, D. B. (1981). Reaction time in Parkinson's disease. *Brain*, *104*, 167–186.

Farrer, M. J. (2006). Genetics of Parkinson disease: Paradigm shifts and future prospects. *Nature Reviews: Genetics*, *7* (4), 306–318.
Franz, E. A., & Miller, J. (2002). Effects of response readiness on reaction time and force output in people with Parkinson's disease. *Brain*, *125* (Pt 8), 1733–1750.
Garnett, E. S., Nahmias, C., & Firnau, G. (1984). Central dopaminergic pathways in hemiparkinsonism examined by positron emission tomography. *Canadian Journal of Neurological Sciences*, *11*, 174–179.
Gauntlett-Gilbert, J., & Brown, V. J. (1998). Reaction time deficits and Parkinson's disease. *Neuroscience and Biobehavioral Reviews*, *22* (6), 865–881.
Golbe, L. I., & Langston, J. W. (1993). The etiology of Parkinson's disease: New directions for research. In J. Jankovic & E. Tolosa (Eds.), *Parkinson's disease and movement disorders* (2nd ed., pp. 93–102). Baltimore: Williams & Wilkins.
Gray, F., Poirier, J., & Scaravilli, F. (1991). Parkinson's disease and parkinsonian syndromes. In S. Duckett (Ed.), *The pathology of the aging human nervous system* (pp. 179–199). Philadelphia: Lea & Febiger.
Hanes, K. R., Andrewes, D. G., & Pantelis, C. (1995). Cognitive flexibility and complex integration in Parkinson's disease, Huntington's disease, and schizophrenia. *Journal of the International Neuropsychological Society*, *1* (6), 545–553.
Hannay, J. H., Howieson, D. B., Loring, D. W., Fischer, J. S., & Lezak, M. D. (2004). Neuropathology for neuropsychologists. In M. D. Lezak, D. B. Howieson, & D. W. Loring (Eds.), *Neuropsychological assessment* (4th ed., pp. 157–285). New York: Oxford University Press.
Hick, W. E. (1952). On the rate of gain of information. *Quarterly Journal of Experimental Psychology*, *4*, 11–26.
Hocherman, S., Moont, R., & Schwartz, M. (2004). Response selection and execution in patients with Parkinson's disease. *Brain Research: Cognitive Brain Research*, *19* (1), 40–51.
Hoover, J. E., & Strick, P. L. (1993). Multiple output channels in the basal ganglia. *Science*, *259*, 819–821.
Hoover, J. E., & Strick, P. L. (1999). The organization of cerebellar and basal ganglia outputs to primary motor cortex as revealed by retrograde transneural transport of herpes simplex virus type. *Journal of Neuroscience*, *19*, 1446–1463.
Houk, J. C. (2001). Neurophysiology of frontal-subcortical loops. In D. G. Lichter & J. L. Cummings (Eds.), *Frontal-subcortical circuits in psychiatric and neurological disorders* (pp. 92–113). New York: Guilford.
Huber, S. J., Christy, J. A., & Paulson, G. W. (1991). Cognitive heterogeneity associated with clinical subtypes of Parkinson's disease. *Neuropsychiatry, Neuropsychology, and Behavioral Neurology*, *4*, 147–157.
Hyman, R. (1953). Stimulus information as a determinant of reaction times. *Journal of Experimental Psychology*, *45*, 188–196.
Inzelberg, R., Plotnik, M., Flash, T., Schechtman, E., Shahar, I., & Korczyn, A. D. (2001). Mental and motor switching in Parkinson's disease. *Journal of Motor Behavior*, *33* (4), 377–385.
Jacobs, D. M., Levy, G., & Marder, K. (2003). Dementia in Parkinson's disease, Huntington's disease, and related disorders. In T. E. Feinberg & M. J. Farah (Eds.), *Behavioral neurology and neuropsychology* (2nd ed.). New York: McGraw-Hill.
Janvin, C. C., Larsen, J. P., Salmon, D. P., Galasko, D., Hugdahl, K., & Aarsland, D. (2006). Cognitive profiles of individual patients with Parkinson's disease and

dementia: Comparison with dementia with Lewy bodies and Alzheimer's disease. *Movement Disorders, 21* (3), 337–342.

Johnson, A. M., Vernon, P. A., Almeida, Q. J., Grantier, L. L., Singarayer, R., & Jog, M. S. (2004). Screening for Parkinson's disease with response time batteries: A pilot study. *BMC Medical Informatics and Decision Making, 4*, 14.

Johnson, R. A., & Wichern, D. W. (2002). *Applied multivariate statistical analysis* (5th ed.). Upper Saddle River, NJ: Prentice Hall.

Kirsch-Darrow, L., Fernandez, H. F., Marsiske, M., Okun, M. S., & Bowers, D. (2006). Dissociating apathy and depression in Parkinson disease. *Neurology, 67* (1), 33–38.

Kutukcu, Y., Marks, W. J., Jr., Goodin, D. S., & Aminoff, M. J. (1998). Cerebral accompaniments to simple and choice reaction tasks in Parkinson's disease. *Brain Research, 799* (1), 1–5.

Lee, A. C., Harris, J. P., & Calvert, J. E. (1998). Impairments of mental rotation in Parkinson's disease. *Neuropsychologia, 36* (1), 109–114.

Lee, C., Grossman, M., Morris, J., Stern, M. B., & Hurtig, H. I. (2003). Attentional resource and processing speed limitations during sentence processing in Parkinson's disease. *Brain and Language, 85* (3), 347–356.

Leenders, K. L., Palmer, A. J., Quinn, N., Clark, J. C., Firnau, G., Garnett, E. S., et al. (1986). Brain dopamine metabolism in patients with Parkinson's disease measured with PET. *Journal of Neurology, Neurosurgery, and Psychiatry, 49*, 855–860.

Lees, A. J. (1994). The concept of bradyphrenia. *Revista de Neurologia (Paris), 150* (12), 823–826.

Lerner, A. J., & Whitehouse, P. J. (2002). Neuropsychiatric aspects of dementias associated with motor dysfunction. In S. C. Yudofsky & R. E. Hales (Eds.), *Textbook of neuropsychiatry and clinical neurosciences* (4th ed.). Washington, DC: American Psychiatric Publishing.

Lezak, M. D., Howieson, D. B., & Loring, D. W. (2004). *Neuropsychological assessment*. New York: Oxford University Press.

Li, M., Kuroiwa, Y., Wang, L., Kamitani, T., Omoto, S., Hayashi, E., et al. (2005). Visual event-related potentials under different interstimulus intervals in Parkinson's disease: Relation to motor disability, WAIS-R, and regional cerebral blood flow. *Parkinsonism and Related Disorders, 11* (4), 209–219.

Lichter, D. G. (2001). Movement disorders and frontal-subcortical circuits. In D. G. Lichter & J. L. Cummings (Eds.), *Frontal-subcortical circuits in psychiatric and neurological disorders* (pp. 260–313). New York: Guilford.

Lichter, D. G., & Cummings, J. L. (2001). Introduction and overview. In D. G. Lichter & J. L. Cummings (Eds.), *Frontal-subcortical circuits in psychiatric and neurological disorders* (pp. 1–43). New York: Guilford.

Lieberman, A. (2006a). Are dementia and depression in Parkinson's disease related? *Journal of Neurol Science, 248* (1–2), 138–142.

Lieberman, A. (2006b). Depression in Parkinson's disease—a review. *Acta Neurologica Scandinavica, 113* (1), 1–8.

Low, K. A., Miller, J., & Vierck, E. (2002). Response slowing in Parkinson's disease: A psychophysiological analysis of premotor and motor processes. *Brain, 125* (Pt 9), 1980–1994.

Luce, R. D. (1986). *Response times: Their role in inferring elementary mental organization*. New York: Oxford University Press.

Mahurin, R. K. (1984). *Differentiation of reaction time performance in Parkinson disease on the basis of motor symptoms.* Unpublished master's thesis, University of Houston, TX.

Mahurin, R. K. (1998). Neural network modeling of basal ganglia function in Parkinson's disease and related disorders. In R. W. Parks, D. S. Levine, & D. L. Long (Eds.), *Fundamentals of neural network modeling: Neuropsychology and cognitive neuroscience* (pp. 331–355). Cambridge, MA: MIT Press.

Mahurin, R. K., Feher, E. P., Nance, M. L., Levy, J. K., & Pirozzolo, F. J. (1993). Cognition in Parkinson's disease and related disorders. In R. Parks, R. Zec, & R. Wilson (Eds.), *Neuropsychology of Alzheimer's disease and other dementias* (pp. 308–349). New York: Oxford University Press.

Mahurin, R. K., & Pirozzolo, F. J. (1986). Chronometric analysis: Clinical applications in aging and dementia. *Developmental Neuropsychology, 2,* 345–362.

Mahurin, R. K., & Pirozzolo, F. J. (1993). Application of Hick's law of response speed in Alzheimer and Parkinson diseases. *Perceptual and Motor Skills, 77* (1), 107–113.

Mayberg, H. S. (1994). Frontal lobe dysfunction in secondary depression. *Journal of Neuropsychiatry and Clinical Neuroscience, 6* (4), 428–442.

Meck, W. H. (1996). Neuropharmacology of timing and time perception. *Brain Research: Cognitive Brain Research, 3* (3–4), 227–242.

Meiran, N., Friedman, G., & Yehene, E. (2004). Parkinson's disease is associated with goal setting deficits during task switching. *Brain and Cognition, 54* (3), 260–262.

Middleton, F. A., & Strick, P. L. (2001). A revised neuroanatomy of frontal-subcortical circuits. In D. G. Lichter & J. L. Cummings (Eds.), *Frontal-subcortical circuits in psychiatric and neurological disorders* (pp. 44–58). New York: Guilford.

Monetta, L., & Pell, M. D. (2006). Effects of verbal working memory deficits on metaphor comprehension in patients with Parkinson's disease. *Brain and Language* (in press).

Montgomery, E. B., Jr., Baker, K. B., Lyons, K., & Koller, W. C. (2000). Motor initiation and execution in essential tremor and Parkinson's disease. *Movement Disorders, 15* (3), 511–515.

Montgomery, E. B., Nuessen, J., Nuessen, G., & Douglas, S. (1991). Reaction time and movement velocity abnormalities in Parkinson's disease under different task conditions. *Neurology, 41,* 1476–1481.

Mortimer, J. A., Pirozzolo, F. J., Hansch, E. C., & Webster, D. D. (1982). Relationship of motor symptoms to intellectual deficits in Parkinson disease. *Neurology, 32* (2), 133–137.

Muller, T., Benz, S., & Bornke, C. (2001). Delay of simple reaction time after levodopa intake. *Clinical Neurophysiology, 112* (11), 2133–2137.

Muller, T., Benz, S., & Przuntek, H. (2000). Choice reaction time after levodopa challenge in Parkinsonian patients. *Journal of Neurological Sciences, 181* (1–2), 98–103.

Muller, T., Benz, S., & Przuntek, H. (2002). Apomorphine delays simple reaction time in Parkinsonian patients. *Parkinsonism and Related Disorders, 8* (5), 357–360.

Muller, T., Eising, E., Kuhn, W., Buttner, T., Coenen, H. H., & Przuntek, H. (1999). Delayed motor response correlates with striatal degeneration in Parkinson's disease. *Acta Neurologica Scandinavica, 100* (4), 227–230.

O'Brien, J. T., Wiseman, R., Burton, E. J., Barber, B., Wesnes, K., Saxby, B., et al. (2002). Cognitive associations of subcortical white matter lesions in older people. *Annals of the New York Academy of Sciences, 977,* 436–444.

Oved, D., Ziv, I., Treves, T. A., Paleacu, D., Melamed, E., & Djaldetti, R. (2006).

Effect of dopamine agonists on fatigue and somnolence in Parkinson's disease. *Movement Disorders, 21,* 1257–1261.

Padovani, A., Costanzi, C., Gilberti, N., & Borroni, B. (2006). Parkinson's disease and dementia. *Neurological Sciences, 27* (Suppl 1), S40–S43.

Partiot, A., Verin, M., Pillon, B., Teixeira-Ferreira, C., Agid, Y., & Dubois, B. (1996). Delayed response tasks in basal ganglia lesions in man: Further evidence for a striato-frontal cooperation in behavioural adaptation. *Neuropsychologia, 34* (7), 709–721.

Pate, D. S., & Margolin, D. I. (1994). Cognitive slowing in Parkinson's and Alzheimer's patients: Distinguishing bradyphrenia from dementia. *Neurology, 44* (4), 669–674.

Pessiglione, M., Czernecki, V., Pillon, B., Dubois, B., Schupbach, M., Agid, Y., et al. (2005). An effect of dopamine depletion on decision-making: The temporal coupling of deliberation and execution. *Journal of Cognitive Neuroscience, 17* (12), 1886–1896.

Phillips, J. G., Schiffter, T., Nicholls, M. E., Bradshaw, J. L., Iansek, R., & Saling, L. L. (1999). Does old age or Parkinson's disease cause bradyphrenia? *Journals of Gerontology: Biological Sciences and Medical Sciences, 54* (8), M404–M409.

Pillon, B., Ertle, S., Deweer, B., Sarazin, M., Agid, Y., & Dubois, B. (1996). Memory for spatial location is affected in Parkinson's disease. *Neuropsychologia, 34* (1), 77–85.

Prasher, D., & Findley, L. (1991). Dopaminergic induced changes in cognitive and motor processing in Parkinson's disease: An electrophysiological investigation. *Journal of Neurology, Neurosurgery, and Psychiatry, 54,* 603–609.

Price, A. L. (2006). Explicit category learning in Parkinson's disease: Deficits related to impaired rule generation and selection processes. *Neuropsychology, 20* (2), 249–257.

Rafal, R. D., Posner, M. I., Walker, J. A., & Friedrich, F. J. (1984). Cognition and the basal ganglia: Separating mental and motor components of performance in Parkinson's disease. *Brain, 107,* 1083–1094.

Rammsayer, T. H. (1994). A cognitive-neuroscience approach for elucidation of mechanisms underlying temporal information processing. *International Journal of Neuroscience, 77* (1–2), 61–76.

Rammsayer, T. H. (1997). Are there dissociable roles of the mesostriatal and mesolimbocortical dopamine systems on temporal information processing in humans? *Neuropsychobiology, 35* (1), 36–45.

Ransmayr, G., Bitschnau, W., Schmidhuber-Eiler, B., Berger, W., Karamat, E., Poewe, W., et al. (1990). Slowing of high-speed memory scanning in Parkinson's disease is related to the severity of Parkinsonian motor symptoms. *Journal of Neural Transmission: Parkinson's Disease and Dementia Section, 2* (4), 265–275.

Rebec, G. V. (2006). Behavioral electrophysiology of psychostimulants. *Neuropsychopharmacology, 31,* 2341–2348.

Rinne, J. O. (2003). Other important dementias. In N. Qizilbash (Ed.), *Evidence-based dementia practice* (pp. 312–329). Oxford, UK: Blackwell.

Rogers, D. (1986). Bradyphrenia in Parkinsonism: A historical review. *Psychological Medicine, 16* (2), 257–265.

Rogers, D., Lees, A. J., Smith, E., Trimble, M., & Stern, G. M. (1987). Bradyphrenia in Parkinson's disease and psychomotor retardation in depressive illness. An experimental study. *Brain, 110* (Pt 3), 761–776.

Roman, M. J., Delis, D. C., Filoteo, J. V., Demadura, T. L., Paulsen, J., Swerdlow, N. R., et al. (1998). Is there a "subcortical" profile of attentional dysfunction? A comparison of patients with Huntington's and Parkinson's diseases on a global–local focused attention task. *Journal of Clinical and Experimental Neuropsychology, 20* (6), 873–884.

Royall, D. R., Mahurin, R. K., & Gray, K. F. (1992). Bedside assessment of executive cognitive impairment: The executive interview. *Journal of the American Geriatric Society, 40* (12), 1221–1226.

Salmon, D. P., Heindel, W. C., & Hamilton, J. M. (2001). Cognitive abilities mediated by frontal-subcortical circuits. In D. G. Lichter & J. L. Cummings (Eds.), *Frontal-subcortical circuits in psychiatric and neurological disorders* (pp. 114–150). New York: Guilford.

Sawamoto, N., Honda, M., Hanakawa, T., Fukuyama, H., & Shibasaki, H. (2002). Cognitive slowing in Parkinson's disease: A behavioral evaluation independent of motor slowing. *Journal of Neuroscience, 22* (12), 5198–5203.

Schapira, A. H. (2006). Etiology of Parkinson's disease. *Neurology, 66* (10 Suppl. 4), S10–S23.

Shannon, C. E. (1948). A mathematical theory of communication. *Bell System Technical Journal, 27*, 379–423.

Shipley, B. A., Deary, I. J., Tan, J., Christie, G., & Starr, J. M. (2002). Efficiency of temporal order discrimination as an indicator of bradyphrenia in Parkinson's disease: The inspection time loop task. *Neuropsychologia, 40* (8), 1488–1493.

Siegert, R. J., Harper, D. N., Cameron, F. B., & Abernethy, D. (2002). Self-initiated versus externally cued reaction times in Parkinson's disease. *Journal of Clinical and Experimental Neuropsychology, 24* (2), 146–153.

Smith, M. C., Goldman, W. P., Janer, K. W., Baty, J. D., & Morris, J. C. (1998). Cognitive speed in nondemented Parkinson's disease. *Journal of the International Neuropsychology Society, 4* (6), 584–592.

Starkstein, S. E., Esteguy, M., Berthier, M. L., Garcia, H., & Leiguarda, R. (1989). Evoked potentials, reaction time and cognitive performance in on and off phases of Parkinson's disease. *Journal of Neurology, Neurosurgery, and Psychiatry, 52*, 338–340.

Strauss, E., Sherman, E. M. S., & Spreen, O. (2006). *A Compendium of neuropsychological tests: Administration, norms, and commentary* (3rd ed.). New York: Oxford University Press.

Strick, P. L., Hoover, J. E., & Mushiake, H. (1993). Evidence for "output channels" in the basal ganglia and cerebellum. In N. Mano, I. Hamada, & M. R. DeLong (Eds.), *Role of the cerebellum and basal ganglia in voluntary movement* (pp. 171–180). Amsterdam: Elsevier.

Tanaka, H., Koenig, T., Pascual-Marqui, R. D., Hirata, K., Kochi, K., & Lehmann, D. (2000). Event-related potential and EEG measures in Parkinson's disease without and with dementia. *Dementia and Geriatric Cognitive Disorders, 11* (1), 39–45.

Taylor, A. E., Saint-Cyr, J. A., & Lang, A. E. (1986). Frontal lobe dysfunction in Parkinson's disease: The cortical focus of neostriatal flow. *Brain, 109*, 845–883.

Teichner, W. H., & Krebs, M. J. (1974). Laws of visual choice reaction time. *Psychological Review, 81*, 75–98.

Troster, A. I., Stalp, L. D., Paolo, A. M., Fields, J. A., & Koller, W. C. (1995). Neuropsychological impairment in Parkinson's disease with and without depression. *Archives of Neurology, 52* (12), 1164–1169.

Uekermann, J., Daum, I., Bielawski, M., Muhlack, S., Peters, S., Przuntek, H., et al.

(2004). Differential executive control impairments in early Parkinson's disease. *Journal of Neural Transmission: Supplement, 68*, 39–51.

Vardy, Y., Bradshaw, J. L., & Iansek, R. (2003). Dual target identification and the attentional blink in Parkinson's disease. *Journal of Clinical and Experimental Neuropsychology, 25* (3), 361–375.

Wang, H., Wang, Y., Wang, D., Cui, L., Tian, S., & Zhang, Y. (2002). Cognitive impairment in Parkinson's disease revealed by event-related potential N270. *Journal of Neurological Sciences, 194* (1), 49–53.

Wang, L., Kuroiwa, Y., Li, M., Kamitani, T., Wang, J., Takahashi, T., et al. (2000). The correlation between P300 alterations and regional cerebral blood flow in non-demented Parkinson's disease. *Neuroscience Letters, 282* (3), 133–136.

Wechsler, D. (1981). *Wechsler Adult Intelligence Scale—Revised manual*. San Antonio, TX: Psychological Corporation.

Weder, B., Azari, N. P., Knorr, U., Seitz, R. J., Keel, A., Nienhusmeier, M., et al. (2000). Disturbed functional brain interactions underlying deficient tactile object discrimination in Parkinson's disease. *Human Brain Mapping, 11* (3), 131–145.

Whittington, C. J., Podd, J., & Stewart-Williams, S. (2006). Memory deficits in Parkinson's disease. *Journal of Clinical and Experimental Neuropsychology, 28* (5), 738–754.

Wilson, R. S., Kaszniak, A. W., Klawans, H. L., & Garron, D. C. (1980). High speed memory scanning in Parkinsonism. *Cortex, 16*, 67–72.

Wolfe, N., Katz, D. I., Albert, M. L., Almozlino, A., Durso, R., Smith, M. C., et al. (1990). Neuropsychological profile linked to low dopamine in Alzheimer's disease, major depression, and Parkinson's disease. *Journal of Neurology, Neurosurgery, and Psychiatry, 53*, 915–917.

Woodward, T. S., Bub, D. N., & Hunter, M. A. (2002). Task switching deficits associated with Parkinson's disease reflect depleted attentional resources. *Neuropsychologia, 40* (12), 1948–1955.

Young, A. B., & Penney, J. B., Jr. (1993). Biochemical and functional organization of the basal ganglia. In J. Jankovic & E. Tolosa (Eds.), *Parkinson's disease and movement disorders* (pp. 1–11). Baltimore: Williams & Wilkins.

Zetusky, W. J., Jankovic, J., & Pirozzolo, F. J. (1985). The heterogeneity of Parkinson's disease: Clinical and prognostic implications. *Neurology, 35*, 522–526.

10 Information processing speed and aging

Timothy A. Salthouse and David J. Madden

This chapter is organized into two sections. The first section consists of a brief examination of the status of a processing speed construct from a psychometric perspective, and the second section is a selective review of potential neurobiological correlates of speed. Although research from psychometric and neurobiological traditions might appear to represent quite different perspectives, we believe that they should be more closely related than is commonly assumed, particularly when, as is the case in this review, they share a common focus on the relation of aging to speed.

Psychometric perspective on information processing speed

Speed is unique in psychological research because it is used both as a measure of performance in specific cognitive tasks, and also as an attribute of individuals. That is, measures of speed frequently serve as a dependent variable in many different types of cognitive tasks, and in this respect speed is an index of task performance somewhat similar to accuracy. However, speed is also considered to be an individual difference characteristic that could affect behavior in a variety of different situations, and in this respect it can be considered similar to other cognitive abilities such as memory or reasoning.

The distinction between the two conceptualizations of speed is particularly pronounced in research on aging because adult age differences in speed are among the largest of any behavioral variables (e.g., Madden, 2001; Salthouse, 1985). Furthermore, to the extent that someone is slow in many different types of tasks, it has been proposed that this characteristic of the individual should be taken into consideration when relying on a measure of speed as a reflection of the individual's susceptibility to various task manipulations. Analytical procedures that might be used for this purpose have been discussed elsewhere (e.g., Faust, Balota, Spieler, & Ferraro, 1999; Madden, 2001; Salthouse & Hedden, 2002), and the primary focus in this section is on how an individual differences construct of speed is best assessed.

Some researchers have assumed that the purest assessment of an individual's speed might be obtained from tasks in which the individual must press one of several keys as rapidly as possible depending on the particular stimulus presented (i.e., reaction time; RT), or from tasks in which decisions are to be made about the identity of briefly presented visual or auditory stimuli (i.e., inspection time). Unfortunately, there is seldom any independent evidence to justify a claim of assessment purity because there is no gold standard against which candidate variables of processing speed can be compared. Moreover, it is not even clear what the best measure might be for such a gold standard because, for example, nerve conduction velocity might be at too low a level, and the speed of executing what are postulated to be elementary cognitive operations might be at too high a level.

Within the psychometric tradition a bootstrap approach is often used to deal with this problem, because decisions about the meaning of variables have been based on analyses of construct validity involving patterns of relations among variables postulated to be the same and variables postulated to be different. That is, many different tests (or tasks) are administered to the same individuals, and then the patterns of interrelations among the variables are examined. When data are available from a wide variety of tests it is often found that speed measures tend to be associated together to form a factor, or theoretical construct, that is distinct from factors derived from other types of cognitive measures.

Examples of this approach are apparent in cognitive test batteries such as the Wechsler Adult Intelligence Scale III (WAIS III; Wechsler, 1997) and the Woodcock-Johnson Tests of Cognitive Abilities III (WJ III; Woodcock, McGrew, & Mather, 2001). Both of these test batteries contain two tests of speed in which the examinee is asked to mark symbols or substitute elements from a code table, or to search for items in an array. A common characteristic of these types of tasks is that the requirements are so simple that errors are infrequent, and consequently most of the variability across people is evident in how quickly the task can be performed. In both exploratory and confirmatory factor analyses these variables have been found to have much stronger relations to each other than they have with variables hypothesized to represent other constructs, such as memory and reasoning. Because there is evidence for both convergent validity, in the form of moderate to strong relations with other measures of the same construct, and discriminant validity, in the form of relatively weak relations with measures hypothesized to represent other constructs, results of this type have been interpreted as establishing the validity of a processing speed construct.

Although a single construct representing processing or perceptual speed is typically found in analyses based on a wide variety of cognitive variables, multiple speed constructs can be distinguished if many measures of speed are included in the same analysis (e.g., Ackerman, Beier, & Boyle, 2002; Babcock, Laguna, & Roesch, 1997). However, it is important to recognize that the finding of several speed constructs is not inconsistent with the existence of a dimension of individual differences corresponding to how quickly someone can carry out simple cognitive operations. Instead, it could merely reflect the application of a finer level of resolution, because multiple constructs would probably be found within any ability domain if many similar measures were available in a moderately large sample.

There is sometimes a tendency to consider almost any type of timed performance as representing a processing speed construct when, in addition to an influence of speed, the variables are likely to reflect a mixture of task-specific factors, such as particular strategies, processes, or knowledge (e.g., Hultsch, Hertzog, Dixon, & Small, 1998; Wilson, Bienias, Evans, & Bennett, 2004). The opposite tendency also exists in that some researchers have claimed that a variable does not reflect processing speed because of a finding that it has significant correlations with another type of variable (e.g., Parkin & Java, 1999). From the current perspective both types of assertions are overstated because they confuse speed as a dependent variable or index of performance in a particular task with speed as an ability that influences performance in many different types of tasks (also see Piccinin & Rabbitt, 1999), and they assume an unrealistic one-to-one correspondence between an observed variable and a theoretical construct. With respect to this latter point, even the best, or "purest," variable probably has multiple influences, and probably represents only a portion of the relevant theoretical construct. The lack of a one-to-one correspondence between variables and constructs is apparent in the results of factor analyses because the square of the standardized regression coefficient from a factor to the variable indicates the proportion of variance in the variable that is associated with the factor, and those coefficients are seldom very close to 1. Moreover, when several factors are included in the analyses, the regression coefficients from other factors to the variable are often significantly greater than 0, indicating that the variable has influences from multiple factors.

Salthouse (2005) recently proposed that a correlation-based procedure could be used to investigate the meaning of individual variables. The procedure involves examining the correlations of the variable with well-accepted constructs that are defined on the basis of the variance common to multiple indicator variables. The rationale is that a variable can be considered to be influenced by a construct to the extent that performance on the variable varies according to the level of that construct in a moderately large sample of adults with a representative range of variation on both the variable and the construct.

There are at least two major requirements of this analytical procedure. First, the indicator variables for the reference constructs should have strong relations to one another, but only weak relations to variables representing other constructs. Unless these conditions hold, the reference constructs may not be well defined, and consequently they would not be informative in determining what other variables represent. And second, the samples of participants should be large enough to allow accurate estimates of the strength of the relations, and not merely to determine whether the relations are significantly different from zero.

A study by Piccinin and Rabbitt (1999) used a variant of this procedure with a measure of performance in a multiple trial substitution task as the target variable. Although they used a growth model to identify both level (i.e., the intercept or starting value) and rate of change (i.e., the slope) parameters, only the level parameter was significantly related to age, and the age correlations were very similar for the measures from each trial (i.e., –.39 to –.42). Unlike the method proposed here, these authors used a single variable to represent each cognitive ability, and thus at least some of the relations they observed may reflect variable-specific influences rather than influences of the hypothesized ability. Nevertheless, the results of their analyses were very similar to those reported below in that the substitution variable had moderate influences from speed and reasoning abilities, but weak influences from memory and vocabulary abilities. Furthermore, as reported by Salthouse (2005), there were no unique age-related influences on the level of the substitution variable after controlling the variance in the other cognitive abilities.

Figure 10.1 illustrates the logic of the proposed procedure, with established cognitive abilities derived from the psychometric tradition serving as reference constructs. It is important to note that almost any set of constructs could be used as the reference constructs in this type of analysis, as long as each construct is defined on the basis of multiple indicator variables that each have moderate to strong relations to each other, and hence can be considered

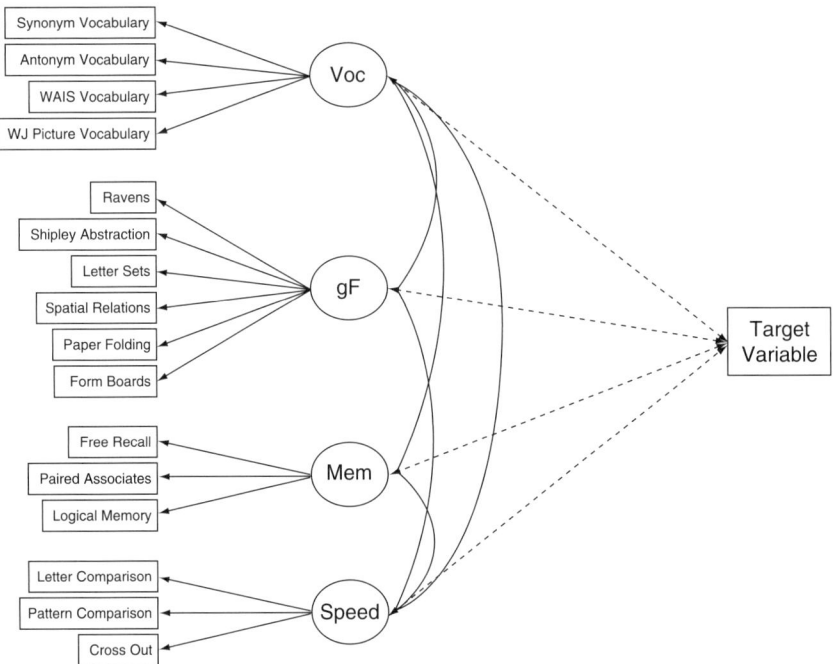

Figure 10.1 Structural model illustrating how the meaning of a variable can be determined by the relative influences of different cognitive abilities on it. "Voc" refers to vocabulary, "gF" to fluid ability, "Mem" to episodic memory, and "Speed" to perceptual speed. See text for details.

to represent the construct. This condition is usually met with psychometric ability constructs because the standardized regression coefficients are typically greater than .70, indicating that the majority of the total variance in each variable was associated with the hypothesized construct.

The analytical procedure can be applied to a variety of variables sometimes considered to represent processing speed, with data aggregated across many studies conducted by Salthouse and colleagues (see Salthouse, 2004, for description of the reference variables and the aggregate data set). Table 10.1

Table 10.1 Standardized regression coefficients for the model portrayed in Figure 10.1

Variable	Reference constructs			
	Speed	Fluid	Mem	Vocab
Trail Making A	.90*	−.20	−.08	.04
Trail Making B	.64*	.12	.06	.00
Stroop Neutral	.77*	−.18	.05	.01
Stroop Congruent	.59*	−.09	.13	−.14
Stroop Incongruent	.53*	.19	.22*	−.13*
DD RT	.43*	−.14	.39*	−.07
DS RT	.54*	−.11	.48*	−.10*
Anti-Cue Congruent RT	.49*	−.09	.20	−.22*
Anti-Cue Incongruent RT	.50*	.01	.09	−.19*
Digit Symbol	.57*	.18*	.13*	−.05
Letter Fluency	.31*	−.01	.12*	.33*
Category Fluency	.31*	−.07	.39*	.18*
Connections—Same	.37*	.33*	.09	−.09
Connections—Alternating	.21*	.09	.07	.07
Maze Tracing Time	.42*	−.07	.24	−.04
Count Back Time	.35*	.22	−.05	.29*
Reading Time—Normal	.53*	−.33*	.21	.34*
Reading Time—Distract.	.43*	.00	.08	.32*

Notes: Trail Making A and B represent the time to connect items in numerical (A) or alternating numerical and alphabetical (B) sequence. The Stroop variables represent the time to name colors of a string of Xs (Neutral), of the words referring to the color (Congruent), or of words referring to a different color (Incongruent). DDRT is a choice reaction time task in which one keypress response is to be made if the pair of digits is the same, and a different keypress response is to be made if the two digits are different. DSRT is a choice reaction time task in which the decision is based on whether the displayed digit and symbol match according to a code table. The two anti-cue variables represent the reaction time to classify a letter when the letter was preceded by a brief flash in the same (Congruent) or opposite (Incongruent) side of the display. The Digit Symbol variable is the number of symbols completed in the WAIS III Digit Symbol Substitution test. Letter fluency is the number of words generated within 60 seconds beginning with a designated letter, and category fluency is the number of words generated within 60 seconds from within a designated category. Connections same and alternating are variants of the Trail Making Test in which items are to be connected according to the same numerical or alphabetical sequence, or according to alternating sequences. Maze tracing time is the time to trace a designated path through a maze, and count back time is the time to count backwards by 3s. The two reading time variables are the rate of reading normal text or text with interpolated distracting material. "Speed" refers to perceptual speed, "Fluid" to fluid ability, "Mem" to episodic memory, and "Vocab" to vacabulary. See text for details.
*$p < .01$

contains the standardized regression coefficients from four reference constructs to different target variables that could each be postulated to be a measure of processing speed. All of the variables measured in units of time have had their signs reflected such that higher values represent faster performance.

It is clear from the entries in the table that few variables are "ability pure," but instead have relations with several different abilities. As might have been expected, the Trail Making A and the Stroop Neutral variables have very strong relations with the perceptual speed construct, which indicates that people with high levels of the three variables used to define the perceptual speed construct in these analyses (see Figure 10.1) tended to be fast in these tasks. However, nearly all of the remaining variables also have significant relations with other ability constructs. For example, the fluency and reading time variables were related to vocabulary ability as well as to speed. Even the RT variables (i.e., Digit Digit RT and Anti-Cue Congruent RT), which some researchers might argue to be among the "purest" speed measures, have significant relations to constructs other than just perceptual speed in these analyses.

Because this analytical procedure is one of the few objective methods of investigating the meaning of a variable, it could be used to help clarify what specific variables actually represent. For example, one researcher might hypothesize that a variable primarily reflects construct A whereas another researcher might hypothesize that it reflects construct B. An advantage of this analytical procedure is that the two positions could be distinguished if reference variables for the two constructs were available. Unfortunately, many currently popular theoretical constructs have not yet been established to possess construct validity, and thus they may not be meaningful as reference constructs in this type of analysis until further research establishes that they have both convergent and discriminant validity.

Most of the variables in Table 10.1 have two or more significant influences, and thus the results summarized in the table also emphasize the importance of relying on several indicator variables to represent a construct when investigating relations among theoretical constructs. Nearly every variable has multiple determinants, but not all of these determinants are equally interesting. However, when a construct is defined on the basis of what several variables have in common, the specific or unique aspects are cancelled and the shared aspects are emphasized. Use of latent constructs therefore not only minimizes the influence of construct-irrelevant aspects, but because only the reliable variance can be shared, it also serves to reduce measurement error. Particularly when attempting to assess the individual difference speed construct, therefore, the additional time and expense to obtain three indicators of each relevant construct will almost always be worth it in terms of improved conceptual and measurement precision. However, multiple measures are desirable even in research concerned with specific theoretical processes, because it is unlikely that any measure is "process pure," and convergence on what is common among several measures may be less dependent on theoretical assumptions than isolation procedures based on subtractive logic.

These studies conducted within the psychometric perspective consider speed as an attribute of individuals that can be assessed at the behavioral level by obtaining converging evidence from the interrelations among different tasks. Neurobiological studies, discussed in the following section, also consider speed to be an attribute of individuals that can be assessed from behavioral measures. From the neurobiological perspective, however, there is greater concern with identifying the properties of the central nervous system that mediate or contribute to variations in speed at the behavioral level.

Neurobiological correlates of speed

What neurobiological variables might be potential correlates of individual differences in speed? There are many candidates for this role, because any variable that is related to both age and speed is a possible mediator. From the psychometric perspective, it would be most informative to focus on speed as an individual differences (ability) construct, because the dependent variable (index) aspect is likely to be highly determined by characteristics of the specific task. Thus, from this perspective, the best approach would be to investigate relations among several variables that have been used to assess perceptual speed.

However, most of the neurobiological research has focused predominantly on speed measures derived from tasks designed to emphasize specific processing stages or components, and has concentrated on Age Group × Task Condition interactions that can often be detected with smaller sample sizes than those required in psychometric research. As a consequence, most neurobiological studies have been primarily concerned with isolating particular information-processing components in individual tasks, rather than with the conceptualization of speed as an individual difference ability defined on the basis of multiple indicators.

Localized activation in neuroimaging

Neuroimaging measures of brain activity during the performance of cognitive tasks have yielded evidence for a variety of age-related differences. Some research in this area uses event-related potentials (ERPs) to measure the distribution of electrical activity across the scalp, and the timing of this activity in relation to cognitive task performance (Bashore, 1993; Bashore, Ridderinkhof, & van der Molen, 1997). These ERP measures indicate the time course of the electrical activity with millisecond resolution, but provide little information regarding the location of the underlying neural events. From whole-brain estimates of neural metabolic function, it has long been known that there is an age-related decline in aspects of resting neural activity, such as cerebral blood flow and oxygen metabolism (Kety, 1956). Both ERPs and the earlier whole-brain measures of blood flow are nontomographic, in that they do not yield a three-dimensional (spatial) assessment of brain activity. In contrast, tomographic measures such as positron emission tomography (PET) and functional magnetic resonance imaging (fMRI) provide information regarding the spatial localization of regional blood flow changes within the brain. In addition, PET and fMRI procedures measure the changes in cerebral blood flow (for specific brain regions), across task conditions, allowing inferences regarding the relation of brain activity to specific task demands (Cabeza, 2001; Madden & Hoffman, 1997; Madden, Whiting, & Huettel, 2005; Raz, 2000, 2005).

Although PET and fMRI can provide valuable data for understanding age-related differences at both neural and behavioral levels, there are several issues that lead to difficulty in the interpretation of results involving people of different ages. For example, it is important to recognize that the data from neuroimaging techniques, such as the level of oxygenated hemoglobin in venous blood (in the case of fMRI), are indirect measures of cerebral blood flow. In turn, cerebral blood flow is an indirect measure of neural activity. There is thus a sense in which the neuroimaging measures are merely another consequence of the critical causal factor, which ultimately may need to be explained in terms of more basic aspects of anatomy or physiology. In addition, interpretations can be complicated because greater activation may represent either more efficient or less efficient processing, and the amount of activation may be related to the amount or composition of brain tissue, both of which may change with age. The coupling between actual neural activity and the hemodynamic properties of the surrounding vasculature (neurovascular coupling) is also dependent on many factors, such as vascular pathology and resting cerebral blood flow, that may change as a function of age (Gazzaley & D'Esposito, 2005). In the case of fMRI, the neurovascular coupling appears to be noisier for older adults than for younger adults, leading to an age-related decline in the signal-to-noise ratio of the measured brain activation (D'Esposito, Zarahn, Aguirre, & Rypma, 1999). However, the time course and amplitude of the fMRI hemodynamic response appear to be qualitatively similar for younger and older adults, allowing some degree of comparison and interpretation (Huettel, Singerman, & McCarthy, 2001).

Several studies have reported that PET and fMRI measures of brain activation correlate with the speed of performance in cognitive tasks, and in some cases this pattern has been found to differ as a function of age. For example, Madden and colleagues (Madden, Turkington, Provenzale, Hawk, Hoffman, & Coleman, 1997) demonstrated that, in a PET analysis of a visual search task, the pattern of brain activation differed significantly between age groups, with younger participants exhibiting greater activation than older adults in ventral occipitotemporal (extrastriate) cortex (Brodmann area [BA] 18), and older participants exhibiting relatively greater activation in medial prefrontal regions (BA 32, 6, and 9). In addition, RT in the search task correlated positively with this regional activation within each age group (i.e., slower responses were associated with higher levels of activation). For younger adults, the correlation was limited primarily to the left extrastriate region (BA 18), although left superior parietal cortex (BA 7) was also involved. For older adults, the correlation involved left medial prefrontal cortex (BA 6) as well as superior parietal cortex (BA 7) bilaterally.

Different patterns of correlation between reaction time and regional brain activation have been observed across different cognitive tasks. Whiting et al. (2003) found that younger and older adults differed significantly in the activation–speed correlation associated with striate and extrastriate cortical regions (BA 17, 37). Among older adults, increasing PET activation in these regions was associated with an increasing effect of word frequency on lexical decision RT (i.e., slower responses to less frequent words), whereas no correlation was evident for younger adults. Madden, Whiting, Provenzale, and Huettel (2004b) reported that, in an fMRI investigation of the detection of individual visual targets, increased activation was associated with faster responses (i.e., a negative correlation between amount of activation and RT). The regional pattern of this correlation differed significantly across age groups, however, and involved deep gray matter structures (thalamus) for older adults but middle frontal gyrus for younger adults. Rypma and D'Esposito (2000) found that for one specific region (dorsolateral prefrontal cortex), the direction of the correlation between activation and RT was actually different for younger and older adults. During the response stage of a working memory task, there was greater activation in dorsolateral prefrontal cortex for younger adults than for older adults. In addition, increasing activation in this region was associated with slower responses for younger adults, but was associated with faster responses for older adults. Rypma and D'Esposito developed a model of the relation between neural activation and response signal strength based on a sigmoid function. The age difference in the pattern of correlation could be represented as a shift in this function with increasing age, with the result that the optimal level of response signal discriminability would occur at lower levels of activation for younger adults, but at higher levels of activation for older adults.

These disparate findings suggest that there is no single brain region that is invariably associated with age-related changes in speed. All of these studies, however, have been based on relatively small samples, and in some cases the apparently different patterns in young and old adults were not evaluated statistically. Most of the studies were also conducted with the goal of isolating information processing demands associated with different cognitive tasks, and it is thus reasonable to expect that the relevant brain regions will vary across the tasks. To identify the brain region(s) that serve as the neurobiological substrate of individual differences in processing speed as a task-independent ability, it will be necessary to examine several different speed measures in the same individuals, and to determine the degree to which age-related differences in brain activation exhibit a similar pattern across those different measures.

Regional volume

Another possible neurobiological substrate of processing speed is amount of brain tissue in specific brain regions. The volume of both gray and white matter declines as a function of increasing adult age, although the trajectories of gray- and white-matter decline differ (Raz, 2000, 2005). Regional variation occurs in age-related volumetric decline, with prefrontal regions exhibiting the steepest rate of decline. Although researchers have devoted substantial effort to interpreting the potential consequences of the differential age-related decline of prefrontal volume, decline is also evident in the volume of other regions including parietal cortex, cerebellum, caudate, and hippocampus (Raz et al., 2005; Resnick, Pham, Kraut, Zonderman, & Davatzikos, 2003). In addition, functions often attributed specifically to the frontal lobe are instead likely to rely on neural networks that are distributed widely throughout the brain (Greenwood, 2000; Mesulam, 1990; Tisserand & Jolles, 2003).

Changes in cortical volume can be difficult to interpret as a potential mediator of age differences in cognitive performance because there are many possible determinants of shrinkage in volume, and function could diminish either before or after a decrease in volume. Nevertheless, there have been several reports of covariation in age effects in cortical volume with those in cognitive performance. For example, Raz and colleagues have used path analysis and hierarchical regression to identify the specific brain regions for which age-related changes in volume might mediate changes in cognitive performance. These cross-sectional studies have revealed that for participants over 60 years of age, a decline in the volume of limbic structures predicted decline in explicit memory (Raz, Gunning-Dixon, Head, & Dupuis, 1998), that age-related decline in performance on a mental imagery task was associated with a reduction in volume of dorsolateral prefrontal cortex (Raz, Briggs, Marks, & Acker, 1999), and that age-related decline in a perceptual-motor skill (pursuit rotor) was statistically mediated by reduction in volume of the cerebellum and putamen (Raz, Williamson, Gunning-Dixon, Head, & Acker, 2000). In an analysis of longitudinal changes in regional brain volume, Rodrigue and Raz (2004) demonstrated that volumetric decline in the entorhinal cortex over a period of 5 years predicted memory performance at the end of the 5-year period.

Few studies have investigated the relation between age-related volumetric decline and age-related changes in perceptual speed. Tisserand, Visser, van Boxtel, and Jolles (2000) found that smaller volume in several brain regions (hippocampus, parahippocampal gyrus, mamillary bodies, third ventricle), and smaller total brain volume, were associated with slower performance on timed neuropsychological tests (Stroop and memory scanning). The relation between volume and speed was eliminated when the effect of age was controlled statistically, suggesting that there was no age-independent effect of brain volume. To extend this approach, it would be of interest to test a model in which the variability in the regional volume measures was controlled before examining the relation between age and speed, which would be the most relevant analysis for identifying the brain volumes as potential mediators of the age–speed relation.

Schretlen et al. (2000) used a similar approach to investigate the degree to which frontal lobe volume mediated age-related differences in fluid intelligence. These authors derived a composite measure of fluid intelligence from a factor analysis of several psychometric measures. Hierarchical regression analyses, in which measures of perceptual speed and working memory were used as statistical mediators, indicated that virtually all of the age-related variance in fluid intelligence was shared with perceptual speed. In separate analyses, the authors examined frontal lobe volume and a measure of executive functioning as mediators of fluid intelligence. In these latter analyses, age remained a significant predictor after frontal lobe volume and executive functioning were controlled statistically, although the age-related variance was reduced substantially. The authors also demonstrated that frontal lobe volume continued to account for a significant amount of variance in fluid ability after age, speed, and executive functioning were entered into the model. The analyses did not include a model in which frontal lobe volume was entered before speed, however, which would be necessary to assess the role of volumetric decline as a potential mediator of age-related changes in speed.

White matter integrity

White matter hyperintensities

A number of researchers have focused on the age-related changes in measures of gray matter structure and function in relation to cognitive performance. Substantial changes also occur in white matter throughout the brain (Resnick et al., 2003), however, and the rate of this volumetric decline appears to increase during later adulthood (Courchesne et al., 2000; Salat, Kaye, & Janowsky, 1999). The decline may differentially target prefrontal regions (Head et al., 2004), but some alteration of white matter structure also occurs in other regions such as the primary visual cortex and the optic nerve (Peters, Moss, & Sethares, 2000; Sandell & Peters, 2001). An important component of these age-related changes is a disintegration of the myelin sheath surrounding the axon, which could impair cognitive performance by slowing neural conduction velocity and disrupting widespread cortical circuits (Peters & Sethares, 2002). This type of reduction in white matter integrity, especially in prefrontal regions, has been proposed as a mechanism responsible for age-related cognitive change (Bartzokis, Sultzer, Lu, Neuchterlein, Mintz, Cummings, 2004; O'Sullivan, Jones, Summers, Morris, Williams, & Markus, 2001).

One method for determining the role of white matter integrity in age-related cognitive changes is to assess the number of white matter lesions visible in structural MRI scans. Small lesions of white matter appear as areas of hyperintensity on T2-weighted or proton density-weighted MRI scans, and the number of these areas of white matter hyperintensity (WMH) tends to increase with age even in asymptomatic individuals. In a meta-analysis of published research on white matter hyperintensities, Gunning-Dixon and Raz (2000) found that an increasing number of WMH areas was associated with decreased performance in several cognitive domains, especially processing speed, executive functioning, and explicit memory. The mean effect size for the relation between WMH and speed, across 16 studies, was $r = .22$. Partialling the influence of age did not have a substantial effect, however, suggesting that the influences of WMH and age on speed may be relatively independent of one another.

DeCarli et al. (1995) pointed out that studies of WMH typically include participants with hypertension and other cardiovascular risk factors. These authors examined correlations of white matter abnormality and cognitive variables in 51 adults between 19 and 91 years of age who were free of hypertension and other cardiovascular risk factors. They found that increasing WMH volume was a significant predictor, independently of age, of smaller brain volumes and lower performance scores across several psychometric measures, especially measures believed to reflect frontal lobe functioning. In addition, individuals with increased WMH volume tended to have lower metabolic activity (as measured by PET) in the frontal lobe, leading DeCarli et al. to conclude that WMH may play a role in age-related cognitive changes.

Leaper et al. (2001) proposed that the negative association between WMH and cognitive performance holds for fluid abilities but not for crystallized abilities. These authors performed MRI scans on 95 individuals, all of whom were 78 years of age and part of a Scottish cohort that also had standardized intelligence testing conducted at age 11. The results indicated a significant negative correlation between WMH and fluid ability (but not crystallized ability) at age 78, which was independent of general intelligence as measured at age 11. In another analysis of this cohort, Deary, Leaper, Murray, Staff, and Whalley (2003) identified a common factor among four tests of reasoning, memory, and speed. Both increasing WMH and the intelligence score at 11 years of age shared variance with the general cognitive factor at age 78, but these effects were independent. Similarly, in a longitudinal study of a Danish cohort, Garde, Mortensen, Krabbe, Rostrup, and Larsson (2000) also found that rated WMH severity was associated with small, though reliable, decline in some fluid abilities between 70 and 80 years of age, and that this pattern was independent of a measure of intelligence at 50 years of age. In a large population-based study of 1077 individuals 60–89 years of age, de Groot et al. (2000) reported that periventricular WMH severity was more closely associated with neuropsychological performance decline than was subcortical WMH severity, and that tests involving speed appeared to be more affected by WMH than were memory tasks. Bigler et al. (2003) noted a similar pattern in a sample of 195 older adults, most of whom exhibited some form of dementia. Thus, the effects of WMH appear across several cognitive domains, and there is some evidence that these effects differentially involve speed, but less direct evidence that WMH shares specifically age-related variance in cognitive performance or speed.

Diffusion tensor imaging

In addition to evaluating the effects of WMH, the recently developed technique of diffusion tensor imaging (DTI) is likely to be informative regarding age-related changes in structural integrity of white matter. This type of imaging measures both the rate and the directionality of the displacement distribution of water molecules across tissue components on a voxel-by-voxel basis. In DTI, fractional anisotropy (FA) provides a voxel-based measure of the functional integrity and specific organization of myelinated axonal fibers. Fractional anisotropy (ranging from 0 to 1.0), represents the degree to which water molecules diffuse in a single direction, which in turn is affected by axonal restrictions and myelin content. Thus, the structural integrity of white matter can be expressed as a continuous variable (with FA and related measures), rather than relying exclusively on lesions visible as hyperintensities in T2-weighted images. As stated previously, the neural networks mediating cognitive performance are widely distributed throughout the brain, and these networks establish connectivity through white matter pathways. The frontal lobe, for example, has extensive connections to posterior cortical regions, and to the basal ganglia and related subcortical structures. Changes in frontal lobe functioning may therefore result from age-related damage at various points in the network (Bashore, 1993; Hicks & Birren, 1970; Rubin, 1999).

The interpretation of FA and other DTI measures is still developing. For some brain regions, notably the corpus callosum, which consists of well-defined white matter pathways, the interpretation is straightforward. Outside of the corpus callosum, however, axons may be crossing from different directions, which would lead to a lower FA even if the individual axons were intact. While acknowledging this caveat, several studies have reported an age-related decline in FA, suggesting a decline in the integrity of white matter pathways (Moseley, 2002; Pfefferbaum, Sullivan, Hedehus, Lim, Adalsteinsson, & Moseley, 2000). This decline appears to have an anterior-to-posterior gradient, such that white matter in the frontal regions of the brain is more vulnerable to age-related decline in FA than more posterior regions (Head et al., 2004; O'Sullivan et al., 2001; Pfefferbaum, Adalsteinsson, & Sullivan, 2005; Sullivan et al., 2001), but there are also exceptions to this trend (Salat et al., 2005).

To what extent do these white matter changes influence age-related changes in speed? Several studies have reported that lower performance on various cognitive measures is associated with decline in white matter integrity as measured from DTI (Moseley, Bammer, & Illes, 2002). Other findings have also linked age-related decline in DTI measures to age-related change in cognitive performance, though indirectly, by demonstrating some correlation between cognitive performance and DTI measures (usually FA) within an older adult sample (O'Sullivan et al., 2001; Sullivan et al., 2001). In general, these studies have demonstrated that decreases in FA are associated with lower performance on various cognitive measures. Only one study has investigated the age-related differences in the cognition–FA relation, by comparing this relation in samples of younger and older adults. Madden, Whiting, Huettel, White, MacFall, and Provenzale (2004a) reported that FA within particular regions was related to a response time measure, such that lower FA (reflecting lower coherence of myelin tracts) was associated with slower responses in a visual target detection task. The regional FA measure that was the best predictor of RT, however, differed significantly between younger and older adults, being associated with the splenium of the corpus callosum for younger adults, but the anterior limb of the internal capsule for older adults (Figure 10.2). An important aspect of these data is that the regions exhibiting an age difference in the correlation between RT and FA were not necessarily those exhibiting the greatest age-related decline in FA, so the correlation change is not simply a consequence of an overall decline in FA. Shenkin, Bastin, MacGillivray, Deary, Starr, and Wardlaw (2003), analyzing the longitudinal Scottish cohort discussed previously, found that lower FA at age 80 was associated with lower scores in general intelligence, but that this association was also evident for intelligence scores obtained at age 11. Thus, FA and related DTI measures may not be isolating the changes in white matter occurring entirely during aging, but may also reflect differences in white matter integrity established at an earlier age.

Other neurobiological variables

The variables mentioned above are obviously not the only possible neurobiological substrates of age-related differences in processing speed. For example, several studies have reported significant age-related decreases in the number of D_2 receptor sites for the neurotransmitter dopamine, even in the absence of significant disease (Bäckman & Farde, 2005). This neurotransmitter operates through three pathways: a nigrostriatal pathway projecting from the substantia nigra to the basal ganglia, a mesolimbic pathway projecting from ventral mesencephalon to limbic regions, and a mesocortical system projecting from the ventral mesencephalon to the neocortex. Significant impairment of these pathways, common in disorders such as Parkinson's disease and Huntington's disease, leads to deficits across multiple cognitive domains, including perceptual speed, attention, episodic memory, and executive functioning. In PET studies of healthy adults, significant correlations have been observed between dopamine D_2 receptor binding and various measures of cognitive functioning (Bäckman et al., 2000; Backman, Nyberg,

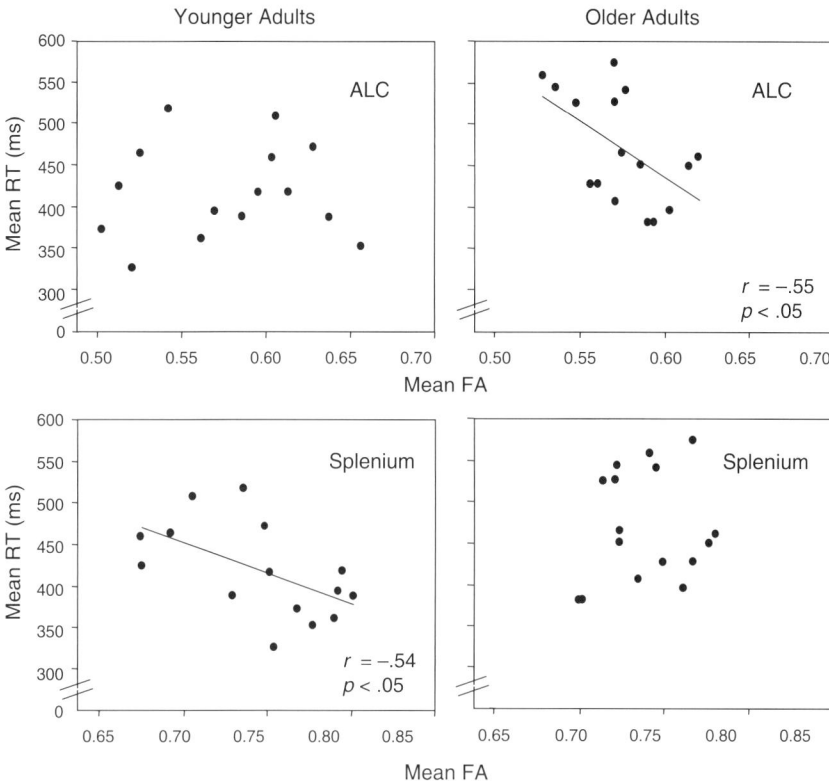

Figure 10.2 Correlation between reaction time (RT) in a visual target detection task and fractional anisotropy (FA) in white matter regions, reprinted with permission from Madden et al. (2004a). ALC = anterior limb of internal capsule; Splenium = splenium of corpus callosum.

Lindenberger, Li, & Farde, 2006; Volkow et al., 1998). Bäckman et al. (2000) used hierarchical regression procedures and demonstrated that individual differences in dopamine D_2 receptor binding for the caudate and putamen accounted for nearly all of the age-related variance in tests of episodic memory and perceptual speed. Computer simulation models also suggest that age-related cognitive changes can be characterized as an effect of decline in dopaminergic transmission (Braver et al., 2001; Li, 2005). Significant relations with both age and different cognitive variables have also been reported with certain hormones (e.g., Aleman et al., 1999; Aleman, de Vries, de Haan, Verhaar, Samson, & Koppeschaar, 2000; Dik, Pluijm, Jonker, Deeg, Lomecky, & Lips, 2003; Papadakis, Grady, Tierney, Black, Wells, & Grunfeld, 1995), and with several cerebral metabolites assessed with magnetic resonance spectroscopy (e.g., Ferguson, et al., 2002; Jung, Brooks, Yeo, Chiulli, Weers, & Sibbitt, 1999; Valenzuela, Sachdev, Wen, Shnier, Brodaty, & Gillies, 2000) raising the possibility that these factors might also be involved in age-related declines in speed.

Conclusions

In this chapter we have briefly reviewed some of the recent research concerned with two different perspectives on speed, both represented by a great deal of research activity at the current time. Although we acknowledge that the two perspectives have not yet been integrated, we hope that this chapter might stimulate efforts in these directions, because we believe that both perspectives would benefit from linking the findings in the two areas. From this review, we suggest that three points are particularly important. First, investigations of the age-related effects of neurobiological variables would benefit from defining speed and cognitive performance on the basis of multiple indicator variables. Second, although it is likely that age-related changes in brain function are differentially greater in some regions, such as prefrontal cortex, the relevant networks for speed and other cognitive processes are widely distributed and include subcortical structures. Thus, it is important to consider the possibility that changes in cognitive performance, and in task-related neural activation, may be the result of disruption at various points in the relevant network. And third, the neural mediators of age-related changes in processing speed are not limited to the volume and activation of gray matter, but also include white matter integrity.

References

Ackerman, P. L., Beier, M. E., & Boyle, M. O. (2002). Individual differences in working memory within a nomological network of cognitive and perceptual speed abilities. *Journal of Experimental Psychology: General, 131*, 567–589.

Aleman, A., de Vries, W. R., de Haan, E. H., Verhaar, H. J. J., Samson, M. M., & Koppeschaar, H. P. F. (2000). Age-sensitive cognitive function, growth hormone and insulin-like growth factor 1 plasma levels in healthy older men. *Neuropsychobiology, 41*, 73–78.

Aleman, A., Verhaar, H. J. J., de Haan, E. H. F., de Vries, W. R., Samson, M. M., Drent, M. L., et al. (1999). Insulin-like growth factor-1 and cognitive function in healthy older men. *Journal of Clinical Endocrinology and Metabolism, 84*, 471–475.

Babcock, R. L., Laguna, K. D., & Roesch, S. C. (1997). A comparison of the factor structure of processing speed for younger and older adults: Testing the assumptions of measurement equivalence across age groups. *Psychology and Aging, 12*, 268–276.

Bäckman, L., & Farde, L. (2005). The role of dopamine systems in cognitive aging. In R. Cabeza, L. Nyberg, & D. Park (Eds.), *Cognitive neuroscience of aging: Linking cognitive and cerebral aging* (pp. 58–84). New York: Oxford University Press.

Bäckman, L., Ginovart, N., Dixon, R. A., Wahlin, T. B., Wahlin, A., Halldin, C., et al. (2000). Age-related cognitive deficits mediated by changes in the striatal dopamine system. *American Journal of Psychiatry, 157*, 635–637.

Bäckman, L., Nyberg, L., Lindenberger, U., Li, S. C., & Farde, L. (2006). The correlative triad among aging, dopamine, and cognition: Current status and future prospects. *Neuroscience and Biobehavioral Reviews, 30* (6), 791–807.

Bartzokis, G., Sultzer, D., Lu, P. H., Nuechterlein, K. H., Mintz, J., & Cummings, J. L. (2004). Heterogeneous age-related breakdown of white matter structural integrity: Implications for cortical "disconnection" in aging and Alzheimer's disease. *Neurobiology of Aging, 25*, 843–851.

Bashore, T. R. (1993). Differential effects of aging on the neurocognitive functions subserving speeded mental processing. In J. Cerella, J. Rybash, W. Hoyer, & M. L. Commons (Eds.), *Adult information processing: Limits on loss* (pp. 37–76). San Diego, CA: Academic Press.

Bashore, T. R., Ridderinkhof, K. R., & van der Molen, M. W. (1997). The decline of cognitive processing speed in old age. *Current Directions in Psychological Science, 6*, 163–169.

Bigler, E. D., Lowry, C. M., Kerr, B., Tate, D. F., Hessel, C. D., Earl, H. D., et al. (2003). Role of white matter lesions, cerebral atrophy, and APOE on cognition in older persons with and without dementia: The Cache County, Utah, study of memory and aging. *Neuropsychology, 17*, 339–352.

Braver, T. S., Barch, D. M., Keys, B. A., Carter, C. S., Cohen, J. D., Kaye, J. A., et al. (2001). Context processing in older adults: Evidence for a theory relating cognitive control to neurobiology in healthy aging. *Journal of Experimental Psychology: General, 130*, 746–763.

Cabeza, R. (2001). Functional neuroimaging of cognitive aging. In R. Cabeza & A. Kingstone (Eds.), *Handbook of functional neuroimaging of cognition* (pp. 331–377). Cambridge, MA: MIT Press.

Courchesne, E., Chisum, H. J., Townsend, J., Cowles, A., Covington, J., Egaas, B., et al. (2000). Normal brain development and aging: Quantitative analysis at in vivo MR imaging in healthy volunteers. *Radiology, 216*, 672–682.

D'Esposito, M., Zarahn, E., Aguirre, G. K., & Rypma, B. (1999). The effect of normal aging on the coupling of neural activity to the BOLD hemodynamic response. *Neuroimage, 10*, 6–14.

de Groot, J. C., de Leeuw, F. E., Oudkerk, M., van Gijn, J., Hofman, A., Jolles, J., et al. (2000). Cerebral white matter lesions and cognitive function: The Rotterdam scan study. *Annals of Neurology, 47*, 145–151.

Deary, I. J., Leaper, S. A., Murray, A. D., Staff, R. T., & Whalley, L. J. (2003). Cerebral white matter abnormalities and lifetime cognitive change: A 67-year follow-up of the Scottish Mental Survey of 1932. *Psychology and Aging, 18*, 140–148.

DeCarli, C., Murphy, D. G., Tranh, M., Grady, C. L., Haxby, J. V., Gillette, J. A., et al. (1995). The effect of white matter hyperintensity volume on brain structure, cognitive performance, and cerebral metabolism of glucose in 51 healthy adults. *Neurology, 45*, 2077–2084.

Dik, M. G., Pluijm, S. M. F., Jonker, C., Deeg, D. J. H., Lomecky, M. Z., & Lips, P. (2003). Insulin-like growth factor I (IGF-1) and cognitive decline in older persons. *Neurobiology of Aging, 24*, 573–581.

Faust, M. E., Balota, D. A., Spieler, D. H., & Ferraro, F. R. (1999). Individual differences in information-processing rate and amount: Implications for group differences in response latency. *Psychological Bulletin, 125*, 777–799.

Ferguson, K. J., MacLullich, A. M. J., Marshall, I., Deary, I. J., Starr, J. M., Seckl,

J. R. et al. (2002). Magnetic resonance spectroscopy and cognitive function in healthy elderly men. *Brain, 125*, 2743–2749.

Garde, E., Mortensen, E. L., Krabbe, K., Rostrup, E., & Larsson, H. B. (2000). Relation between age-related decline in intelligence and cerebral white-matter hyperintensities in healthy octogenarians: A longitudinal study. *Lancet, 356*, 628–634.

Gazzaley, A. H., & D'Esposito, M. (2005). Bold functional MRI and cognitive aging. In R. Cabeza, L. Nyberg, & D. Park (Eds.), *Cognitive neuroscience of aging: Linking cognitive and cerebral aging* (pp. 107–131). New York: Oxford University Press.

Greenwood, P. M. (2000). The frontal aging hypothesis evaluated. *Journal of the International Neuropsychological Society, 6*, 705–726.

Gunning-Dixon, F. M., & Raz, N. (2000). The cognitive correlates of white matter abnormalities in normal aging: A quantitative review. *Neuropsychology, 14*, 224–232.

Head, D., Buckner, R. L., Shimony, J. S., Williams, L. E., Akbudak, E., Conturo, T. E., et al. (2004). Differential vulnerability of anterior white matter in nondemented aging with minimal acceleration in dementia of the Alzheimer type: Evidence from diffusion tensor imaging. *Cerebral Cortex, 14*, 410–423.

Hicks, L. H., & Birren, J. E. (1970). Aging, brain damage, and psychomotor slowing. *Psychological Bulletin, 74*, 377–396.

Huettel, S. A., Singerman, J. D., & McCarthy, G. (2001). The effects of aging upon the hemodynamic response measured by functional MRI. *Neuroimage, 13*, 161–175.

Hultsch, D. F., Hertzog, C., Dixon, R. A., & Small, B. J. (1998). *Memory change in the aged*. New York: Cambridge University Press.

Jung, R. E., Brooks, W. M., Yeo, R. A., Chiulli, S. J., Weers, D. C., & Sibbitt, W. L. (1999). Biochemical markers of intelligence: A proton MR spectroscopy study of normal human brain. *Proceedings of the Royal Society of London, B, 266*, 1375–1379.

Kety, S. S. (1956). Human cerebral blood flow and oxygen consumption as related to aging. *Journal of Chronic Diseases, 3*, 478–486.

Leaper, S. A., Murray, A. D., Lemmon, H. A., Staff, R. T., Deary, I. J., Crawford, J. R., et al. (2001). Neuropsychologic correlates of brain white matter lesions depicted on MR images: 1921 Aberdeen birth cohort. *Radiology, 221*, 51–55.

Li, S.-C. (2005). Neurocomputational perspectives linking neuromodulation, processing noise, representational distinctiveness, and cognitive aging. In R. Cabeza, L. Nyberg, & D. Park (Eds.), *Cognitive neuroscience of aging: Linking cognitive and cerebral aging* (pp. 354–379). New York: Oxford University Press.

Madden, D. J. (2001). Speed and timing of behavioral processes. In J. E. Birren & K. W. Schaie (Eds.), *The handbook of the psychology of aging* (5th ed., pp. 288–312). San Diego, CA: Academic Press.

Madden, D. J., & Hoffman, J. M. (1997). Application of positron emission tomography to age-related cognitive changes. In K. R. R. Krishnan & P. M. Doraiswamy (Eds.), *Brain imaging and clinical psychiatry* (pp. 575–613). New York: Marcel Dekker.

Madden, D. J., Turkington, T. G., Provenzale, J. M., Hawk, T. C., Hoffman, J. M., & Coleman, R. E. (1997). Selective and divided visual attention: Age-related changes in regional cerebral blood flow measured by $H_2^{15}O$ PET. *Human Brain Mapping, 5* (6), 389–409.

Madden, D. J., Whiting, W. L., & Huettel, S. A. (2005). Age-related changes in neural activity during visual perception and attention. In R. Cabeza, L. Nyberg, & D. Park (Eds.), *Cognitive neuroscience of aging: Linking cognitive and cerebral aging* (pp. 157–185). New York: Oxford University Press.

Madden, D. J., Whiting, W. L., Huettel, S. A., White, L. E., MacFall, J. R., & Provenzale, J. M. (2004a). Diffusion tensor imaging of adult age differences in cerebral white matter: Relation to response time. *Neuroimage, 21,* 1174–1181.

Madden, D. J., Whiting, W. L., Provenzale, J. M., & Huettel, S. A. (2004b). Age-related changes in neural activity during visual target detection measured by fMRI. *Cerebral Cortex, 14,* 143–155.

Mesulam, M. M. (1990). Large-scale neurocognitive networks and distributed processing for attention, language, and memory. *Annals of Neurology, 28,* 597–613.

Moseley, M. (2002). Diffusion tensor imaging and aging—a review. *NMR in Biomedicine, 15,* 553–560.

Moseley, M., Bammer, R., & Illes, J. (2002). Diffusion-tensor imaging of cognitive performance. *Brain & Cognition, 50,* 396–413.

O'Sullivan, M., Jones, D. K., Summers, P. E., Morris, R. G., Williams, S. C., & Markus, H. S. (2001). Evidence for cortical "disconnection" as a mechanism of age-related cognitive decline. *Neurology, 57,* 632–638.

Papadakis, M. A., Grady, D., Tierney, M. J., Black, D., Wells, L., & Grunfeld, C. (1995). Insulin-like growth factor 1 and functional status in healthy older men. *Journal of the American Geriatrics Society, 43,* 1350–1355.

Parkin, A. J., & Java, R. I. (1999). Deterioration of frontal lobe function in normal aging: Influences of fluid intelligence versus perceptual speed. *Neuropsychology, 13,* 539–545.

Peters, A., Moss, M. B., & Sethares, C. (2000). Effects of aging on myelinated nerve fibers in monkey primary visual cortex. *Journal of Comparative Neurology, 419,* 364–376.

Peters, A., & Sethares, C. (2002). Aging and the myelinated fibers in prefrontal cortex and corpus callosum of the monkey. *Journal of Comparative Neurology, 442,* 277–291.

Pfefferbaum, A., Adalsteinsson, E., & Sullivan, E. V. (2005). Frontal circuitry degradation marks healthy adult aging: Evidence from diffusion tensor imaging. *Neuroimage, 26,* 891–899.

Pfefferbaum, A., Sullivan, E. V., Hedehus, M., Lim, K. O., Adalsteinsson, E., & Moseley, M. (2000). Age-related decline in brain white matter anisotropy measured with spatially corrected echo-planar diffusion tensor imaging. *Magnetic Resonance in Medicine, 44,* 259–268.

Piccinin, A. M., & Rabbitt, P. M. A. (1999). Contribution of cognitive abilities to performance and improvement on a substitution coding task. *Psychology and Aging, 14,* 539–551.

Raz, N. (2000). Aging of the brain and its impact on cognitive performance: Integration of structural and functional findings. In F. I. M. Craik & T. A. Salthouse (Eds.), *Handbook of aging and cognition* (2nd ed., pp. 1–90). Mahwah, NJ: Lawrence Erlbaum Associates, Inc.

Raz, N. (2005). The aging brain observed in vivo: Differential changes and their modifiers. In R. Cabeza, L. Nyberg, & D. Park (Eds.), *Cognitive neuroscience of aging: Linking cognitive and cerebral aging.* (pp. 19–57). New York: Oxford University Press.

Raz, N., Briggs, S. D., Marks, W., & Acker, J. D. (1999). Age-related deficits in generation and manipulation of mental images: II. The role of dorsolateral prefrontal cortex. *Psychology and Aging, 14,* 436–444.

Raz, N., Gunning-Dixon, F. M., Head, D., & Dupuis, J. H. (1998). Neuroanatomical correlates of cognitive aging: Evidence from structural magnetic resonance imaging. *Neuropsychology, 12,* 95–114.

Raz, N., Lindenberger, U., Rodrigue, K. M., Kennedy, K. M., Head, D., Williamson, A., et al. (2005). Regional brain changes in aging healthy adults: General trends, individual differences and modifiers. *Cerebral Cortex, 15,* 1676–1689.

Raz, N., Williamson, A., Gunning-Dixon, F., Head, D., & Acker, J. D. (2000). Neuroanatomical and cognitive correlates of adult age differences in acquisition of a perceptual-motor skill. *Microscopy Research and Technique, 51,* 85–93.

Resnick, S. M., Pham, D. L., Kraut, M. A., Zonderman, A. B., & Davatzikos, C. (2003). Longitudinal magnetic resonance imaging studies of older adults: A shrinking brain. *Journal of Neuroscience, 23,* 3295–3301.

Rodrigue, K. M., & Raz, N. (2004). Shrinkage of the entorhinal cortex over five years predicts memory performance in healthy adults. *Journal of Neuroscience, 24,* 956–963.

Rubin, D. C. (1999). Frontal-striatal circuits in cognitive aging: Evidence for caudate involvement. *Aging, Neuropsychology, and Cognition, 6,* 241–259.

Rypma, B., & D'Esposito, M. (2000). Isolating the neural mechanisms of age-related changes in human working memory. *Nature Neuroscience, 3,* 509–515.

Salat, D. H., Kaye, J. A., & Janowsky, J. S. (1999). Prefrontal gray and white matter volumes in healthy aging and Alzheimer disease. *Archives of Neurology, 56,* 338–344.

Salat, D. H., Tuch, D. S., Greve, D. N., van der Kouwe, A. J., Hevelone, N. D., Zaleta, A. K., et al. (2005). Age-related alterations in white matter microstructure measured by diffusion tensor imaging. *Neurobiology of Aging, 26,* 1215–1227.

Salthouse, T. A. (1985). Speed of behavior and its implications for cognition. In J. E. Birren & K. W. Schaie (Eds.), *Handbook of the psychology of aging* (2nd ed., pp. 400–426). New York: Van Nostrand Reinhold.

Salthouse, T. A. (2004). Localizing age-related individual differences in a hierarchical structure. *Intelligence, 32,* 541–561.

Salthouse, T. A. (2005). Relations between cognitive abilities and measures of executive functioning. *Neuropsychology, 19,* 532–545.

Salthouse, T. A. & Hedden, T. (2002). Interpreting reaction time measures in between-group comparisons. *Journal of Clinical and Experimental Neuropsychology, 24,* 858–872.

Sandell, J. H., & Peters, A. (2001). Effects of age on nerve fibers in the rhesus monkey optic nerve. *Journal of Comparative Neurology, 429,* 541–553.

Schretlen, D., Pearlson, G. D., Anthony, J. C., Aylward, E. H., Augustine, A. M., Davis, A., et al. (2000). Elucidating the contributions of processing speed, executive ability, and frontal lobe volume to normal age-related differences in fluid intelligence. *Journal of the International Neuropsychological Society, 6,* 52–61.

Shenkin, S. D., Bastin, M. E., MacGillivray, T. J., Deary, I. J., Starr, J. M., & Wardlaw, J. M. (2003). Childhood and current cognitive function in healthy 80-year-olds: A DT-MRI study. *NeuroReport, 14,* 345–349.

Sullivan, E. V., Adalsteinsson, E., Hedehus, M., Ju, C., Moseley, M., Lim, K. O., et al. (2001). Equivalent disruption of regional white matter microstructure in ageing healthy men and women. *NeuroReport, 12,* 99–104.

Tisserand, D. J., & Jolles, J. (2003). On the involvement of prefrontal networks in cognitive ageing. *Cortex, 39,* 1107–1128.

Tisserand, D. J., Visser, P. J., van Boxtel, M. P., & Jolles, J. (2000). The relation between global and limbic brain volumes on MRI and cognitive performance in healthy individuals across the age range. *Neurobiology of Aging, 21,* 569–576.

Valenzuela, M. J., Sachdev, P. S., Wen, W., Shnier, R., Brodaty, H., & Gillies, D. (2000). Dual voxel proton magnetic resonance spectroscopy in the healthy elderly: Subcortical-frontal axonal N-Acetylaspartate levels are correlated with fluid cognitive abilities independent of structural brain changes. *Neuroimage, 12,* 747–756.

Volkow, N. D., Gur, R. C., Wang, G. J., Fowler, J. S., Moberg, P. J., Ding, Y. S., et al. (1998). Association between decline in brain dopamine activity with age and cognitive and motor impairment in healthy individuals. *American Journal of Psychiatry, 155,* 344–349.

Wechsler, D. (1997). *Wechsler Adult Intelligence Scale—Third Edition.* San Antonio, TX: The Psychological Corporation.

Whiting, W. L., Madden, D. J., Langley, L. K., Denny, L. L., Turkington, T. G., Provenzale, J. M., et al. (2003). Lexical and sublexical components of age-related changes in neural activation during visual word identification. *Journal of Cognitive Neuroscience, 15,* 475–487.

Wilson, R. S., Bienias, J. L., Evans, D. A., & Bennett, D. A. (2004). Religious orders study: Overview and change in cognitive and motor speed. *Aging, Neuropsychology and Cognition, 11,* 280–303.

Woodcock, R. W., McGrew, K. S., & Mather, N. (2001). *Woodcock-Johnson III Tests of Cognitive Abilities.* Itasca, IL: Riverside Publishing Co.

11 Everyday life applications and rehabilitation of processing speed deficits: Aging as a model for clinical populations

Karlene K. Ball and David E. Vance

Introduction

Many individuals experience declines in their ability to function effectively and independently with advancing age. In particular, sensory, perceptual, and cognitive functions may deteriorate in later life for some individuals, and it is widely believed that declines in these functions contribute to a corresponding decline in the ability to perform everyday activities. While much is now known about cognitive and sensory aging, less is known about the functional consequences, as well as the underlying reasons for declining abilities on everyday tasks. Furthermore, research aimed at the development of interventions to prevent, delay, or reverse disabilities that can affect older adults is relatively recent. With current trends toward increased longevity in the population, the potential for maintaining functional abilities into older age is of particular importance. Enhancement of basic sensory and cognitive functions into older age may help individuals sustain their personal autonomy by prolonging their abilities to perform instrumental activities of daily living. Furthermore, the high degree of interindividual variation in function among older adults, along with varying degrees of intraindividual plasticity in function, points to the influence of environment and life history factors in this area. It also suggests that these functions are subject to some degree of control. This chapter will discuss the importance of processing speed in the performance of everyday activities, and the development of interventions geared toward improving speed of processing and the everyday activities that rely on this ability. While the focus of this chapter is on aging, it is hoped that the issues, concepts, and techniques discussed can be viewed more broadly to potentially apply to clinical populations where deficits in information processing speed significantly affect everyday life activities. Many of these clinical populations are described in detail in other chapters in this book.

Speed of processing and aging

While there are numerous theories and models as to how human information processing takes place, they all agree that there must be sensory coding, some form of storage of information, and a system for retrieval and modification of stored information. Furthermore, the process of attention is used to allocate cognitive resources to either external or internal stimuli. Research continues to elaborate the structures and processing of such a system in both young and older individuals. Aging effects have been evaluated at all stages of the system (usually focusing on only one stage at a time), as well as on attention, processing strategies, and other higher level cognitive functions. Although this literature is too extensive to thoroughly review, there appears to be a common thread, that of reduced processing speed, which emerges repeatedly as a mechanism associated with at least some of the age-related declines in cognitive functioning (e.g., Baudouin, Vanneste, & Isingrini, 2004; Brigman & Cherry, 2002; Fisk & Warr, 1998; MacDonald, Hultsch, Strauss, & Dixon, 2003; Zimprich & Martin, 2002).

Age-related changes in processing speed have been recognized for some time in many disciplines. For example, there has been consensus among visual scientists that the temporal resolving power of the visual system declines with age (Botwinick, 1984; Sekuler, Kline, & Dismukes, 1983). Typically, older adults have been found to require longer delays between stimuli before both are seen as separate percepts (Kline & Orme-Rogers, 1978). This type of processing speed loss has also been demonstrated in studies of critical flicker fusion (Brozek & Keys, 1945; Coppinger, 1955; Misiak, 1947), complementary afterimages (Kline & Nestor, 1977) and masking (Kline & Birren, 1975; Kline & Szafran, 1975). The explanation typically advanced for these findings is that the aging visual nervous system recovers from the effects of stimulation more slowly than younger systems (i.e., older individuals require more processing time, in general, than younger adults).

Birren (1974) was one of the first to theorize that generalized slowing of abilities underlies age-related decline, at least in part. As part of the normal aging process, the speed with which older adults process information declines (Salthouse, 1985, 1990, 1993; Schaie, 1989, 1994). In fact, several recent longitudinal studies have confirmed that slower speed of processing accounts for a significant proportion of age-related cognitive decline (Finkel, Mintzer, Dysken, Krishnan, Burt, & McRae, 2004; Lemke & Zimprich, 2005; Zimprich & Martin, 2002).

Speed of processing has been defined as the rate at which information, once made available to the senses, is processed and understood at the cognitive level (Ball, Vance, Edwards, & Wadley, 2004). Adequate speed of processing ability allows individuals to respond quickly and efficiently to a variety of simple and complex stimuli, thus providing one of the functional capabilities to permit successful negotiation of the environment. In many cases, adequate speed of processing has survival benefits, such as allowing a driver to perceive dangerous situations in a timely manner in order to successfully avoid impact.

Assessing speed of processing

Speed of processing is difficult to measure because like other psychological events, it is not directly observable. Therefore, tests that approximate this ability are used to quantify it. All of these measurers are time dependent, in terms of the length of time required to complete a task, the presentation time of a stimulus to be perceived, or the number of correct responses within a fixed time interval.

Measurement issues

Speed of processing, like other cognitive abilities, has many assessment constraints. First, many measures tap multiple cognitive domains. For example, the WAIS Digit Symbol Substitution Test assesses speed of processing along with mental flexibility and psychomotor ability. Similarly, Trails B assesses speed of processing along with attention switching and psychomotor ability, and is frequently classified as a measure of executive function. Practically all cognitive tests possess this spillover effect, where multiple cognitive domains are being used to perform a task. Second, speed of processing is an inexact term; it has many meanings. For example, it can be interpreted as sensory speed—the speed at which sensory data are carried to the brain. It can be classified as central speed of processing—the speed at which higher order cognitive abilities process sensory data and determine a response. Cerella, Poon, and Williams (1980) referred to this as central or computational processing, while all other processing is referred to as peripheral or sensorimotor processing. Then there is response speed—the speed at which the appropriate response is performed. All three or a combination thereof can be considered speed of processing. Finally, task characteristics of speed of processing can result in differential outcomes. For example, speed of processing tasks that have a verbal component have been found to demonstrate less age-related decline than speed of processing tasks that involve more spatial information (Salthouse, 2000). In this case a highly learned skill, verbalization, may mask any underlying differences in processing speed. Similarly, reaction time tasks may accentuate age differences in processing speed because of changes in muscle control, arthritis, and other conditions that affect the ability of the individual to complete a movement.

Tests of cognition, like speed of processing, are also prone to an array of individual, physiological, and environmental influences that affect the validity and reliability of such measures. Individual characteristics such as education and mood can affect the outcome of tests of speed of processing. Those who are less educated and more depressed generally perform more poorly on cognitive measures (Benedict, Dobraski, & Godlstein, 1999; Collie, Shafiq-Antonacci, Maruff, Tyler, & Currie, 1999). With approximately 10% of older adults exhibiting depressive symptoms (Jefferson & Greist, 1993), this is an important consideration when assessing cognitive ability.

Physiological processes also impact cognitive performance. May and Hasher (1998) found that circadian rhythms are an important consideration because older adults performed better on cognitive measures during times that corresponded more in synchrony with their arousal state. Poor hydration can impact cognitive functioning, such as slowed psychomotor processing speed (Suhr, Hall, Patterson, & Niinisto, 2004). Also prescription medications, benzodiazepine use, or polypharmacy, which is common in older adults, can also detrimentally impact cognition (Linjakumpu, Hartikainen, Klaukka, Veijola, Kivela, & Isoaho, 2002). Such factors are also important considerations when examining cognitive ability.

Environmental and cultural factors are important too, especially since many measures have historical biases. For example, Park, Nisbett, and Hedden (1999) reported that people reared in different cultures actually process information differently. In addition, historical biases can influence test performance. For example, because younger adults have been exposed to more testing situations, they are generally more test savvy than their older counterparts, which gives them an advantage when participating in cognitive research. For example, most younger adults are more sophisticated in taking cognitive tests that require multiple-choice responses, process-of-elimination, computer testing, and timed tests. Thus tests that utilize such procedures may unintentionally place older adults at a disadvantage, resulting in relatively poorer performance. Unfortunately, it is difficult to measure these cognitive abilities without using such testing procedures. One method of solving these measurement issues is to collect for each individual a large number of measures in multiple domains. Such a battery of tests may then permit assessment of a wide range of factors so that the variability in responses may be assigned to appropriate factors through statistical analysis. One obvious disadvantage of such an approach is that older adults fatigue more easily, which in turn induces a different measurement problem.

Speed of processing and everyday functioning

The majority of research evaluating aging effects on cognitive function has been laboratory based. While such research is important for understanding the aging process, many have argued that laboratory deficits may not show up in the day-to-day functioning of elderly adults because of various compensation strategies. We now review the research that explores the link between cognitive aging and everyday measures of cognitive competence.

Declines in everyday activities such as instrumental activities of daily living (IADL) and activities of daily living (ADL) are a common concern with aging and chronic illness. This concern arises because it increases dependency, decreases autonomy, and compromises quality of life (Aguero-Torres, Thomas, Winbald, & Fratiglioni, 2002; Murtagh & Hubert, 2004). Advancing age is one of the most significant predictors of impairment in everyday functioning (Barberger, Fabrigoule, Rouch, Letenneur, & Dartigues,

1999; Steen, Sonn, Hanson, & Steen, 2001). Barberger and Fabrigoule (1997) remarked that functional ability and cognitive impairment exhibit similar patterns of increasing prevalence with age. With the robust relationship between aging and cognition, it is understandable why both are associated with everyday functioning.

All cognitive abilities are essential for everyday functioning (Dodge, Kadowaki, Hayakawa, Yamakawa, Sekikawa, & Ueshima, 2005). For example, in a study of cognitively intact older adults ($N = 100$), Smits, Deeg, and Jonker (1997) found that fluid intelligence and everyday memory were independently associated with IADL disability. However, speed of processing may be particularly important for the following reasons. First, as mentioned earlier, declines in speed of processing may impact other cognitive abilities such that the collective decline in cognitive ability results in poorer everyday functioning. Second, many everyday activities have a time component necessary for proficiency. Thus those who can quickly detect an object in the road will be more likely to avoid an accident, and those who process information at a slower rate will experience more trouble with such reaction-dependent responses. Similarly, those who can process a menu of options on the telephone may complete their call and obtain the information they desire, while those who cannot process the information in a timely manner may hang up in frustration.

Another arena of everyday function that has been studied relative to cognitive abilities is the use of computers and other new technologies. Several researchers have sought to determine how age-related differences in cognitive abilities are linked to performance on computer tasks. This is particularly relevant as data show that persons are remaining in the work force longer (Panek, 1997). There has also been an increased prevalence of computers in the workplace. Czaja (2001) reported that more than half of all workers utilize a computer in their job, and it is likely that this proportion will continue to increase. Also, computer systems are found in many different settings, performing a variety of tasks, and are no longer used only by technical specialists.

In general, studies have found that age, along with computer experience and cognitive abilities, predict computer task performance (Czaja and Sharit, 1993; Gomez, Egan, & Devlin, 1986; Rosson, 1983; Salthouse, 1996; Vincente, Hayes, & Willies, 1987). However, it has also been demonstrated that once computer experience and certain cognitive variables are accounted for, age no longer predicts performance. Czaja, Sharit, Nair, and Rubert (1998) conducted a large-scale study in order to investigate the relationships of a number of variables including age, cognitive abilities, and computer experience to performance on computer tasks. One portion of this study examined participants' performance (time per task) on a data entry task. This task is highly relevant as it is a commonly performed task in a wide range of industry settings (e.g., item processing, order entry), and many people are asked to perform the task. In addition, performance on a data entry task emphasizes speed (processing and motor). In this study, 110 participants were recruited in three age groups, younger (20–39 years), middle-aged (40–59 years), and older (60–75 years). They were provided with extensive training and practice (9 hours over 3 days) on a data entry task that involved the simulated entry of trip records for a trucking company. Those persons currently or previously employed in a data entry job were excluded. An extensive cognitive battery was administered, with tasks measuring processing speed, attention, visuospatial skills, abstraction, language, memory, and motor skills. In addition, a computer experience questionnaire was completed by all participants. The dependent variable was the number of trip records entered into the computer per hour during the last day of practice. An age-group analysis of variance revealed that the older participants input significantly less data than the younger and middle-aged participants. However, additional analyses revealed that age difference in work output was mediated by other variables. In stepwise regression analyses, Czaja et al. (1988) found visuospatial skills (Digit Symbol Substitution), computer experience, processing speed (Posner Letter Matching Task, Sternberg Short Term Memory Search Task, Figural Visual Scanning and Discrimination, Two Choice Visual Reaction Time Task), and motor skills (Purdue Pegboard Test, Trail Making Test A) accounted for 51% of the variance in the data entry task. After those variables were entered into the regression, age did not account for performance differences. In agreement with these findings, Salthouse (1996) also found that a large proportion of age-related variance in a synthetic work task was explained by speed of processing.

One of the primary areas in which declines in speed of processing have been studied extensively is mobility. Close to 20% of adults over the age of 65 experience difficulty with mobility (Guralnik, Fried, & Salive, 1996). Mobility impairments compromise autonomy and everyday functioning, resulting in decreased quality of life. Declines in speed of processing have been found to impact several aspects of mobility, including driving, crashes, gait, and falling.

One measure of speed of processing that has been studied extensively relative to a variety of measures of everyday performance, and in particular mobility, is the Useful Field of View (specifically the UFOV® test—Visual Awareness, Inc.). Visual information processing speed, as measured by this test, reliably predicts driving competency (Ball & Owsley, 1993; Ball, Owsley, Sloane, Roenker, & Bruni, 1993; Owsley, Ball, et al., 1998; Owsley, McGwin, & Ball, 1998). Older drivers with slower processing speed have been found to be at least twice as likely as older adults with faster speed of processing to incur an at-fault crash over the subsequent three to four years (Ball et al., 2006). Processing speed measured in this manner has also been related to an elevated risk for falls (Sims, McGwin, Pulley, & Roseman, 2001; Staplin, Gish, & Wagner, 2003), and reduced life space and driving space (Stalvey, Owsley, Sloane & Ball, 1999; Owsley, Stalvey, Wells, & Sloane, 1999). It has also been associated with performance of mobility tasks such as transitioning from sitting to standing as well as balance and gait (Owsley & McGwin, 2004) and functional reach (Riolo, 2003). Additionally, speed of processing measured with this test has been related to the performance of other IADLs such as the ability to quickly and accurately look up phone numbers, count out change, find a particular item on a crowded shelf, and read food and medication labels (Owsley, Sloane, McGwin, & Ball, 2002). Furthermore, faster speed of processing has been associated with maintained health status with advancing age (Hultsch, Hammer, & Small, 1993; Rosnick, Small, Borenstein Graves, & Mortimer, 2004). Considering the strong association between speed of processing, everyday performance, and health status, speed of processing training has also been studied relative to its potential to sustain and/or enhance everyday functioning among older adults.

Remediating speed of processing declines

The speed of processing training described here (Visual Awareness, Inc.), involves trainer-guided practice of computer-based exercises (target detection, identification, discrimination, and localization) presented very quickly and followed by a masking pattern (Ball et al., 2002; Ball, Beard, Roenker, Miller, & Griggs, 1988; Sekuler & Ball, 1986). Speed of processing training is ability specific, with the primary aim of improving mental processing speed such that increasingly more complex information can be processed within briefer periods of time. Reaction time is not measured and is not a factor in the training protocol. Rather, display speed, ranging from 17 to 500 ms is the primary manipulation made during training. In addition to stimulus duration, difficulty of the training tasks is increased by gradually increasing the number and complexity of the task demands, such as requiring simultaneous visual and auditory identification tasks. Unlike other cognitive training programs, such as memory or reasoning training (Ball et al., 2002; Rebok, Montaglione, & Bendlin, 1998; Willis & Schaie, 1986), speed of processing training tasks are non-verbal. Memory and reasoning training techniques, similar to Kramer and colleagues' dual-task training (Kramer, Larish, & Strayer, 1995; Kramer, Larish, Weber, & Bardell, 1999), primarily target strategies for improving performance. In contrast, speed training as described here uses practice to improve a basic, primary cognitive ability. Kramer and colleagues' dual-task training involves performance of two different tasks simultaneously (monitoring and alphabet–arithmetic tasks). Their training technique primarily aims to improve one's ability to manage and coordinate multiple tasks by varying the priority emphasis that trainees assign to each of the tasks. Such training would be quite attentive in nature. Speed training, on the other hand, requires the preattentive processing of targets throughout the visual field while simultaneously performing an attentive primary task in central vision, and there is not sufficient time during the tasks for participants to switch attention. Interestingly, while age-related declines are commonly reported for attentive tasks, preattentive or parallel processing of information has been thought to be relatively stable with age (Hasher & Zachs, 1979; Hoyer & Plude, 1980). Deficits on this measure, however, occur for a subset of older adults, and the prevalence of speed of processing deficits increases with age (Ball, Roenker, & Bruni, 1990). Variable priority dual-task training is similar to speed training in that both involve a hybrid training procedure which includes both part-task and whole-task training (Kramer et al., 1995). In speed training, as the complexity of training tasks increases, the more complex tasks include components of earlier training tasks. Thus speed training is hypothesized to build the trainees' capacity to perform everyday speeded tasks.

Support for the hypothesis that speed of processing training can positively impact everyday performance for older adults experiencing cognitive slowing has been found in several studies (Edwards, Wadley, Myers, Roenker, Cissell, & Ball, 2002; Edwards, Wadley, Vance, Roenker, & Ball, 2005; Roenker, Cissell, Ball, Wadley, & Edwards, 2003) summarized in Table 11.1. Older adults who underwent speed of processing training exhibited safer on-road driving performance in the driving study (Roenker et al., 2003) as compared to a simulator-trained group, and more efficient and accurate performance of Timed IADLs in the UAB Training, Accelerate, and SKILL studies (Edwards et al., 2002; Edwards et al., 2005) as compared to a social and computer contact control group.

Recently, a large-scale randomized, controlled, single-blind trial (ACTIVE) evaluated whether three cognitive training protocols (memory, reasoning, and speed of processing) improved mental abilities and daily functioning in a volunteer sample of 2832 persons aged 65 to 94 (Jobe et al., 2001). Participants were randomized to 10 sessions of group training for memory, reasoning, or speed of processing, or to a no-contact control group. Primary outcome measures included tests of cognitive function and cognitively demanding everyday functioning. Results of phase one of the ACTIVE study demonstrated that each intervention improved the targeted cognitive ability, and that these cognitive improvements were durable to 2 years ($p < .001$). Eighty-seven percent of speed-, 74% of reasoning-, and 26% of memory-trained participants demonstrated reliable cognitive improvement at immediate post-test. Four-session booster training at the end of the first year enhanced training gains in the speed ($p < .001$) and reasoning ($p < .001$) training groups (speed boost 92%, no boost 68%; reasoning boost 73%, no boost 49%), which were maintained at 2-year follow-up ($p < .001$ and $< .01$ respectively). Results supported the effectiveness and durability of the cognitive training interventions in improving targeted cognitive abilities. Training effects were of a magnitude equal to the amount of decline expected in nondemented elderly over 4- to 14-year intervals. Because of minimal functional decline across all groups over a 2-year period, longer follow-up is required to observe training effects on the maintenance of everyday function. With respect to health-related quality of life (HRQoL), however, defined as clinically relevant drops (i.e., $> .5$ SD), on four or more of the eight SF-36 scales

Table 11.1 Summary of studies examining speed of processing training in the elderly

Study	N	Inclusion criteria	Ages	Education range	Training mode & duration	Follow-up period	Transfer of training (effect size)
UAB training	97	Community-dwelling	61–95	6th grade to Ph.D.	Group, 5 weeks	N/A	UFOV (.62), TIADL
Accelerate	159	Community-dwelling MMSE ≥ 25 Visual acuity ≥ 20/40 Contrast sensitivity ≥ 1.35 Poor UFOV	65–92	8th grade to Ph.D.	Group & individual, varied	N/A	UFOV (1.87), TIADL
SKILL	126	Community-dwelling MMSE ≥ 23 Visual acuity ≥ 20/80 Contrast sensitivity ≥ 1.35 Poor UFOV	63–87	8th grade to Ph.D.	Group & individual, 5 weeks	N/A	UFOV (1.94), TIADL
Driving	104	Community-dwelling Visual acuity ≥ 20/40 Poor UFOV	55–86	Not known	Individual, 2 weeks	18 months	UFOV (2.50), Road Sign Test Driving Performance
ACT-VE	2832	Community-dwelling MMSE ≥ 23 Visual acuity ≥ 20/70	65–94	4th grade to Ph.D.	Group, 5 weeks	2 years	UFOV (1.463), UFOV (.867–2 yrs)
Home-based training	266	Community-dwelling MMSE ≥ 23 Visual acuity ≥ 20/40 Poor UFOV	65–91	5th grade to Ph.D.	Individual, 5 weeks	N/A	UFOV (1.74)

Notes: UAB = University of Alabama at Birmingham; SKILL = Staying Keen in Later Life; ACTIVE = Advanced Cognitive Training for Independent and Vital Elderly; UFOV = Useful Field of View test; TIADL = Timed Instrumental Activities of Daily Living test; MMSE = Mini-Mental Status Exam; N/A = not applicable.

between baseline and the 24-month follow-up, speed of processing trained participants were less likely to have extensive HRQoL decline (AOR = 0.643; p = .004 compared to controls. Thus although all three training groups (speed, memory, and reasoning) improved in cognitive ability, only speed of processing protected against extensive, clinically relevant decline in HRQoL at 24 months. These results are consistent with the idea that cognitive training can prevent decline, since trained participants were less likely, or at least slower, to experience decline relative to the control groups (Wolinsky, Unverzagt, Smith, Jones, Wright, & Tennstedt, in press).

In a separate investigation, Roenker and colleagues (2003) evaluated the effects of training-related improvements in processing speed on the driving performance of older adults. Older adults participated either in a speed training program (n = 48), a driving skills training program performed in a driving simulator (n = 22), or a low-risk reference group (n = 25). Before training, immediately after training or an equivalent time delay, and after an 18-month delay, each participant was evaluated in a driving simulator and completed a 14-mile open road driving evaluation. As illustrated in Figures 11.1 and 11.2, speed training not only improved the Useful Field of View, but also reduced response time to traffic signs presented in the driving simulator, as well as the number of dangerous maneuvers made during the driving evaluation. The simulator-trained group improved on two driving performance measures: turning into the correct lane and proper signal use.

The persistence of these effects over an 18-month test interval was also evaluated. The benefits of speed training were still present 18 months after training, while the benefits of simulator training were not.

In order to further evaluate transfer of speed of processing training to everyday abilities, several different outcome measures have been used. One

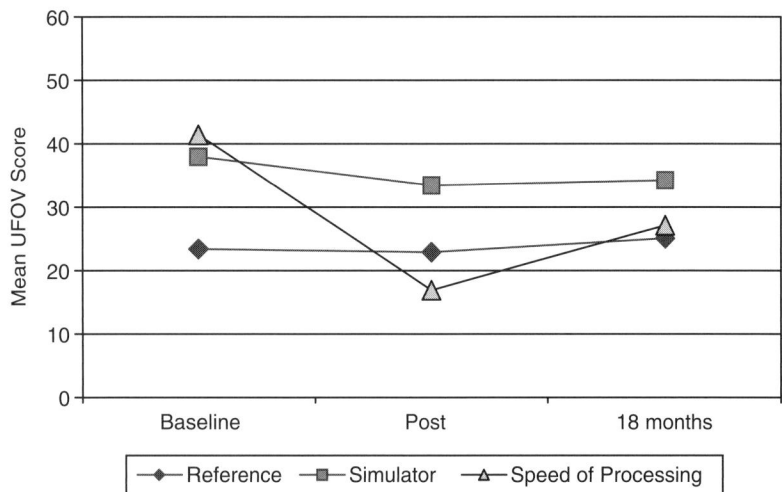

Figure 11.1 Useful Field of View performance across time by group.

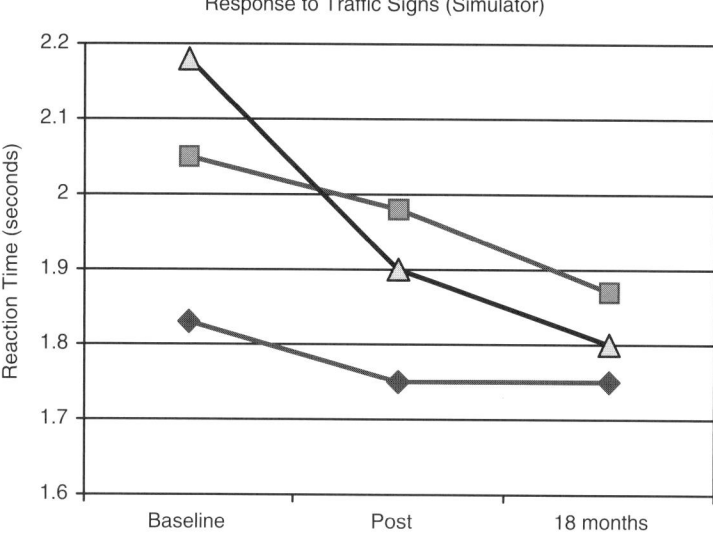
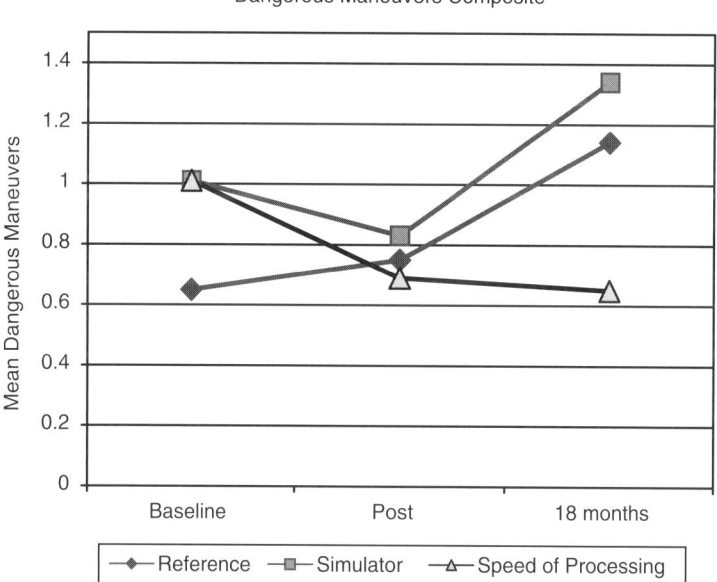

Figure 11.2 Simulator—response to traffic signs and dangerous maneuvers across time by group.

way of evaluating everyday function involves a measure of complex reaction time, referred to as "The Road Sign Test" (Ball et al., 2002; Edwards et al., 2002; Roenker et al., 2003). This measure has been used in a driving simulator (Roenker et al., 2003), and has also been adapted as a computerized measure of everyday speed that has been used in several past and ongoing studies, including ACTIVE. In both versions of the Road Sign Test, participants view road signs (pedestrians, bicycle, right and left turn arrows) with and without a red slash. They are instructed to disregard signs with a red slash (distractors), and to respond as quickly as possible, using a computer mouse, to signs without a slash (targets). In the computerized version of the test, required reactions are moving the mouse to the left (in response to a left turn sign) or right (in response to a right turn sign), and clicking a button on the mouse (in response to a bicycle or pedestrian sign). Prior to the test trials, all participants practice clicking and moving the mouse until proficiency is demonstrated. In the Driving Simulator version of the test, participants react to turn signals by turning the steering wheel in the proper direction, and react to bicycle or pedestrian signs by pressing the brake pedal. This measure includes two conditions in which either three or six signs are displayed on the screen at a time, and each condition includes 12 trials. Stimuli remain on the display until a correct response is made. The average reaction time is calculated across all trials.

Speed of processing training was found to transfer to enhanced Road Sign Test performance, as administered in a Driving Simulator (Roenker et al., 2003). Individuals who underwent speed of processing training showed quicker reaction times (about 277 ms faster, on average) for Road Sign Test performance at immediate post-test relative to their baseline performance, and this improvement was maintained for at least 18 months. For a vehicle moving at 55 mph, this improvement of 277 ms translates into a 22-foot shorter stopping distance (Roenker et al., 2003). Interestingly, when the Road Sign Test was administered via computer and required reactions with a mouse, transfer of speed of processing training was not immediately evident in other studies (Edwards et al., 2002; Edwards et al., 2005). On the other hand, these studies also had smaller effect sizes for cognitive training gain.

Another measure of everyday speed is the Timed Instrumental Activities of Daily Living test (TIADL; Owsley et al., 2002). The TIADL involves laboratory measurement of five timed tasks that simulate everyday instrumental activities of daily living. Like the Road Sign Test, this has been classified as an everyday speed measure (Ball et al., 2002). Tasks include: finding a telephone number of a specific individual in the telephone directory; finding and correctly counting out $0.67 cents from a group of coins; finding and reading the ingredients on a food can label; finding two food items in an array of food items simulating a crowded pantry shelf; and finding and reading the directions on a medicine container. Time in seconds required to complete each task is recorded. If the participant does not complete the task within the pre-set time limit, testing for that particular task discontinues. For the tasks completed with minor errors, a penalty is added to completion time. The times for each of the tasks are transformed into z-scores, which are then equally weighted to form a composite.

Several studies in Table 11.1 found that transfer of speed of processing training led to improved performance on the TIADL test. Participants who underwent speed of processing training completed the TIADL tasks more efficiently and more accurately as compared to controls. Transfer effects were greatest in the studies where cognitive gains were also higher.

Further research has demonstrated that speed of processing training can potentially be self-administered. This self-administered training involves the use of videotapes and a workbook rather than a trainer and personal computer. Wadley and colleagues (Wadley, Benz, Ball, Roenker, Edwards, & Vance, 2006) adapted this home-based training from the speed of processing training laboratory protocol discussed above. In the home-based speed of processing training, older participants were oriented by the examiner to relevant training procedures and materials including eight videotapes, a manual containing written instructions (including the order in which to use the tapes, the importance of deciding viewing times, etc.), multiple scoring sheets, and diary pages on which to record the data of each session and any difficulties or distractions encountered during that session. The video practice and training trials contain the same range of display durations as well as basic training tasks (speed of processing, divided attention, and selective attention) that are used in the laboratory-based training protocol. The participant views each trial on the tape, is given a short period to record his or her response on the scoring forms, and then receives feedback about the correct answer. The narrator explains that if a participant has failed to master a block of trials on the first attempt, he or she should rewind the tape to a clearly marked flag (e.g., BLOCK 2) in order to repeat that block until mastery is achieved before advancing to the next block. The participant is also instructed that if he or she fails to achieve mastery of a block after three attempts, he or she should repeat the preceding block of training trials before moving ahead. Participants were instructed to spend two 1-hour sessions a week for 5 weeks to approximate the standard laboratory training protocols. To test the effectiveness of this home-based speed of processing training protocol, participants aged 65 and older who exhibited slower processing speed at baseline were assigned to one of four groups: laboratory speed of processing training, home-based speed of processing training, internet control group, and no-contact control group. Participants who underwent home-based speed of processing training improved their processing speed significantly more than either control group. Their gains in speed of processing were 74% as great as those who underwent the laboratory speed of processing training, indicating that those with poor processing speed can improve their processing speed at home using such widely available technology.

The body of work in speed of processing training indicates that different versions and timing of this training are effective in improving performance.

However, additional work is needed. First, such studies have recruited people who are functional enough to drive to the testing/training facilities. Thus those with reduced speed of processing who are more likely to avoid such driving situations would likely benefit from training; however, no studies to date have targeted this group of at-risk adults. Second, other interventions known to improve cognitive function (e.g., exercise or medications) should be evaluated in combination with cognitive training to evaluate the impact of multi-component approaches.

Importance of training for clinical populations

Although there are age-related cognitive declines associated with speed of processing, such declines may be more pronounced in certain clinical populations. Thus targeting those populations for speed of processing evaluation and training may result in improved functioning, which translates into improved functioning in everyday tasks. There are several clinical populations that may be sensitive to speed of processing impairments, including those with mild cognitive impairment (MCI), dementia, diabetes, cardiovascular disease, multiple sclerosis, traumatic brain injury and those aging with HIV, just to name a few (DeLuca, Chelune, Tulsky, Lengefelder, & Chiaravalloti, 2004; Fillit et al., 2002; Madigan, DeLuca, Diamond, Tramontano, & Averill, 2000). Two examples are provided.

Mazer and colleagues (Mazer, Sofer, Korner-Bitensky, Gelinas, Hanley, & Wood-Dauphinee, 2003) examined the use of speed of processing training on driving performance in adults with stroke. They assigned participants to one of two treatment arms, either a speed of processing training condition or a traditional computerized visuoperception training condition. An occupational therapist blind to the treatment assignment administered the evaluations. No significant differences were found between the groups on any of the outcomes. However, in the adults with right-side lesions who received speed training, there was a twofold increase (52.4% vs 28.6%) in the success rate of the on-road driving evaluation. This suggests that speed of processing training may be helpful in restoring some cognitive and everyday functioning in those with select impairments.

Neuropsychological performance is being closely examined in those with HIV. Heaton and colleagues (1995) found that neuropsychological impairments were likely to be expressed in slower speed of information processing, among other domains. Reger, Welsh, Razani, Martin, and Boone (2002) conducted a meta-analysis on the cognitive declines in HIV. In their analysis of 41 studies, they found that information processing speed, along with motor functioning, were among the cognitive domains demonstrating the greatest decline from early to late stages of infection. Examining the cognitive sequelae is becoming especially germane as more people are aging with this disease (Vance, 2004; Vance & Robinson, 2004). Because speed of processing training has been developed and used in older adults who experience declines in such ability, similar technology may be applied to those with HIV who might be experiencing similar declines (Vance & Burrage, 2006).

Conclusion

As the population ages, the study of cognitive aging, and an understanding of the impact of cognitive function on everyday activities, continue to grow in importance. Such importance stems primarily from the links being established between cognition and many vital activities of daily living such as working, the use of technology, mobility, driving, and falling. Fortunately, training studies indicate that at least some cognitive functions can be improved in older adults, that improved performance endures for a period of years, and that improved cognition is associated with improved performance in everyday functioning in certain circumstances. This provides hope to those who are experiencing cognitive declines as a result of either age-related causes or other causes such as disease status, medication side effects, polypharmacy, or depression.

With respect to speed of processing training specifically, future research should explore the potential of this intervention in clinical populations where impaired information processing speed is one of the major sequelae. Clearly, impaired processing speed also affects everyday life activities in such clinical groups, and intervention studies aimed at improving speed of processing are needed. For example, MCI represents a group at high risk for functional declines that threaten independence. Pharmacological treatments are currently being widely examined in clinical trials in this population to evaluate their impact on the progression of cognitive decline and subsequent dementia diagnosis. Exploring the potential of cognitive training concurrently in this population would help researchers gain an understanding of whether or not functional abilities, such as driving, might be maintained for longer periods of time. Future research and interventions in this area will also need to focus on a mechanism to identify those experiencing speed of processing declines. AAA (American Automobile Association) has recently released a self-assessment product, "Roadwise Review," to help older adults evaluate their functional abilities at home. Along the same line, an ongoing project is currently investigating the effectiveness of training software that can be self-administered in a variety of settings (senior centers, doctors' offices, etc.), but as yet such widespread training options are unavailable. Further research could also provide a clearer understanding of what "dose" of speed of processing training is required initially, as well as a timeline for booster sessions to maximize training benefit. Although those with initial speed of processing decline seem to immediately benefit most, it is still unclear whether those performing well initially may also benefit longitudinally. Finally, it is now clear that processing speed is not a singular entity, since different types of speed of processing have been identified (Chiaravalloti, Christodoulou, Demaree, & DeLuca, 2003). Research needs to further examine how these aspects of processing speed are related to various real-world problems. For example, visual speed of processing may be more important for driving, while motor speed of processing may be more important for writing and falling.

More studies such as ACTIVE, which include long-term follow-up, evaluation of cognitive training gains on daily functioning, and large numbers of older participants, are needed. Ideally, these studies should begin to evaluate combinations of interventions known individually to provide benefit. For example, combining different cognitive training programs themselves, or combining them with exercise, nutritional supplements, and/or medications could strengthen the benefits of cognitive training for older adults.

In conclusion, most of the cognitive training research in the area of processing speed indicates that there is benefit from training. Older adults seem to benefit from many approaches to improve their basic cognitive abilities. Since cognitive decline can translate into real-world impairment, and speed of processing decline in particular can impact public safety and quality of life, it is important for older adults to realize that a decline need not immediately be considered irreversible, or even inevitable.

Notes

The Center for Translational Research on Aging and Mobility is supported by an Edward R. Roybal Center grant #5 P30 AG022838. Karlene Ball has a financial involvement (stock ownership and consultant) with Visual Awareness, Inc. This company owns the patent to the "Useful Field of View Visual Attention Analyzer," as well as the UFOV® speed of processing training program described in the chapter.

References

Aguero-Torres, H., Thomas, V. S., Winbald, B., & Fratiglioni, L. (2002). The impact of somatic and cognitive disorders on the functional status of the elderly. *Journal of Clinical Epidemiology*, 55 (10), 1007–1012.

Ball, K. K., Beard, B. L., Roenker, D. L., Miller, R. L., & Griggs, D. S. (1988). Age and visual search: Expanding the useful field of view. *Journal of the Optical Society of America. A, Optics, Image Science, and Vision*, 5 (12), 2210–2219.

Ball, K., Berch, D. B., Helmers, K. F., Jobe, J. B., Leveck, M. D., Marsiske, M., et al. for the ACTIVE Study Group (2002). Effect of cognitive training interventions with older adults: A randomized controlled trial. *Journal of the American Medical Association*, 288, 2271–2281.

Ball, K., & Owsley, C. (1993). The useful field of view test: A new technique for evaluating age-related declines in visual function. *Journal of the American Optometric Association*, 64 (1), 71–79.

Ball, K., Owsley, C., Sloane, M. E., Roenker, D. L., & Bruni, J. R. (1993). Visual attention problems as a predictor of vehicle crashes in older drivers. *Investigative Ophthalmology and Visual Science*, 34 (11), 3110–3123.

Ball, K. K., Roenker, D. L., & Bruni, J. R. (1990). Developmental changes in attention and visual search throughout adulthood. In J. Enns (Ed.), *Advances in Psychology* (Vol. 69, pp. 489–508). Amsterdam: North-Holland.

Ball, K. K., Vance, D. E., Edwards, J. E., & Wadley, V. W. (2004). Aging and the brain (pp. 795–809). In M. Rizzo & P. J. Eslinger (Eds.), *Principles and practice of behavioral neurology and neuropsychology*. Philadelphia: Saunders.

Ball, K. K., Roenker, D. L., Wadley, V. G., Edwards, J. D., Roth, D. L., McGwin, G. J., et al. (2006). Can high-risk older drivers be identified through performance-based measures in a Department of Motor Vehicles setting? *Journal of the American Geriatrics Society, 54* (1), 77–84.

Barberger, G. P., & Fabrigoule, C. (1997). Disability and cognitive impairment in the elderly. *Disability and Rehabilitation, 19*, 175–193.

Barberger, G. P., Fabrigoule, C., Rouch, I., Letenneur, L., & Dartigues, J. F. (1999). Neuropsychological correlates of self-reported performance in instrumental activities of daily living and prediction of dementia. *Journal of Gerontology, 54* (5), P293–P303.

Baudouin, A., Vanneste, S., & Isingrini, M. (2004). Age-related cognitive slowing: The role of spontaneous tempo and processing speed. *Experimental Aging Research, 30* (3), 225–239.

Benedict, R. H., Dobraski, M., & Godlstein, M. Z. (1999). A preliminary study of the association between changes in mood and cognition in a mixed geriatric psychiatry sample. *Journal of Gerontology, 54*, 94–99.

Birren, J. E. (1974). Translations in gerontology—from lab to life. Psychophysiology and speed of response. *American Psychologist, 29* (11), 808–815.

Brigman, S., & Cherry, K. E. (2002). Age and skilled performance: Contributions of working memory and processing speed. *Brain & Cognition, 50* (2), 242–256.

Botwinick, J. (1984). *Aging and behavior* (3rd ed.). New York: Springer.

Brozek, J., & Keys, A. (1945). Changes in flicker–fusion frequency with age. *Journal of Consulting and Clinical Psychology, 9*, 87–90.

Cerella, J., Poon, L. W., & Williams, D. M. (1980). Age and the complexity hypothesis. In L. Poon (Ed.), *Aging in the 1980s: Psychological issues* (pp. 332–340). Washington, DC: American Psychological Association.

Chiaravalloti, N. D., Chirstodoulou, C., Demaree, H. A., & DeLuca, J. (2003). Differentiating simple versus complex processing speed: Influence on new learning and memory performance. *Journal of Clinical and Experimental Neuropsychology, 25* (4), 489–501.

Collie, A., Shafiq-Antonacci R., Maruff, P., Tyler, P., & Currie, J. (1999). Norms and the effects of demographic variables on a neuropsychological battery for use in healthy ageing in Australian population. *Australia and New Zealand Journal of Psychiatry, 33*, 568–578.

Coppinger, N. W. (1955). The relationship between critical flicker frequency and chronological age for varying levels of stimulus brightness. *Journal of Gerontology, 10*, 48–52.

Czaja, S. J. (2001). Technological change and the older worker. In J. E. Birren & K. W. Schaie (Eds.), *Handbook of the psychology of aging* (pp. 547–568). New York: Academic Press.

Czaja, S. J., & Sharit, J. (1993). Age differences in the performance of computer-based work. *Psychology and Aging, 8* (1), 59–67.

Czaja, S. J., Sharit, J., Nair, S. N., & Rubert, M. (1998). Understanding sources of user variability in computer-based data entry performance. *Behaviour and Information Technology, 17* (5), 282–293.

DeLuca, J., Chelune, G. J., Tulsky, D., Lengenfelder, J. & Chiaravalloti, N. D. (2004). Is processing speed or working memory the primary information processing deficit in multiple sclerosis? *Journal of Clinical and Experimental Neuropsychology, 26,* 550–562.

Dodge, H. H., Kadowaki, T., Hayakawa, T., Yamakawa, M., Sekikawa, A., & Ueshima, H. (2005). Cognitive impairment as a strong predictor of incident disability in specific ADL-IADL tasks among community-dwelling elders: The Azuchi Study. *Gerontologist, 45* (2), 222–230.

Edwards, J. D., Wadley, V. G., Myers, R. S., Roenker, D. L., Cissell, G. M., & Ball, K. K. (2002). Transfer of a speed of processing intervention to near and far cognitive functions. *Gerontology, 48,* 329–340.

Edwards, J. E., Wadley, V. G., Vance, D. E., Roenker, D. L., & Ball, K. K. (2005). The impact of speed of processing training on cognitive and everyday performance. *Aging and Mental Health, 9,* 1–10.

Fillit, H. M., Butler, R. N., O'Connell, A. W., Albert, M. S., Birren, J. E., Cotman, C. W., et al. (2002). Achieving and maintaining cognitive vitality with aging. *Mayo Clinic Proceedings, 77* (7), 681–696.

Finkel, S. I., Mintzer, J. E., Dysken, M., Krishnan, K. R., Burt, T., & McRae, T. (2004). A randomized, placebo-controlled study for the efficacy and safety of sertaline in the treatment of the behavioral manifestations of Alzheimer's disease in outpatients treated with donepezil. *International Journal of Geriatric Psychiatry, 19* (1), 9–18.

Fisk, J. E., & Warr, P. B. (1998). Associative learning and short-term forgetting as a function of age, perceptual speed, and central executive functioning. *Journals of Gerontology, 53* (2), P112–P121.

Gomez, L. M., Egan, D. E., & Devlin, S. J. (1986). Learning to use a text-editor: Some learner characteristics that predict success. *Human Computer Interaction, 2,* 1–23.

Guralnik, J. M., Fried, L. P., & Salive, M. E. (1996). Disability as a public health outcome in the aging population. *Annual Review of Public Health, 17,* 25–46.

Hasher, L., & Zachs, R. (1979). Visual conspicuity, visual search, and fixation tendencies of the eye. *Vision Research, 17,* 91–97.

Heaton, R. K., Grant, I., Butters, N., White, D. A., Kirson, D., Atkinson, J. H., et al. (1995). The HNRC 500—neuropsychology of HIV infection at different disease stages. *Journal of the International Neuropsychological Society, 1* (3), 231–251.

Hoyer, W., & Plude, D. (1980). Attentional and perceptual processes in the study of cognitive aging. In L. W. Poon (ed.), *Aging in the 1980s: Psychological issues* (pp. 227–238). Washington, DC: American Psychological Association.

Hultsch, D. F., Hammer, M., & Small, B. J. (1993). Age differences in cognitive performance in later life: Relationships to self-reported health and activity life style. *Journal of Gerontology, 48* (1), 1–11.

Jefferson, J. W., & Greist, J. H. (1993). *Depression and older people: Recognizing hidden signs and taking steps toward recovery*. Madison, WI: Pratt Pharmaceuticals.

Jobe, J. B., Smith, D. M., Ball, K. K., Tennstedt, S. L., Marsiske, M., Willis, S. L., et al. (2001). ACTIVE: A cognitive intervention trial to promote independence in older adults. *Controlled Clinical Trials, 22,* 453–479.

Kline, D. W., & Birren, J. E. (1975). Age differences in backward dichoptic masking. *Experimental Aging Research, 1,* 17–25.

Kline, D., & Nestor, S. (1977). Persistence of complementary afterimages as a function of adult age and exposure duration. *Experimental Aging Research, 3,* 191–201.

Kline, D., & Orme-Rogers, C. (1978). Examination of stimulus persistence as the basis for superior visual identification performance among older adults. *Journal of Gerontology, 33,* 76–81.

Kline, D. W., & Szafran, J. (1975). Age difference in backward monoptic visual noise masking. *Journal of Gerontology, 30,* 307–311.

Kramer, A., Larish, J. F., & Strayer, D. L. (1995). Training for attentional control in dual task settings: A comparison of young and old adults. *Journal of Experimental Psychology: Applied, 1* (1), 50–76.

Kramer, A. F., Larish, J. L., Weber, T. A., & Bardell, L. (1999). Training for executive control: Task coordination strategies and aging. In D. Gopher & A. Koriat (Eds.), *Attention and performance XVII: Cognitive regulation of performance: Interaction of theory and application.* London: MIT Press.

Lemke, U., & Zimprich, D. (2005). Longitudinal changes in memory performance and processing speed in old age. *Aging, Neuropsychology, and Cognition, 12,* 57–77.

Linjakumpu, T., Hartikainen, S., Klaukka, T., Veijola, J., Kivela, S. L., & Isoaho, R. (2002). Use of medications and polypharmacy are increasing among the elderly. *Journal of Clinical Epidemiology, 55* (8), 809–817.

MacDonald, S. W., Hultsch, D. F., Strauss, E., & Dixon, R. A. (2003). Age-related slowing of digit symbol substitution revisited: What do longitudinal age changes reflect? *Journal of Gerontology, 58* (3), P187–P194.

Madigan, N., DeLuca, J., Diamond, B. J., Tramontano, G., and Averill, A. (2000). Speed of information processing in traumatic brain injury: A modality-specific impairment? *Journal of Head Trauma Rehabilitation, 15,* 943–956.

May, C. P., & Hasher, L. (1998). Synchrony effects in inhibitory control over thought and action. *Journal of Experimental Psychology: Human Perception and Performance, 24,* 363–379.

Mazer, B. L., Sofer, S., Korner-Bitensky, N., Gelinas, I., Hanley, J., & Wood-Dauphinee, S. (2003). Effectiveness of a visual attention retraining program on the driving performance of clients with stroke. *Archives of Physical Medicine & Rehabilitation, 84* (4), 541–550.

Misiak, H. (1947). Age and sex differences in critical flicker frequency. *Journal of Experimental Psychology, 37,* 318–332.

Murtagh, K. N., & Hubert, H. B. (2004). Gender differences in physical disability among an elderly cohort. *American Journal of Public Health, 94* (8), 1406–1411.

Owsley, C., Ball, K., McGwin, G., Jr., Sloane, M. E., Roenker, D. L., White, M. F., et al. (1998). Visual processing impairment and risk of motor vehicle crash among older adults. *Journal of the American Medical Association, 279* (14), 1083–1088.

Owsley, C., & McGwin, G., Jr. (2004). Association between visual attention and mobility in older adults. *Journal of the American Geriatric Society, 52* (11), 1901–1906.

Owsley, C., McGwin, G., Jr., & Ball, K. K. (1998). Vision impairment, eye disease, and injurious motor vehicle crashes in the elderly. *Ophthalmic Epidemiology, 5,* 101–113.

Owsley, C., Sloane, M., McGwin, G., Jr., & Ball, K. (2002). Timed Instrumental Activities of Daily Living tasks: Relationship to cognitive function and everyday performance assessments in older adults. *Gerontology, 48,* 254–265.

Owsley, C., Stalvey, B., Wells, J., & Sloane, M. E. (1999). Older drivers and cataract: Driving habits and crash risk. *The Journals of Gerontology. Series A, Biological Sciences and Medical Sciences, 54A*, M203–M211.

Panek, P. E. (1997). The older worker. In A. D. Fisk, & W. A. Rogers (Eds.), *Handbook of human factors and the older adult* (pp. 363–394). San Diego, CA: Academic Press.

Park, D. C., Nisbett, R., & Hedden, T. (1999). Aging, culture, and cognition. *Journal of Gerontology, 54*, 75–84.

Rebok, G. W., Montaglione, C. J., & Bendlin, G. (1988). Effects of age and training on memory for pragmatic implication in advertising. *Journal of Gerontology, 43* (3), 75–78.

Reger, M., Welsch, R., Razani, J., Martin, D. J., & Boone, K. B. (2002). A meta-analysis of the neuropsychological sequelae of HIV infection. *Journal of the International Neuropsychological Society, 8* (3), 410–424.

Riolo, L. (2003). Attention contributes to functional reach test scores in older adults with history of falling. *Physical and Occupational Therapy in Geriatrics, 22*, 15–29.

Roenker, D. L., Cissell, G. M., Ball, K. K., Wadley, V. G., & Edwards, J. D. (2003). Speed-of-processing and driving simulator training result in improved driving performance. *Human Factors, 45* (2), 218–233.

Rosnick, C. B., Small, B. J., Borenstein Graves, A., & Mortimer, J. A. (2004). Health predictors of cognition in the Charlotte County Healthy Aging Study. *Aging, Neuropsychology and Cognition, 11*, 89–99.

Rosson, M. B. (1983). Patterns of experience in text editing. In R. N. Smith, R. W. Pew, & A. Jonda (Eds.), *Proceedings of the AM CHI 83 Human Factors in Computing Systems Conference* (pp. 171–175), December 12–15, 1983, Boston, MA.

Salthouse, T. A. (1985). Speed of behavior and its implications for cognition. In J. E. Birren & K. W. Schaie (Eds.), *Handbook of the psychology of aging* (2nd ed., pp. 400–426). New York: Van Nostrand Reinhold.

Salthouse, T. A. (1990). Cognitive competence and expertise in aging. In J. E. Birren & K. W. Schaie (Eds.), *Handbook of the psychology of aging* (3rd ed., pp. 310–319). San Diego, CA: Academic Press.

Salthouse, T. A. (1993). Speed mediation of adult age differences in cognition. *Developmental Psychology, 29* (4), 722–738.

Salthouse, T. A. (1996). The processing-speed theory of adult age differences in cognition. *Psychological Review, 10*, 403–428.

Salthouse, T. A. (2000). Aging and measures of processing speed. *Biological Psychology, 54*, 35–54.

Schaie, K. W. (1989). Perceptual speed in adulthood: Cross-sectional and longitudinal studies. *Psychology & Aging, 4* (44), 443–453.

Schaie, K. W. (1994). The course of adult intellectual development. *American Psychologist, 49*, 304–313.

Sekuler, R., & Ball, K. (1986). Visual localization: Age and practice. *Journal of the Optical Society of America. A, Optics, Image Science, and Vision, 3* (6), 864–867.

Sekuler, R., Kline, D., & Dismukes, K. (1983). Aging and human visual function. *Optometry and Vision Science, 60* (6), 547.

Sims, R., McGwin, G., Pulley, L., & Roseman, J. M. (2001). Mobility impairments in crash-involved older drivers. *Journal of Aging and Health, 13* (3), 430–438.

Smits, C. H., Deeg, D. J., & Jonker, C. (1997). Cognitive and emotional predictors of disablement in older adults. *Journal of Aging and Health, 9* (2), 204–221.

Stalvey, B. T., Owsley, C., Sloane, M. E., & Ball, K. K. (1999). The Life Space

Questionaire: A measure of the extent of mobility of older adults. *The Journal of Applied Gerontology, 18* (4), 460–478.
Staplin, L. K., Gish, K. W., & Wagner, E. K. (2003). MaryPODS revisited: Updated crash analysis and implications for screening program implementation. *Journal of Safety Research, 34,* 389–397.
Steen, G., Sonn, U., Hanson, A. B., & Steen, B. (2001). Cognitive function and functional ability. A cross-sectional and longitudinal study at ages 85 and 95 in a non-demented population. *Aging—Clinical and Experimental Research, 13* (2), 68–77.
Suhr, J. A., Hall, J., Patterson, S. M., & Niinisto, R. T. (2004). The relation of hydration status to cognitive performance in healthy older adults. *International Journal of Psychophysiology, 53* (2), 121–125.
Vance, D. E. (2004). Cortical and subcortical dynamics of aging with HIV infection. *Perceptual and Motor Skills, 98,* 647–655.
Vance, D. E., & Burrage, J. W. Jr. (2006). Promoting successful cognitive aging in adults with HIV: Strategies for intervention. *Journal of Gerontological Nursing, 32* (11), 34–41.
Vance, D. E., Dawson, J., Wadley, V. G., Edwards, J. D., Roenker, D. L., Rizzo, M., et al. (2007). The Accelerate Study: The longitudinal effect of speed of processing training on cognitive performance of older adults. *Rehabilitation Psychology, 52* (1), 89–96.
Vance, D. E., & Robinson, F. P. (2004). Reconciling successful aging with HIV: A biopsychosocial overview. *Journal of HIV/AIDS and Social Services, 3* (1), 59–78.
Vincente, K. J., Hayes, B. C. & Willies, R. C. (1987). Assaying and isolating individual differences in searching a hierarchical file system. *Human Factors, 29,* 349–359.
Wadley, V. G., Benz, R. L., Ball, K. K., Roenker, D. L., Edwards, J. D., & Vance, D. E. (2006). Development and evaluation of home-based speed of processing training for older adults. *Archives of Physical Medicine and Rehabilitation, 87,* 757–763.
Willis, S. L., & Schaie, K. W. (1986). Training the elderly on the ability factors of spatial orientation and inductive reasoning. *Psychology and Aging, 1* (3), 239–247.
Wolinsky, F. D., Unverzagt, F. W., Smith, D. M., Jones, R., Wright, E., & Tennstedt, S. L. (in press). The effects of the ACTIVE cognitive training trial on clinically relevant declines in health-related quality of life. *Journals of Gerontology: Social Sciences.*
Zimprich, D., & Martin, M. (2002). Can longitudinal changes in processing speed explain longitudinal age changes in fluid intelligence? *Psychology & Aging, 17* (4), 690–695.

12 Information processing speed: How fast, how slow, and how come?

John DeLuca

> Intelligence is quickness to apprehend as distinct from ability, which is capacity to act wisely on the thing apprehended.
> (Alfred North Whitehead, from Bartlett, 1968)

Since antiquity, philosophers and scientists have focused their studies of the mind on its faculties. The speed with which mental operations occur received little to no attention. In modern science, processing speed (PS) was first studied by Galton in the late 1800s and operationally defined as reaction time, a conceptualization that continued for about 40–50 years. But during this period, the actual speed of higher level operations was not considered as important as understanding the basic or fundamental operations of the mind itself. The waning of such fundamentalism resulted in information PS vanishing from scientific study, only to be rediscovered during the later part of the twentieth century (see chapter 1 of this volume).

Even with the renewed interest in studying information PS during the last 30 years, why is it that today we still do not have an accepted working model of human information PS that is integrated into larger theories of cognitive operations of the brain? As seen in chapter 1, the one exception is the study of intelligence, but no clear consensus appears on the horizon despite over 100 years of inquiry. There are often fleeting allusions to PS in some theoretical discussions of other human mental faculties, particularly with respect to developmental theories (see Cowan, Elliot, Saults, Nugent, Bomb, & Hismjatullina, 2006). Theoretical perspectives on working memory have perhaps developed like few other cognitive constructs over the last 40 years. However, in Baddeley's recent review of the human working memory, PS is mentioned only once, and only as an aside (Baddeley, 2003). Baddeley himself recognizes that he has not incorporated PS in his theoretical formulations of working memory (Personal communication, 2006). In reality, clinical and cognitive science today lack an integrative model of perhaps one of the most elemental yet essential workings of the human mind; the speed with which mental operations is conducted.

Throughout the various chapters of this volume there are numerous examples of how PS is a fundamental operation of the human brain, how it is affected by neurological insult, and how it affects higher cognitive processes. It is perhaps the most sensitive mental construct to insults of the brain in humans. So why is its relative neglect from a theoretical perspective so pervasive?

Defining processing speed

One reason why PS has been neglected from broader cognitive theories of cognition is its definition. More specifically, the construct of PS itself was rarely defined, and when it was, it was usually defined operationally or methodologically, mostly as reaction time. In reality, the study of human information PS requires its own conceptual definition. I propose the following definition: *the time required to execute a cognitive task or the amount of work that can be completed within a finite period of time.*

Related to problems in definition, PS also suffers from construct contamination. That is, there really are no good measures of "pure" PS; it must be coupled with other cognitive constructs. In fact, PS is inextricably intertwined with other mental operations, operations that have themselves either received more scientific attention, or seem more "important." For example, PS, working memory, and attention are frequently confused and used interchangeably, both conceptually and in the tests used in their assessment. For example, Spreen and Straus (1998) describe the Symbol Digit Modalities Test (SDMT) as a test assessing "visual scanning, tracking and motoric speed" (p. 253). Yet on page 255 it states that the SDMT has been shown to be one of the best measures of information PS. Although few if any neuropsychological instruments are "process pure," the cross-contamination between PS, working memory, and attention is particularly notable and problematic.

A second issue regarding its definition is the fact that PS has traditionally been conceptualized as a unitary concept. Thus for over 100 years since Galton a unitary model of PS served psychology well, but only in examining PS as an elemental human operation that influences higher cognitive functions. We know today that human information PS is multidimensional and may have several components. For instance, Cattell (1971) provided empirical evidence for the existence of at least seven forms of "mental speed." The multidimensional nature of PS is a point made by several authors throughout this book. A recent study illustrates this point. Using factor analysis, Chiaravalloti, Christodoulou, Demaree, and DeLuca (2003) identified two components of PS; simple and complex. Simple PS was based on reaction time performance, while complex PS required higher level processing efficiency, including divided attention (i.e., PASAT), and loaded orthogonally on its own factor. Importantly, complex PS, and not simple PS, was associated with performance on higher cognitive functions (i.e., learning and memory). These data suggest that simple and complex PS measure distinct aspects of cognitive processes. Simple PS thus may not be closely associated with higher cognitive functions as some suggest (Lezak, Howiesen, & Loring, 2004), but it is complex PS where the association is primarily observed. Examination of such a hypothesis is an important area of future research.

Processing speed in clinical populations: General conclusions

Are there any general conclusions that can be drawn from the research discussed in the current book? The following is an attempt to integrate some of these general points.

Processing speed and other cognitive constructs

The most consistent findings among all of the chapters in this volume is the fact that PS has a significant influence on higher order cognitive constructs such as working memory, episodic memory, executive functions, reasoning, problem solving, visual spatial skills, and academic skills such as reading and arithmetic. This finding is so pervasive as to be essentially unequivocal.

The key question now is how may slowed PS actually affect other cognitive mechanisms? Recognizing the multidimensional nature of PS, Salthouse (1996, p. 404) writes:

> the speed with which an individual performs a cognitive activity is not simply a function of the processes required in that activity but also a reflection of his or her ability to rapidly carry out many different types of processing operations.

As has been described in chapters throughout this book, Salthouse proposed two distinct mechanisms in which complex PS affects higher cognition: a *limited time mechanism*, and a *simultaneity mechanism*. The limited time mechanism states that slower speed of executing many processing operations means that less processing can be completed in a given amount of time. The underlying principal for the limited time mechanism is that the "necessary operations may not be completed if the processing is slow" (Salthouse, 1996, p. 406). Specifically, the time to perform later operations is significantly restricted when one spends a large portion of available time executing the early operations of a task. The simultaneity mechanism refers to the notion that products from early processing may no longer be available by the time later processing is completed. That is, when the rate of executing operations is slow, this results in less relevant information because this information is impoverished or degraded by the time other simultaneous information processing is completed. Importantly, at least in the aging literature, this degradation has been shown to be a function of slower speed of processing and not the rate of information loss or decay in working memory (Salthouse, 1996).

While Salthouse (1996) makes a strong case for how these two mechanisms are responsible for the relationship between speed of processing and quality and/or accuracy of higher level cognitive operations in aging, it is natural to suspect that these same two mechanisms may also be responsible for a large part of the variance in clinical populations. Indeed, as outlined throughout this book, there is mounting evidence to support this very relationship. For example, there is ample evidence that slowed PS can affect learning and memory (e.g., DeLuca, Schultheis, Madigan, Christodoulou, & Averill, 2000; Gaudino, Chiaravalloti, DeLuca, & Diamond, 2001; Salthouse, 1996). Thus, for episodic memory, it is hypothesized that slowed complex PS diminishes the strength of encoding (as a result of the two mechanisms described above), resulting in a cascade of deficient learning leading to poor recall and recognition, which ultimately affects everyday life functional activity (DeLuca, Chelune, Tulsky, Lengenfelder, & Chiaravalloti, 2004; Kail, 1998).

New proposed model of working memory incorporating processing speed

This brings us back to the need to incorporate PS into current theoretical models of cognitive processes. Perhaps the most well formulated and studied is Baddeley's model of working memory (WM), which as stated above, has not incorporated a PS component. Briefly, working memory is a limited-capacity system for both storage (or maintenance) and manipulation of information. Storage or maintenance occurs in two (or three, see Baddeley, 2003) slave systems—the phonological loop and the visuospatial sketchpad. The central executive is an attentional control system that conducts the manipulation of this stored material. One proposed model for incorporating PS into the working memory model, the WM-PS model, is illustrated in Figure 12.1. This model incorporates two important constructs from the PS literature. The first is the incorporation of the *limited time mechanism* and the *simultaneity mechanism* of Salthouse (1996). It is clear that these PS

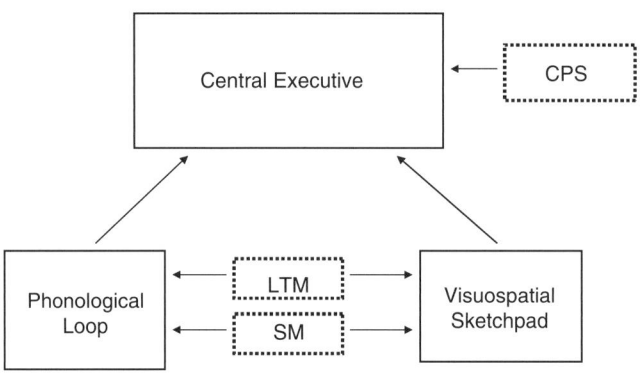

LTM = Limited Time Mechanism
SM = Simultaneity Mechanism
CPS = Complex Processing Speed

Figure 12.1 The working memory–processing speed (WM-PS) model.

mechanisms can affect working memory accuracy, and may have a particular influence on the operation of the slave systems of working memory.

The second construct incorporates the notion of complex PS and its effect on higher cognitive processes. Because Chiaravalloti et al. (2003) showed that only complex PS and not simple PS influenced higher cognitive operations, one can hypothesize that the central executive of Baddeley's working memory model can be particularly influenced by this complex PS construct.

This initial model is not designed to be explanatory. Rather, it is an initial attempt to formulate a working hypothesis from which data can be generated and the model updated accordingly from future research.

Processing speed and working memory are correlated but separable

Several chapters in this volume have discussed how PS is intricately intertwined with higher cognitive constructs. So does PS simply have a moderating effect on higher cognitive constructs or can it be conceptualized as a fundamental or core cognitive entity with an independent influence on performance? One of the difficulties in differentiating PS from other cognitive constructs, such as working memory, is that one construct is purportedly assessed (using current neuropsychological instruments), but is often interpreted as assessing another construct. For example, on the SDMT, patients are asked to complete the task in a given amount of time. As such, patients can be impaired on the SDMT either because of slowed PS, or because errors are made, presumably as a result of problems in working memory and/or attention, or even manual-motor difficulties on the written version of the test.

One thing we know absolutely from over 100 years of research is the existence of what has been referred to as the speed–accuracy trade-off. That is, the speed required to complete a task can be such that accuracy of performance is compromised, and vice versa. However, it is also known that this relationship is neither absolute, nor linear. For instance, recent work with clinical populations clearly shows that PS and working memory accuracy can have separate or "independent" effects on performance (Martin, Donders, & Thompson, 2000). DeLuca et al. (2004) showed that persons with multiple sclerosis (MS) who are relative early in the course of their disease (i.e., relapsing–remitting course) display clinically significant problems primarily in PS and not in working memory accuracy. However, as the disease progresses (i.e., to a secondary-progressive course), performance decrements in both PS and working memory accuracy become apparent, albeit to a greater degree in PS. Several studies have shown that when working memory accuracy is held constant between clinical samples and healthy controls (e.g., 50% correct), persons with MS or traumatic brain injury (TBI) still display significantly worse PS performance (Demaree, DeLuca, Gaudino, & Diamond, 1999; Madigan, DeLuca, Diamond, Tramontano, & Averill 2000), a finding also observed in aging (Diamond et al., 2000). Lengenfelder, Bryant, Diamond, Kalmar, Moore, and DeLuca (2006) found that at a lower working memory load, 100% of persons with MS were able to achieve performance accuracy levels equivalent to healthy control participants, but required more time (i.e., impaired PS) to do so. In contrast, at a higher working memory load, impairments in both accuracy and PS emerged in 30% of the participants with MS. Taken together, these data clearly show that, although interactive, PS can have an influence on performance that is independent of other cognitive constructs.

With these findings in mind, what can be predicted based on the WM-PS model illustrated in Figure 12.1? First, in this model, PS can have relatively independent influences from working memory performance. That is, PS can be impaired yet have little impact on working memory performance, and vice versa. Perhaps this is why speed is not contained in Baddeley's current model of working memory. However, there comes a point where the speed—accuracy trade-off kicks in and strains one element (PS or working memory accuracy), and begins to affect the performance of the other construct. What remains unclear is exactly how the two truly interact. This interaction between PS and other higher level cognitive constructs is a critical area of focus for future research in clinical rehabilitation science.

Processing speed is especially sensitive to insult to the brain

If PS is associated with higher cerebral functioning, then insults to the brain should result in decreased performance on tests of PS. This notion has received unanimous support throughout the book in discussion of childhood disorders, schizophrenia, MS, TBI, schizophrenia, depression, Huntington's disease, Parkinson's disease, reading disability, autism, and attention-deficit/hyperactivity disorder. In fact, the evidence is now virtually universal and unequivocal that PS is the most sensitive cognitive construct to cerebral damage. Even regarding "normal" development and aging, it is clear that PS is the primary cognitive construct that can define alterations or challenges to individual performance. For instance, Kail (chapter 5, p. 119) states:

> Given the popular view that atypical development is often a delayed or slower form of typical development, PS is likely to be among those basic processes that contribute to atypical development.

Given the known sensitivity of PS to brain damage, it is now incumbent on researchers and clinicians to develop effective methods for rehabilitation. The chapter by Ball and Vance (chapter 11) illustrates how this effort is in its infancy in clinical rehabilitation science.

Neural substrate of processing speed

Lastly, although a fair amount of research has been conducted investigating the neural processes associated with PS, we are only beginning to understand the potential biological substrate of the information PS in humans. It is likely that new functional neuroimaging techniques (such as diffusion tensor imaging) will hold great promise for this quest. However, as has been stated in several chapters, no single brain region has been, or is likely to be, identified as the neural substrate for PS. Rather, a neural network of complex interconnectivity with multiple regions of the brain will probably be observed, for something as seemingly simple and basic as information PS (see Salthouse & Madden, chapter 10; and Dickenson & Gold, chapter 6, in this volume). Thus, for instance, diminished PS has been associated with neurotransmitter activity (e.g., diminished cholinergic function, reduced D_2 receptor sites for dopamine and altered glutamate activity), white matter integrity (e.g., increased number of white matter intensities), diminished glucose metabolism, and decreased nerve conduction velocities (e.g., evoked potentials, event-related potentials or ERPs, electroencephalogram or EEG). While this accumulated evidence points to specific mechanisms associated with PS in humans, none alone is capable of explaining the totality and complexity of PS.

The most advanced and well accepted theoretical model of the biological substrates of PS is the "neural efficiency model," most often associated with the study of intelligence (Jensen, 1982; Vernon, 1983, 1987). This model states that a faster central nervous system allows for more rapid processing of information, and is related to more efficient cognitive information processing and higher intelligence. Faster PS allows more information to be processed before it is lost through decay or interference (see Salthouse mechanisms above), and is therefore more efficient (Jensen, 1993). As stated by several authors in this volume (e.g., Posthuma & de Geus, chapter 4; Dickenson & Gold, chapter 6, and Salthouse & Madden, chapter 10), there is now significant scientific support for this contention, although the association is not always strong or universal. For example, recent studies clearly show that brain nerve conduction velocities are positively correlated with cognitive performance, but this relationship is not strong and is influenced by various factors such as age and gender (e.g., Reed, Vernon, & Johnson, 2004).

Despite the enthusiasm regarding recent support for a model first suggested by Galton in 1883, one must recognize that recent physiological support for a neural efficiency hypothesis is moderate at best, and there appear to be mediating factors (e.g., sex) that may limit this relationship (see Neubauer, Fink, & Schrausser, 2002). Nonetheless, cumulatively, the data clearly show that speed of processing is a result of neural processes that are related to enhanced cognitive and intellectual functioning in humans. It is also clear that an insult to the brain, even mild in intensity, also has a direct impact, resulting in slowed information PS. Where the logic breaks down is that while PS is clearly reduced following brain damage, it does not necessarily result in decreased intelligence. For example, persons with MS who display PS as the primary cognitive impairment typically do not show intellectual decline, as measured by verbal intelligence. In reality, this should not be surprising, even to advocates of the neural efficiency hypothesis, since the correlations between intelligence and PS are typically around .3, or .5 at the most, thus accounting for only 9 to 25% of the variance.

Taken together, the findings across numerous studies of PS and the brain converge on the conclusion that there is some sort of global, biologically driven mechanism that limits the speed with which information is processed. Determining more precisely what that mechanism(s) is remains a major challenge for future investigators.

Concluding remarks

Information PS is one of the most basic operations of the human mind. There are numerous examples throughout this book of how PS is essential for efficient human functioning, both in higher cortical functioning (neural and cognitive) and in everyday life operations. PS is now finally recognized as a clinically significant entity in its own right (see chapter 1), being one of the more sensitive aspects of cognitive processing following damage to the brain. Just as scientists seek to understand the tiniest particles known (e.g., atoms) so that we can have a greater understanding of broader aspects of our world and universe, so we should strive to do the same in our understanding of the human mind; and PS is the road to this discovery. While much has been learned in over 100 years of inquiry about human information PS, there is far more to know than is known now. It is clear that unlocking the secrets of PS over the next several decades can have significant benefits for our understanding of the human mind and brain, and in neuropsychological rehabilitation.

References

Baddeley, A. (2003). Working memory: Looking back and looking forward. *Nature Reviews: Neuroscience*, *4*, 829–839.
Bartlett, J. (1968). *Familiar quotations*. Boston: Little, Brown and Company.
Cattell, R. B. (1971). *Abilities: Their structure, growth, and action*. Boston: Houghton-Mifflin.
Chiaravalloti, N., Christodoulou, C., Demaree H., & DeLuca J. (2003). Differentiating simple vs. complex processing speed: Influence on new learning and memory performance. *Journal of Clinical and Experimental Neuropsychology*, *25*, 489–501.
Cowan, N., Elliot, E. M., Saults, J. S., Nugent, L. D., Bomb, P., & Hismjatullina, A. (2006). Rethinking speed theories of cognitive development: Increasing the rate of recall without affecting accuracy. *Psychological Science*, *17*, 67–73.
DeLuca, J., Chelune, G. J., Tulsky, D., Lengenfelder, J., & Chiaravalloti, N. D. (2004). Is processing speed or working memory the primary information processing deficit in multiple sclerosis? *Journal of Clinical and Experimental Neuropsychology*, *26*, 550–562.
DeLuca, J., Schultheis, M. T., Madigan, N. K., Christodoulou, C., & Averill, A.

(2000). Acquisition vs retrieval deficits in traumatic brain injury: Implications for memory rehabilitation. *Archives of Physical Medicine and Rehabilitation*, 81, 1327–1333.

Demaree, H. A., DeLuca, J., Gaudino, E. A., & Diamond, B. J. (1999). Speed of information processing as a key deficit in multiple sclerosis: Implications for rehabilitation. *Journal of Neurology, Neurosurgery, and Psychiatry*, 67, 661–663.

Diamond, B. J., DeLuca, J., Rosenthal, D., Vlar, R., Davis, K., Lucas, G., et al. (2000). Information processing in older versus younger adults: Accuracy vs speed. *International Journal of Rehabilitation and Health*, 5, 55–64.

Gaudino, E., Chiaravalloti, N., DeLuca, J., & Diamond, B. J. (2001). A comparison of memory performance in relapsing–remitting, primary progressive and secondary progressive multiple sclerosis. *Neuropsychiatry, Neuropsychology and Behavioral Neurology*, 14, 32–44.

Jensen, A. R. (1982). Reaction times and psychometric g. In H. J. Eysenck (Ed.), *A model for intelligence*. Berlin: Springer-Verlag.

Jensen, A. R. (1993). Why is reaction time correlated with psychometric g? *Current Directions in Psychological Science*, 2, 53–56.

Kail, R. (1998). Speed of information processing in patients with multiple sclerosis. *Journal of Clinical and Experimental Neuropsychology*, 20, 98–106.

Lengenfelder, J., Bryant, D., Diamond, B. J., Kalmar, J. H., Moore, N. B., & DeLuca, J. (2006). Processing speed interacts with working memory efficiency in multiple sclerosis. *Archives of Clinical Neuropsychology*, 21, 229–238.

Lezak, M. D., Howiesen, D. B., & Loring, D. W. (2004). *Neuropsychological Assessment* (4th ed.). New York: Oxford University Press.

Madigan, N., DeLuca, J., Diamond, B. J., Tramontano, G., & Averill, A. (2000). Speed of information processing in traumatic brain injury: A modality-specific impairment? *Journal of Head Trauma Rehabilitation*, 15, 943–956.

Martin, T. A., Donders, J., & Thompson, E. (2000). Potential of and problems with new measures of psychometric intelligence after traumatic brain injury. *Rehabilitation Psychology*, 45, 402–408.

Neubauer, A. C., Fink, A., & Schrausser, D. G. (2002). Intelligence and neural efficiency: The influence of task content and sex on the brain–IQ relationship. *Intelligence*, 30, 515–536.

Reed, T. E., Vernon, P. A., & Johnson, A. M. (2004). Confirmation of correlation between brain nerve conduction velocity and intelligence level in normal adults. *Intelligence*, 32, 563–572.

Salthouse, T. A. (1996). The processing-speed theory of adult age differences in cognition. *Psychological Review*, 103, 403–428.

Spreen, O., & Strauss, E. (1998). *A compendium of neuropsychological tests: Administration, norms and commentary* (2nd ed.). New York: Oxford University Press.

Vernon, P. A. (1983). Speed of information processing and general intelligence. *Intelligence*, 7, 53–70.

Vernon, P. A. (Ed.). (1987). *Speed of information-processing and intelligence*. Norwood, NJ: Ablex.

Author index

Abernethy, D. 206
Ablin, A. 111
Abukmeil, S. S. 135
Achiron, A. 21, 155, 156, 161
Acker, J. D. 230
Ackerman, P. L. 222
Adalsteinsson, E. 233, 234
Adams, C. 144
Adams, H. F. 174, 175
Adams, J. H. 174
Adams, K. M. 33
Adams, R. L. 39
Ader, H. J. 144, 154, 156, 160
Ades, H. W. 33
Adler, L. E. 144
Afridi, S. 200
Agid, Y. 195, 205, 207, 212
Aguero-Torres, H. 246
Aguirre, G. K. 228
Ahmed, A. 36
Akbudak, E. 231, 233
Alaoui, P. 173
Albert, M. L. 195, 207
Albert, M. S. 256
Albert, R. H. 21
Aleman, A. 125, 128, 140, 235
Alexander, G. E. 196, 197
Alexander, M. P. 180, 200
Alexander, R. W. 38
Alfonso, V. C. 16
Allan, K. M. 35
Allan, L. M. 207
Allen, G. L. 58
Alloy, L. B. 66
Almasy, L. 87
Almeida, A. J. 84
Almeida, Q. J. 202
Almozlino, A. 207
Alphs, L. D. 125
Al-Schihabi, M. T. 186
Amador, S. C. 205
Amador, X. 141
Ambrus, J., Jr. 54, 55, 68
Amieva, H. 162, 165

Aminoff, M. J. 201, 202
Anaki, D. 200
Anchisi, A. M. 135
Andrade, J. 175
Andreasen, N. C. 125, 127, 129, 130, 131, 139, 144
Andreou, P. 89
Andrews, D. G. 198
Angelakis, E. 85
Angleitner, A. 34, 89, 90
Aniskiewicz, A. S. 68
Ankey, C. D. 12
Anokhin, A. P. 85
Ansel, M. 127, 136
Anthony, J. C. 231
Appelboim, N. 21, 155, 156
Arbuckle, J. L. 81
Arbuthnott, K. 39
Archibald, C. J. 21, 30, 54, 63, 68, 69, 155, 160, 161, 164
Arezzo, J. C. 144
Arimone, Y. 162, 165
Army Individual Test Battery 39
Arndt, S. 127, 129, 130, 131, 139
Arnett, P. A. 63, 66, 154, 162
Arnold, A. M. 144
Asarnow, R. R. 173
Asherson, P. 91
Asikainen, I. 174, 187
Aston-Jones, G. 87
Atkinson, J. H. 256
Auer, L. M. 85
Augustine, A. M. 231
Auth, T. L. 154
Averill, A. 21, 22, 29, 55, 61, 68, 175, 176, 178, 180, 181, 185, 256, 268, 269
Axelrod, B. N. 38, 39
Ayarbe, S. D. 156
Aylward, E. H. 231
Azari, N. P. 200
Azouvi, P. 37, 176, 182

Baaré, W. F. C. 91
Babcock, R. L. 32, 222

Bäckman, L. 234
Badcock, J. C. 84
Baddeley, A. D. 30, 54, 55, 56, 89, 113, 114, 156, 175, 181, 265, 268
Baddlely, B. T. 175
Bagert, B. 167
Baguley, I. 173, 174, 175, 176, 181, 183
Bain, J. D. 38, 174, 179
Bajszar, G. M. 66
Baker, K. B. 202
Baker, L. A. 89
Ball, D. 43
Ball, K. K. 41, 42, 43, 244, 248, 249, 250, 252, 254, 255
Balota, D. A. 221
Bammer, R. 234
Barak, O. 176
Barak, Y. 21, 155, 156, 161
Barat, M. 173
Barber, B. 199
Barberger, G. P. 246, 247
Barbieri-Berger, S. 18, 30, 42, 63, 154, 155, 161
Barch, D. M. 142, 235
Bardell, L. 249
Barett, P. 29
Barker, G. J. 153
Barker-Collo, S. L. 20, 155, 162
Barnes, M. 118
Barnes, T. R. 140, 144
Baron, R. M. 58
Barrett, G. 87
Barrett-Connor, E. 65
Barrett-Woodbridge, M. 21
Barroso, J. 161, 166
Barry, N. S. 59
Bartels, C. 174, 175
Bartels, M. 91
Barth, J. 174, 175, 187
Bartok, J. 54
Bartzokis, G. 231
Basar, E. 85
Basar-Eroglu, C. 85
Bashore, T. R. 227, 233
Basile-Sculz, R. 127, 136
Bastin, M. E. 234
Batchelor, J. 38, 183
Bates, J. A. 129, 130, 139
Bates, T. C. 35
Battersby, J. C. 153
Baty, J. D. 203
Baudouin, A. 244
Baum, C. M. 162
Bawden, H. N. 117
Baxendale, S. 140
Bayles, K. A. 205
Bazana, P. G. 36
Beall, J. A. 176
Beard, B. 43
Beard, B. L. 249
Bearden, C. E. 135

Beatty, W. W. 154
Beauchamp, N. J., Jr. 144
Becker, J. T. 29, 137
Bedard, M. A. 207
Beebe, G. W. 154
Beekman, A. T. 201
Beglinger, L. 181
Behrmann, M. 206
Beier, M. E. 222
Belanger, H. G. 174
Beldowicz, D. 54, 62, 155
Bell, L. 129, 130, 139
Bellack, A. S. 125, 127, 129, 130, 136, 142
Belleville, S. 203
Bendlin, G. 249
Benedek, G. 55
Benedict, R. H. 54, 55, 68, 165, 245
Benmoyal-Segal, L. 200
Bennett, D. A. 223
Bennett, P. J. 42
Bentler, P. M. 81
Benton, A. L. 65, 67
Benz, R. L. 255
Benz, S. 208
Berch, D. B. 43, 249, 254
Bergamaschi, R. 155, 163
Berger, W. 204
Bernardin, L. 66, 153, 154, 164
Berns, S. M. 127, 136
Berry, E. L. 206
Berthier, M. L. 201
Besson, J. A. 207
Beth, R. E. 38
Bherer, L. 203
Bickford, P. 144
Bielawski, M. 205
Bieliauskas, L. A. 33
Bienias, J. L. 223
Bigelow, L. B. 142
Bigler, E. D. 21, 174, 175, 176, 180, 181, 233
Bilder, R. M. 127, 129, 130, 139
Biloa-Tang, M. 135
Binder, J. R. 66, 154
Binder, K. S. 58
Binder, L. M. 174
Binneman, B. 129, 130
Binns, M. A. 180
Bird, L. 127, 136
Birren, J. E. 126, 233, 244, 256
Bissessur, S. 200
Bitschnau, W. 204
Black, D. 235
Blamire, A. M. 84
Blanco, C. 154
Blecker, C. R. 166
Bleiberg, J. 40
Bleijenberg, G. 62
Blumbergs, P. C. 174
Blumhardt, L. D. 87
Bly, B. M. 54, 62, 156

Bo, L. 153
Bo, P. 134
Bogner, J. 185
Bokura, H. 206
Boll, T. J. 29, 38, 178
Bomb, P. 265
Bonavita, S. 161
Bond, M. 173
Bondi, M. W. 205
Bonnaud, V. 205
Bonnet, M. 162, 165
Boodoo, G. 12
Boomsma, D. I. 81, 84, 85, 86, 87, 88, 89, 91, 92
Boone, K. B. 38, 39, 256
Bor, D. 36
Borenstein Graves, A. 249
Borger, N. A. 89
Boring, E. G. 33
Boringa, J. B. 144, 154, 156, 160
Borkenau, P. 34, 89, 90
Bornke, C. 208
Boronow, J. J. 127
Borroni, B. 199, 201, 212
Bosone, D. 155, 163
Bosson, J. L. 135
Botwinick, J. 244
Bouchard, T. J. 9, 12, 89, 91
Boudineau, M. 162, 165
Bouffett, E. 111
Bougerol, T. 135
Bouquet, C. A. 205
Bowden, S. C. 21
Bowers, D. 201
Bowes, S. G. 202, 205
Bowey, J. A. 114
Boykin, A. W. 12
Boyle, M. O. 222
Bradshaw, J. L. 84, 202, 204, 205
Brand, C. R. 35
Braren, M. 86
Brassington, J. C. 153
Braver, T. S. 158, 235
Brebion, G. 59, 141
Brebner, J. 33, 34, 35
Breese, C. R. 144
Brekke, J. S. 127, 136
Brennan, M. 65
Breteler, M. M. 200
Brettle, R. P. 87
Brewer, N. 108
Brezsnyak, M. P. 107
Briggs, S. D. 230
Brigman, S. 244
Brinley, J. F. 104
Brittain, J. L. 29, 178
Brodaty, H. 235
Brody, N. 12
Broe, G. A. 174, 176
Bronstein, Y. L. 200

Brooks, W. M. 235
Brookshire, B. 118
Brouwer, W. H. 175, 176, 180, 181, 182, 184, 185, 186, 187
Brown, G. C. 21
Brown, R. G. 201
Brown, V. J. 89, 203
Brozek, J. 244
Bruni, J. R. 248, 250
Bryan, J. 57
Bryant, D. 21, 22, 37, 38, 55, 68, 157, 158, 159, 160, 161
Bryant, P. 116
Buccafusca, M. 161
Buchanan, R. W. 125, 127, 129, 130, 136, 142
Buchsbaum, M. 34, 144
Bucik, V. 64
Buck, P. 39
Buckner, R. L. 231, 233
Bud, D. N. 205
Burks, J. S. 33
Burmeister, I. A. 60
Burn, D. J. 207
Burns, N. R. 11, 35
Burns, T. 87, 88
Burt, C. 7
Burt, T. 244
Burton, E. J. 199
Burwell, R. D. 59
Buschke, H. 58, 61, 62
Busenbark, D. 156
Bushke, H. 37
Bussel, B. 37, 176, 182
Bustini, M. 136, 141
Butler, R. N. 256
Butters, M. A. 55
Butters, N. 256
Buttner, T. 208
Byerley, W. 144
Byrne, M. 135

Cabeza, R. 228
Cahn, D. 65
Calder, S. A. 207
Callaway, E. 34
Callies, A. 62
Calne, D. B. 203
Calvert, J. E. 204
Cameron, F. B. 206
Campbell, K. B. 87
Canfield, R. L. 107
Cannon, T. D. 61, 135
Cansino, S. 87
Cantagello, A. 181, 182
Cappelleri, J. C. 21, 68, 155, 164
Capruso, D. X. 111
Cardon, L. R. 82, 91
Carey, C. L. 127
Carlson, S. R. 87, 88, 92
Carone, D. A. 165

Carpenter, P. A. 115
Carpenter, W. T., Jr. 125
Carroll, J. B. 16, 58, 136
Carruthers, K. 140
Carter, C. S. 142, 235
Caryl, P. G. 11, 92
Caskey, B. J. 107
Catlin, R. 41
Cattell, J. 5, 18
Cattell, R. B. 35, 266
Catts, H. W. 116
Caulkins, M. E. 137
Cavallucci, C. 175
Ceci, S. J. 12
Celius, E. G. 162
Censits, D. M. 139
Cerella, J. 56, 245
Cerretano, R. 155, 163
Chaiken, S. R. 34
Chakeres, D. 163
Chapman, J. P. 70
Charlett, A. 202, 206
Chatel, D. M. 33
Chatfield, D. A. 55, 174
Chaytor, N. 57
Chelune, G. J. 31, 38, 54, 68, 79, 91, 156, 157, 158, 161, 163, 256, 257, 268, 269
Cherny, S. 91
Cherry, K. E. 244
Chi, M. T. H. 103
Chiaravalloti, N. 18, 19, 20, 29, 31, 37, 38, 43, 54, 62, 63, 67, 68, 69, 79, 91, 154 156, 157, 158, 161, 163, 176, 177, 256, 257, 268, 269
Chisum, H. J. 231
Chiswick, A. 87
Chiulli, S. J. 235
Chorlian, D. B. 87
Chouinard, S. 207
Chow, T. W. 200
Christal, R. E. 56
Christensen, B. K. 127
Christian, J. C. 85, 87
Christie, G. 84, 204
Christodoulou, C. 18, 19, 20, 29, 30, 31, 37, 42, 43, 54, 62, 63, 67, 68, 69, 154, 156, 161, 175, 176, 177, 257, 268
Christou, C. 115
Christy, J. A. 207
Chuah, Y. M. L. 114
Cicerone, K. D. 54, 61, 185
Cienfuegos, A. 144
Cifu, D. X. 173
Cirillo, M. A. 58
Cissell, G. M. 42, 43, 250, 252, 254
Citterio, A. 155, 163
Clafferty, R. 135
Clapp, I. E. 163
Clark, C. R. 127
Clark, J. C. 200
Clark, L. N. 200

Clayes, G. 2
Clement, P. F. 55
Cluydts, R. 62
Coenen, H. H. 208
Cohen, J. A. 87
Cohen, J. D. 132, 134, 142, 158, 235
Cohen, R. A. 30, 42, 86
Colbert, J. 126
Cole, M. A. 55, 175, 181, 182
Coleman, R. E. 228
Coles, M. 86, 88
Collie, A. 245
Collins, L. F. 34, 37
Collins, M. W. 34, 41
Comijs, H. C. 201
Conturo, T. E. 231, 233
Cook, D. J. 129
Cook, S. E. 60
Cooks, J., 174,
Coon, V. E. 29, 57
Cooper, C. J. 11, 35
Cooper, J. A. 202, 208
Coppinger, N. W. 244
Coppola, R. 85
Corey-Bloom, J. 65
Coslett, H. B. 175
Costanzi, C. 199, 201, 212
Cosway, R. 135
Cotman, C. W. 256
Couillet, J. 182
Courchesne, E. 231
Coursey, R. D. 125, 127, 136
Court, J. H. 34
Courtney, S. M. 166
Cousins, P. 111
Covington, J. 231
Cowan, N. 115, 143, 265
Cowles, A. 231
Coyle, J. T. 144
Coyle, P. K. 37
Crawford, J. A. 111
Crawford, J. R. 20, 35, 207, 232
Creech, B. 127, 136
Crossen, J. R. 29
Crouch, J. 187
Crow, T. J. 125, 129, 130, 135
Crutcher, M. D. 196, 197
Cui, L. 201
Cumming, G. 132, 134
Cummings, J. L. 195, 196, 197, 201, 231
Cunnington, R. 202
Curran, C. 174, 183, 185
Curran, S. 91
Currie, J. 245
Curtiss, G. 55, 174, 175
Cycowicz, Y. M. 86
Czaja, S. J. 247, 248
Czernecki, V. 207
Czobor, P. 127, 136

Dabrowski, J. J. 37
Daneluzzo, E. 136, 141
Daneman, M. 115
Dartigues, J. F. 246
Das, M. 129, 130
Das-Small, E. A. 56
Daum, I. 205
Davatzikos, C. 230, 231
David, A. S. 59
Davidson, P. S. 200
Davie, C. A. 66, 153
Davis, A. 3, 231
Davis, H. P. 66
Davis, K. 57, 269
Davis, K. L. 144
Dawson, J. 257
De Caro, M. F. 161
de Geus, E. J. 84, 85, 86, 87, 88, 89, 91, 92
de Groot, J. C. 232
de Groot, V. 155
de Haan, E. H. 125, 128, 140, 235
de Jong, P. F. 56
de Lau, L. M. 200
de Leeuw, F. E. 232
De Sonneville, L. M. 144, 154, 155, 156, 160
de Vree, B. 62
de Vries, W. R. 235
Deary, I. J. 8, 9, 10, 11, 20, 29, 34, 35, 36, 84, 87, 92, 136, 204, 232, 234, 235
Debecker, J. 86
DeCarli, C. 232
Deecke, L. 88
Deeg, D. J. 201, 235, 247
Deelman, B. G. 181, 183, 184
Defontaines, B. 195, 201
DeFries, J. C. 91
D'Elia, L. F. 29, 38, 39
Delis, D. C. 59, 203
DeLisi, L. E. 129, 130, 134, 135, 139
Deloche, G. 181, 182
Deloire, M. S. 162, 165
DeLong, M. R. 197
DeLuca, J. 18, 19, 20, 21, 22, 29, 30, 31, 37, 38, 42, 43, 54, 55, 57, 61, 62, 63, 66, 67, 68, 69, 79, 91, 154, 155, 156, 157, 158, 159, 160, 161, 162, 163, 175, 176, 177, 178, 180, 181, 185, 186, 256, 257, 268, 269
Demadura, T. L. 203
Demaree, H. A. 18, 19, 20, 29, 30, 31, 37, 42, 43, 54, 57, 62, 63, 66, 67, 68, 69, 91, 127, 134, 156, 158, 161, 176, 177, 257, 269
Demery, J. A. 55, 174, 175, 181, 182
Demetriou, A. 115
Dempster, F. N. 56, 113
Denney, D. R. 54, 126, 144, 154, 162
Dennis, M. 117
Denny, L. L. 229
Der, G. 10, 11, 34, 36
Desmedt, J. E. 86
Desmond, J. E. 36

DeSousa, E. A. 21
D'Esposito, M. 175, 181, 182, 228, 229
Detterman, D. K. 89
Devlin, S. J. 247
Deweer, B. 195, 201
Diamond, B. J. 18, 21, 22, 29, 30, 38, 42, 54, 55, 57, 61, 62, 63, 66, 67, 68, 91, 154, 156, 158, 159, 160, 161, 176, 178, 180, 181, 185, 257, 269
Diamond, S. 3, 5
Dickerson, F. 127
Dickins, J. 202, 204
Dickinson, D. 125, 127, 136, 137, 138
Dien, J. 86
Dik, M. G. 235
Dikmen, S. 174
Ding, Y. S. 235
Dingemans, P. M. 59
Dirmen, D. 17
Dismukes, K. 244
Dixit, N. K. 55, 175, 181, 182
Dixon, L. B. 125
Dixon, R. A. 233, 234, 235, 244
Dixon, R. M. 84
Djaldetti, R. 200
Dobbs, A. R. 60
Dobbs, R. J. 202, 204
Dobraski, M. 245
Dobson, S. H. 58
Dodge, H. H. 247
Dolske, M. C. 38
Donchin, E. 86, 88
Donders, F. C. 33, 43, 89, 202
Donders, J. 1, 15, 21, 29, 40, 181, 269
Donovan-Lepore, A. M. 127, 136
Donovick, P. J. 176
Dopfer, R. 111
Dougall, N. 36
Douglas, S. 202
Drachman, D. A. 86, 87
Dragcvic, M. 84
Drent, M. L. 235
Drozd, S. 129, 130
Dubois, B. 195, 201, 205, 207
Duchesne, N. 207
Dugas, M. 87
Duley, J. F. 59
Duly, D. 135
Duncan, J. 36
Duncombe, M. E. 204
Dupuis, J. H. 230
Durso, R. 207
Dykman, B. 66
Dysken, M. 244

Earl, H. D. 233
Eaton, W. O. 112
Ebert, A. D. 174, 175
Ebmeier, K. P. 36, 207
Edelstein, S. 65

Edwards, D. F. 162
Edwards, J. D. 42, 43, 248, 250, 252, 254, 255, 257
Edwards, J. E. 244, 250, 254
Egaas, B. 231
Egan, D. E. 247
Egan, M. F. 129, 130, 135
Egan, V. G. 20, 87
Eisenberg, H. 174, 175
Eising, E. 208
Ekstrom, R. B. 17
Elias, J. W. 209
Eling, P. A. T. M. 184
Ellingson, R. J. 85
Elliott, C. D. 15, 17
Elliott, E. M. 115, 265
Engberg, A. W. 174, 183
Engel, R. 87
Engel, R. A. 18, 30, 42, 63, 154, 161
Englander, J. 173
Engle, R. W. 115
Eriksen, B. A. 89
Eriksen, C. W. 89
Ertle, J. P. 87
Ertle, S. 195
Esteguy, M. 201
Evans, D. A. 223
Evans, D. R. 145
Evarts, E. V. 203
Ewing, F. M. E. 36
Ewing-Cobbs, L. 118
Exton-Smith, A. N. 87
Eysenck, H. J. 7, 8, 29

Fabrigoule, C. 246, 247
Fahy, J. F. 179
Faiss, J. H. 156, 161, 162
Falkenstein, M. 88
Fancher, R. E. 7
Faraone, S. V. 129, 130, 131
Farde, L. 234, 235
Farina, D. 161
Farrer, M. J. 200
Fasotti, L. 184
Faust, M. E. 221
Fearnside, M. R. 38, 183
Feher, E. P. 201
Fein, D. 58, 91
Feldman, J. F. 91
Feldman, R. G. 195
Feldmann, G. M. 17
Felmingham, K. L. 174, 175, 176, 181, 183
Fenton, G. W. 85
Ferguson, A. N. 114
Ferguson, K. J. 235
Fernandez, H. F. 201
Ferraro, F. R. 221
Ferrer, E. 107, 108
Ferrer-Caja, E. 107, 108

Feuer, D. 9, 89
Field, H. L. 164
Field, M. 34
Fields, J. A. 200
Fields, R. B. 60
Fielstein, E. M. 38
Filley, C. M. 163
Fillit, H. M. 256
Filoteo, J. V. 203
Finch, S. 132, 134
Findley, L. 202
Fink, A. 64, 271
Finkel, S. I. 244
Finlayson, M. A. J. 184
Firnau, G. 200
Fischer, J. S. 201
Fischl, B. 12, 36
Fisher, C. B. 65
Fisher, L. M. 126
Fisk, G. D. 186
Fisk, J. D. 21, 30, 63, 68, 155, 161
Fisk, J. E. 65, 244
Fjell, A. M. 12, 36
Flanagan, D. P. 16
Flash, T. 205
Flavell, J. H. 112
Flegal, K 167
Fleming, M. 175
Fletcher, J. M. 7, 118
Fogle, T. 39
Foong, J. 66
Forbes, P. 106
Ford, G. 10, 11, 36
Ford, J. M. 86
Fork, M. 174, 175
Forney, D. L. 173
Forstot, M. 62
Foster, J. K. 206
Fowler, J. S. 235
Frank, J. 3
Frank, Y. 86
Franklin, G. M. 33, 163
Franz, E. A. 206
Fratiglioni, L. 246
Frazier, T. W. 127, 134
French, J. W. 17
Fried, L. P. 248
Friedberg, F. 37
Friedman, D. 86
Friedman, G. 205
Friedman, J. I. 144
Friedman, S. 87
Friedrich, F. J. 195, 208
Frier, B. M. 20, 36, 84
Frith, C. 202
Fry, A. F. 55, 56, 79, 106, 113
Fu, F. H. 34
Fukuyama, H. 29, 204
Fuld, P. A. 62
Fuller, K. H. 29

Fulton, J. C. 164
Funkenstein, H. H. 41

Gabrieli, J. D. E. 36
Gaeta, H. 86
Gaines, J. 165
Galletly, C. A. 127
Galton, F. 29, 43
Ganguli, M. 60
Garay, E. 30, 43
Garcia, H. 201
Garde, E. 144, 232
Garmoe, W. S. 40
Garnett, E. S. 200
Garron, D. C. 204
Garver, K. E. 31, 106
Gary, H. 174, 175
Gathercole, S. E. 56
Gaudino, E. A. 18, 20, 21, 29, 30, 42, 54, 62, 63, 68, 91, 154, 156, 158, 161, 162, 268, 269
Gauntlett-Gilbert, J. 89, 203
Gay, N. 54
Gazzaley, A. H. 228
Geffen, G. M. 84, 87, 89, 92
Geffen, L. B. 84, 87, 89, 92
Gelinas, I. 256
Gennarelli, T. A. 175
Genova, H. M. 163
Gentry, J. R. 175
Gevins, A. 87
Giardini, A. 134
Giedd, J. 111
Gil, R. 205
Gilbert, B. 203
Gilberti, N. 199, 201, 212
Gilboa, A. 176
Gillette, J. A. 232
Gillies, D. 235
Ginovart, N. 234, 235
Gish, K. W. 248
Gladsjo, J. A. 58, 127, 136, 137
Glahn, D. 61
Glicksohn, J. 64
Gloor, P. 84, 85
Glover, G. H. 36
Goddard, N. 36
Godersky, J. C. 175
Godlstein, M. Z. 245
Golbe, L. I. 200
Gold, J. M. 125, 127, 129, 130, 136, 137, 138, 142
Goldberg, R. W. 125
Goldberg, T. E. 129, 130, 135, 142
Goldman, R. S. 129, 130, 139, 143
Goldman, W. P. 203
Goldstein, J. M. 129, 130, 131
Gomez, L. M. 247
Gonzalez, R. 127
Goodin, D. S. 201, 202
Goodwin, F. K. 126

Goodwin, G. M. 36, 87, 92
Gordon, P. A. 153
Gorman, J. M. 141
Goswami, U. 116
Gottesman, I. I. 85, 145
Gould, S. J. 10
Goverover, Y. 163
Grady, C. L. 232
Grady, D. 235
Grafman, J. 66, 154, 155, 161
Graham, D. I. 174
Grant, I. 256
Grant, J. 84
Grantier, L. L. 202
Gray, F. 200
Gray, K. F. 209
Green, A. 173, 174, 175, 176, 181, 183
Greenwood, P. M. 230
Greist, J. H. 245
Greve, D. N. 233
Grieb-Neff, P. 185
Griggs, D. S. 249
Grigsby, J. 156
Grochowski, S. 143
Gron, G. 179, 180
Gronwall, D. 19, 37, 54, 155, 177
Grossman, M. 164, 205
Grossman, R. I. 164, 175
Grubich, C. 174, 175
Grunfeld, C. 235
Gscheidle, T. 129, 130, 135
Gunning-Dixon, F. M. 230, 232
Gur, R. C. 135, 137, 235
Gur, R. E. 135
Guralnik, J. M. 248
Gurdijan, E. S. 175
Gustafsson, J. E. 35
Gutchess, A. H. 186
Guttmann, C. R. 156, 165

Hackley, S. A. 88
Haddock, C. K. 131, 132
Hadley, T. 135
Hahn, M. 162
Hale, S. 55, 56, 79, 106, 109, 113
Hall, J. 249
Hall, L. K. 107, 115, 116, 118
Halldin, C. 234, 235
Halliday, M. S. 113
Halligan, E. M. 60
Halper, J. 20, 21, 162
Halpern, E. 40
Hamagami, F. 107, 108
Hamby, S. L. 59
Hamer, R. M. 127
Hames, K. 154
Hamilton, J. M. 198
Hamilton, R. J. 85
Hamilton, Z. 115
Hammer, M. 249

Hamsher, K. 65, 67
Hanakawa, T. 29, 204
Hanes, K. R. 198
Hanley, J. 256
Hannay, J. H. 201
Hansch, E. C. 206
Hansell, N. K. 87, 92
Hansen, J. C. 88
Hanson, A. B. 247
Hanson, D. R. 145
Harman, H. H. 17
Harper, D. N. 206
Harris, J. 200
Harris, J. P. 204
Harrison, P. L. 16
Harrow, M. 126
Hart, T. 185
Hartikainen, S. 246
Hartl, R. 41
Hartlage, S. 66
Hartman, M. 141
Harvey, N. S. 208
Harvey, P. D. 144
Hasher, L. 246, 250
Hasher, L. 250
Haslam, A. S. 38
Haslam, C. 38, 183
Haughton, V. M. 164
Haukka, J. 61
Hauser, U. 156
Hawk, T. C. 228
Hawkins, K. A. 1, 21, 40
Hawkins, S. 38, 183
Haxby, J. V. 232
Hayakawa, T. 247
Hayashi, E. 202
Hayes, B. C. 247
Hayward, M. 87
Head, D. 230, 231, 233
Heaton, R. 127, 136, 137
Heaton, R. K. 33, 58, 163, 256
Hedden, T. 32, 221, 246
Hedehus, M. 233, 234
Hedges, L. V. 129, 131
Heibronner, R. L. 39
Heindel, W. C. 198
Heinrichs, R. W. 125, 132, 133, 140, 142
Heinze, H. J. 156
Helisalmi, S. 85
Helmers, K. F. 43, 249, 254
Henderson, N. B. 87
Henley, M. 202, 207
Henry, G. K. 39
Hepburn, D. A. 20, 36
Herbener, E. S. 129, 130, 139
Herbst, K. L. 86
Hermens, D. 85
Hernandez, M. A. 161, 166
Herndon, R. M. 153, 163
Hertzberg, H. 111

Hertzog, C. 223
Herzog, H. 36
Hessel, C. D. 233
Hetherington, C. R. 184
Hevelone, N. D. 233
Hick, W. E. 211
Hicks, L. H. 233
Hicks, R. E. 64
Hiehle, J. F. 175
Higginson, C. I. 66, 162
High, W. M. 174, 187
Hijman, R. 125, 128, 140
Hill, E. 39
Hill, S. K. 129, 130, 139
Hillary, F. G. 54, 62, 156, 163
Hiller, J. E. 174
Hillier, S. L. 174
Hillyard, S. A. 88
Hirata, K. 201, 202
Hismjatullina, A. 265
Hitch, G. 54
Hitch, G. J. 30, 113, 175
Ho, C. S.-H 116
Ho, H. Z. 89
Hocherman, S. 203
Hodges, A. 135
Hof, P. R. 144
Hoff, A. L. 129, 130, 135, 139
Hoffman, J. M. 228
Hofman, A. 232
Hohnsbein, J. 88
Hohol, M. J. 156, 165
Holly, M. 87
Holthausen, E. A. E. 59
Honda, M. 29, 204
Hood, A. 205
Hoofien, D. 176
Hoormann, J. 88
Hoover, J. E. 196, 197
Hopkins, D. G., 59,
Horn, J. L. 87, 16, 35
Horne, N. 54, 126, 144, 154, 162
Horon, R. 139
Horrobin, D. F. 145
Houk, J. C. 198, 199
Houtler, B. D. 39
Howard, L. 87
Howiesen, D. B. 267
Howieson, D. B. 201, 209, 267
Hoyer, W. 250
Hoyer, W. J. 127
Hu, C.-G. 116
Huber, S. J. 163, 207
Hubert, H. B. 246
Hudziak, J. J. 91
Huettel, S. A. 234, 235, 228, 229
Hugenholtz, H. 21
Hughes, C. 129, 130
Huijbregts, S. C. 155
Huk, W. J. 111

Hulme, C. 113
Hulshoff Pol, H. E. 91
Hulstijn, W. 127, 134, 140
Hultsch, D. 249
Hultsch, D. F. 223, 244
Hume, W. 85
Humphreys, M. S. 174, 179
Humphries, T. 86
Hunt, E. 90
Hunter, H. 36
Hunter, M. A. 205
Hunter, R. 92
Huntly, B. J. P. 36, 84
Hurst, R. W. 175
Hurtig, H. I. 205
Hutchison, C. W. 36
Huttenlocher, P. R. 111
Hyde, T. M. 129, 130, 135
Hyman, R. 211

Iacono, W. G. 85, 87, 88, 92
Iannone, V. N. 125, 127, 137, 138
Iansek, R. 84, 202, 204, 205
Illes, J. 234
Inzelberg, R. 205
Isingrini, M. 244
Isoaho, R. 246
Iverson, G. 34, 41
Izor, R. 205

Jablensky, A. 84
Jackson, R. 11, 35
Jacobs, D. M. 198, 205
Jadad, A. R. 129
Jaeger, J. 127, 136
Jakab, M. 165
Jamison, K. R. 126
Janer, K. W. 203
Janka, Z. 55
Jankovic, J. 206
Janowsky, J. S. 231
Janvin, C. C. 209
Jausovec, K. 87
Jausovec, N. 87
Java, R. I. 223
Javitt, D. C. 143, 144
Jefferson, J. W. 245
Jenkins, L. 109
Jennett, B. 173, 174
Jensen, A. R. 8, 10, 12, 13, 29, 79, 83, 136, 271
Jeste, D. V. 58, 127, 136, 137
Jobe, J. B. 43, 250
Joebe, J. B. 249, 254
Joerding, J. A. 109
Jog, M. 84
Jog, M. S. 202
Jogems-Kosterman, B. J. 134, 140
John, E. R. 86
Johnson, A. M. 84, 202, 271
Johnson, M. B. 15, 16, 17

Johnson, R. A. 209
Johnson, S. K. 18, 29, 30, 42, 54, 62, 63, 155
Johnston, K. M. 34
Jokic, C. 37
Jolles, J. 59, 230, 232
Jones, A. 129
Jones, B. P. 135
Jones, D. K. 233
Jones, H. 59
Jones, N. R. 21
Jones, R. 252
Jonides, J. 158
Jonker, C. 201, 235, 247
Jordan, N. 202, 208
Jöreskog, K. 81
Jovik, C. 176, 182
Joy, S. 58, 91
Joynson, R. B. 7
Ju, C. 233, 234
Juhel, J. 114
Jung, R. E. 235
Jungreis, C. 144

Kadowaki, T. 247
Kahn, R. S. 91, 125, 128, 140
Kail, R. 21, 32, 56, 57, 101, 102, 103, 106, 107, 108, 109, 110, 113, 114, 115, 116, 118, 143, 155, 161, 268
Kaleta, D. A. 153
Kalkers, N. F. 155
Kalman, B. 21
Kalmar, J. H. 20, 21, 22, 37, 38, 55, 68, 157, 158, 159, 160, 161, 162
Kalnin, A. 156
Kamin, L. J. 7
Kamitani, T. 201, 202
Kander, D. R. 175
Kane, M. J. 115
Kane, R. L. 40
Kantor, L. 9
Kaplan, E. 58, 59, 91, 154
Kaplan, E. F. 41
Karamat, E. 204
Karlins, E. 200
Karmiloff-Smith, A. 84
Kaste, M. 174, 187
Kaszniak, A. W. 204, 205
Katsanis, J. 87, 88, 92
Katz, D. I. 207
Kausch, D. G. 30, 42
Kaye, J. A. 231, 235
Keefe, R. S. 127
Keel, A. 200
Kelemen, O. 55
Keller, C. V. 115
Keller, T. A. 115
Kelley, S. M. 54, 63, 67, 68
Kemp, B. J. 33
Kendler, K. S. 135
Kennedy, J. E. 55

Kennedy, J. L. 127
Kennedy, K. M. 230
Kennedy, P. M. 156
Kenway, E. 183
Keri, S. 55
Kerr, B. 233
Keshavan, M. S. 129, 130, 139
Kesler, S. R. 174, 17
Kessler, H. R. 30, 42
Kety, S. S. 227
Keys, A. 244
Keys, B. A. 65, 66, 235
Keyser-Marcus, L. 173
Khoury, S. J. 156, 165
Kieseppa, T. 61
Kikinis, R. 156, 165
Kim, H. 54, 63, 67, 68
Kinsbourne, M. 64
Kinsella, G. 21, 22, 173, 175, 176, 177, 179, 184
Kirasic, K. C. 58
Kirkwood, M. 106
Kirpatrick, B. 125
Kirsch-Darrow, L. 201
Kirson, D. 256
Kishiyama, S. S. 167
Kivela, S. L. 246
Klauber, J. 187
Klaukka, T. 246
Klawans, H. L. 204
Klimesch, W. 85
Kline, D. 244
Kline, R. B. 138
Knights, R. M. 117
Knobler, R. L. 164
Knorr, E. 64
Knorr, U. 200
Kobayashi, S. 206
Kochi, K. 201, 202
Koenig, T. 201, 202
Koga, Y. 101
Kok, A. 86
Kolev, V. 85
Koller, W. C. 200, 202
Kolodny, J. 36
Kononen, M. 85
Kopell, B. S. 86
Kopp, B. 156, 161, 162
Koppeschaar, H. P. F. 235
Köpruner, V. 85
Korczyn, A. D. 205
Koren, D. 129, 130, 131
Kornblum, S. 142
Korner-Bitensky, N. 256
Körnhuber, H. H. 88
Kosinski, R. J. 33, 34
Kovacs, F. 184
Krabbe, K. 232
Kraemer, H. C. 86
Kraft, G. I. 153

Kramer, A. 149, 250
Kramer, J. H. 59, 111
Kramer, N. 29, 30, 62, 63, 68
Kraus, J. F. 173
Kraut, M. A. 230, 231
Kravcisin, N. 156
Krebs, M. J. 211
Kremen, W. S. 129, 130, 131
Kreutzer, J. S. 173, 174, 175, 183, 184, 185
Krikorian, R. 54
Krishnan, K. R. 244
Krupp, L. B. 37
Kubicki, M. 144
Kuhn, W. 208
Kumari, V. 129, 130
Kundel, A. 156, 161, 162
Kuney, S. 85
Kuntsi, J. 89, 91
Kuperman, S. 87
Kurland, L. T. 154
Kuroiwa, Y. 201, 202
Kurtzke, J. F. 154
Kushner, M. 139
Kuslansky, G. 61
Kutas, M. 88
Kutukcu, Y. 201, 202
Kyllonen, P. C. 56

La Marche, J. A. 29, 178
Lacey, J. F. 115
Lader, M. H. 85
Ladish, C. 87
Laguna, K. D. 222
Lam, C. S. 21
LaMarche, J. A. 38
Lamberty, G. J. 33
Landro, N. I. 162
Lane, D. M. 127
Lang, A. E. 206
Langan, S. J. 20, 36, 92
Lange, G. 29, 54, 62, 156
Langer, T. 111
Langley, L. K. 229
Langston, J. W. 200
Larish, J. F. 149, 250
LaRocca, N. G. 154
Larrabee, G. J. 174
Larson, M. J. 55, 175, 181, 182
Larsson, H. B. 232
Lathrop, G. H. 85
Lauer, K. 30, 42
Laughlin, S. 111
Laurent, A. 135
Lautenschlager, G. 32
Laux, L. F. 127
Lavie, M. 155, 156
Lawrence, B. 109
Lazar, N. A. 31, 106
Lazarus, R. 173, 174
Lazeron, R. H. 144, 154, 156, 160

Leahy, B. J. 21
Leaper, S. A. 232
Leathem, J. 20, 38
Lebowitz, B. K. 174
Leclercq, M. 181, 182
Leclerq, M. 182
Lecours, A. R. 111
Lee, A. C. 204
Lee, C. 205
Lee, D. H. 12
Lee, M. A. 84
Leech, E. E. 173, 176
Leenders, K. L. 200
Lees, A. J. 195, 207
Lefkowitz, D. 144
Lehman, A. F. 125
Lehmann, D. 201, 202
Lehtovirta, M. 85
Leiguarda, R. 201
Lemke, U. 244
Lemmon, H. A. 232
Lemmon, V. W. 153
Lencz, T. 127, 136
Lengenfelder, J. 22, 31, 38, 54, 55, 68, 79, 91, 154, 157, 158, 159, 160, 161, 163, 186, 256, 268, 269
Lenzenweger, M. F. 34
Leo, G. J. 153, 154, 155, 156, 164
Leonard, S. 144
Lerner, A. J. 200
Lesser, I. M. 39
Letenneur, L. 246
Leveck, M. D. 43, 249, 254
Levin, H. E. 174, 175
Levin, H. S. 111, 117, 118, 173, 187
Levy, G. 198, 205
Levy, J. K. 201
Lewis, M. D. 153
Lezak, M. D. 29, 59, 142, 173, 174, 201, 209, 267
Li, M. 201, 202
Li, S.-C. 232, 234
Li, T. K. 85, 87
Lichtenstein, P. 91
Lichter, D. G. 196, 198
Liddle, P. F. 125
Lieberman, A. 200, 201
Lieberman, J. A. 143
Liederman, E. 144
Light, R. 173
Lim, K. O. 233, 234
Lima, S. D. 109
Lindenberger, U. 230, 234
Linjakumpu, T. 246
Lips, P. 235
Lipton, R. B. 61
Littler, J. E. 113
Litvan, I. 154, 155, 161
Liu, W. C. 156
Llinás, R. R. 84, 85

Llorente, A. M. 29
Logan, W. J. 86, 87
Logie, R. 113
Logie, R. H. 175
Lomecky, M. Z. 235
Long, C. J. 34, 37, 179
Longstreth, W. T., Jr. 144
Lopes da Silva, F. H. 84, 85
Lopez, E. 173
Lopez, S. L. 41
Loring, D. W. 201, 209, 267
Lovell, M. R. 34, 41
Lovera, J. 167
Low, K. A. 202
Lowry, C. M. 233
Lu, P. H. 231
Lubar, J. F. 85
Lublin, F. D. 153, 164
Lucas, G. 57, 269
Luce, R. D. 34, 202
Luchetta, T. 66, 154
Luciano, M. 84, 87, 89, 91, 92
Luck, S. J. 86
Lucking, S. 29
Luna, B. 31, 106
Lundervold, A. 12, 36
Lusczcz, M. A. 57
Lykke Mortensen, E. 144
Lykken, D. T. 9, 85, 89
Lynch, M. 80
Lynch, S. G. 54, 126, 144, 154, 162
Lyons, K. 202

May, J. 89
Mabbott, D. J. 111
MacDonald, J. W. 161, 165
MacDonald, R. 180
MacDonald, S. W. 244
MacFall, J. R. 234, 235
MacGillivray, T. J. 234
MacGregor, L. A. 37
Mackin, G. A. 156, 165
MacLeod, K. J. 36, 84
MacLeod, K. M. 36
MacLullich, A. M. J. 235
Madden, D. J. 221, 228, 229, 234, 235
Madigan, N. K. 21, 22, 29, 55, 61, 68, 175, 176, 178, 180, 181, 185, 256, 268, 269
Maggiore, C. 165
Mahadik, S. P. 145
Mahurin, R. K. 197, 201, 202, 207, 209, 211
Maier, S. E. 144
Malapani, C. 195, 201
Malec, J. F. 174, 187
Malhotra, A. K. 127
Malone, M. A. 86, 87
Mamelak, M. 42
Manavis, J. 174
Mangan, G. L. 35
Manil, J. 86

Manly, T. 175
Mannermaa, A. 85
Mannon, L. J. 164
Manolio, T. A. 144
Marchioni, E. 155, 163
Marco, E. J. 135
Marcotte, T. D. 127
Marder, K. 198, 205
Margolin, D. I. 203
Marks, W. 179, 230
Marks, W. J., Jr. 201, 202
Markus, H. S. 233
Marlier, N. 37, 176, 182
Maroon, J. C. 34, 41
Marsden, C. D. 201
Marsh, N. V. 153
Marshall, A. 36
Marshall, I. 36, 235
Marshall, L. F. 187
Marshall, P. S. 62
Marshall, W. H. 33
Marsiske, M. 43, 201, 249, 250, 254
Martin, D. J. 256
Martin, M. 244
Martin, N. G. 81, 84, 87, 89, 92
Martin, S. 87
Martin, T. A. 1, 21, 29, 40, 181, 269
Martin, Y. 182
Martinez, J. M. 154, 155, 161
Maruff, P. 245
Marwitz, J. H. 185
Masson, F. 173
Masson, H. 207
Masur, D. M. 37
Matano, A. 181, 182
Matarazzo, J. D. 40
Mather, N. 222
Mathias, J. L. 21, 176
Mattei, P. 136, 141
Matthay, K. K. 111
Maurelli, M. 155, 163
Maurette, P. 173
Maurizio, A. M. 129, 130, 135
May, C. 246
Mayberg, H. S. 200
Mayberry, M. T. 114
Mazaux, J. M. 173
Mazer, B. L. 256
McAdams, L. A. 58, 127, 136, 137
McArthur, D. L. 173
McBride-Chang, C. 116
McCabe, D. C. 54, 55, 68
McCann, H. 141
McCardle, J. J. 107, 108
McCarthy, G. 228
McClain, L. 64
McClean, A. 174
McClearn, G. E. 91
McCleary, C. 173
McCrimmon, R. J. 36, 84

McDonald, B. C. 161, 165
McDonald, W. I. 153
McDowell, S. 175, 181, 182
McFarland, K. 38, 174, 179
McFarlane, A. C. 127
McGarry-Roberts, P. A. 87
McGrew, K. S. 13, 222
McGue, M. 9, 87, 88, 89, 91, 92
McGwin, G. 42, 248, 249, 254
McKeith, I. G. 207
McKenney, P. D. 125
McLean, A. J. 174
McMahon, R. P. 125, 127, 129, 130, 136, 142
McNary, S. W. 125
McRae, T. 244
Meadows, M. E. 86
Meck, W. H. 199
Meier, W. 111
Meiran, N. 205
Mejia-Santana, H. 200
Melamed, E. 200
Melchior, H. 166
Mennemeier, M. 186
Menon, D. K. 55, 174
Merzbach, U. C. 3
Mesulam, M. M. 84, 85, 230
Metz, L. M. 54, 69, 160, 164
Metzer, J. 174
Meyer, M. 36
Michiels, V. 62
Middleton, F. A. 196, 197
Miller, B. L. 39
Miller, C. A. 109
Miller, D. H. 66, 153
Miller, E. N. 29
Miller, G. A. 70
Miller, G. W. 64
Miller, J. 206
Miller, L. T. 56, 106
Miller, R. 43, 249
Miller, W. R. 126
Millis, S. R. 183, 184
Minden, S. L. 66
Mintz, J. 231
Mintzer, J. E. 244
Mirsky, A. F. 135
Mishara, A. L. 129
Misiak, H. 244
Mitchell, D. R. 164
Mitchell, R. F. 90
Mitrushina, M. N. 38, 39
Mittl, R. L. 175
Moberg, P. J. 235
Mohamed, S. 127, 129, 130, 131, 139
Moher, D. 129
Moher, M. 129
Molloy, S. 207
Monetta, L. 200
Montaglione, C. J. 249
Montgomery, E. B. 202

Montgomery, G. W. 91
Moonis, M. 86
Moont, R. 203
Moore, D. J. 58, 127, 136, 137
Moore, N. B. 20, 21, 22, 55, 158, 159, 160, 161, 162
Morales, R. V. 116
Morant, G. M. 101
Morgen, K. 166
Mork, S. 153
Morris, J. 205
Morris, J. C. 203
Morris, R. G. 233
Morrison, T. 162
Mortensen, E. L. 232
Morthland, M. 38
Mortimer, J. A. 206, 249
Morzorati, S. 85, 87
Moscovitch, M. 175, 181, 182, 200
Moseley, M. 233, 234
Moss, M. B. 231
Mourant, R. 186
Mrazek, L. 36
Muhlack, S. 205
Mulder, E. J. C. 88, 89
Mulkern, R. V. 144
Muller, K. 187
Muller, T. 208
Mulsant, B. H. 55
Munoz-Cespedes, J. M. 181, 182
Murphy, D. G. 232
Murray, A. D. 232
Murtagh, K. N. 246
Mushiake, H. 196
Mutch, W. J. 207
Myers, R. S. 43, 250, 254
Myerson, J. 109

Naatanen, R. 88
Nageishi, Y. 87
Nagler, B. 154
Nahmias, C. 200
Nakajima, Y. 87
Nalthan, P. J. 36
Nance, M. L. 201
Napolitano, B. 86
Natelson, B. H. 29, 30, 54, 61, 62, 63, 68, 155
Neale, M. C. 81, 82, 85, 86, 91, 92
Nebes, R. D. 55, 60
Nefzger, M. D. 154
Neisser, U. 12
Nelson, H. E. 140, 144
Nelson, L. M. 33, 163
Nestor, P. G. 144
Nestor, S. 244
Nettelbeck, T. 11, 34, 35, 111, 117
Neubauer, A. 34
Neubauer, A. C. 64, 89, 90, 271
Ng, K. 174
Ni, X. 127

Nicholls, M. E. 84, 204
Nick, T. G. 174, 183, 184, 187
Nicolson, R. I. 206
Niendam, T. A. 135
Nienhusmeier, M. 200
Nieto, A. 161, 166
Nieuwenhuis, S. 87
Niinisto, R. T. 249
Nimmo-Smith, I. 66
Nisbett, R. 246
Nittono, H. 87
Nitzan, D. 64
Nocentini, U. 161
Noesworthy, M. 111
Noll, D. C. 158
Norton, J. A., Jr., 8,
Norwig, J. 41
Noskin, O. 57
Novack, T. 183, 184, 186
Nuechterlein, K. H. 135, 231
Nuessen, J. 202
Nugent, L. D. 115, 265
Nyberg, L. 234
Nybo, T. 187
Nystrom, L. E. 158

Ober, B. A. 59
O'Brien, J. T. 199, 207
O'Connell, A. W. 256
O'Connor, S. 85, 87
O'Donnell, B. F. 86, 87
O'Donnell, J. P. 37
Oestreicher, J. M. 37
Oken, B. S. 167
Okun, M. S. 201
O'Leary, D. 127, 129, 130, 131, 139
O'Leary, D. S. 144
Olivares, T. 161, 166
Olkin, I. 129, 131
Olsen, S. 125
Olson, R. K. 91
Olver, J. H. 174, 183, 185
Omoto, S. 202
O'Neill, C. J. 204
Opudkerk, M. 232
Orav, J. 156, 165
Orme-Rogers, C. 244
Osmon, D. C. 11, 35
O'Sullivan, M. 233
Oved, D. 200
Owsley, C. 248, 249, 254
Owsley, C. 42, 43

Padovani, A. 199, 201, 212
Pakalnis, A. 163
Paleacu, D. 200
Palmer, A. J. 200
Palmer, B. W. 58, 127, 136, 137
Panek, P. E. 247
Pantelis, C. 140, 144, 198

Paolo, A. M. 200
Papadakis, M. A. 235
Paradiso, S. 144
Parente, F. 127
Parente, M. 165
Park, D. C. 32, 186, 246
Park, H. 144
Park, N. W. 175, 181, 182
Park, Y. 103, 106, 113
Parkin, A. J. 223
Parmenter, B. A. 54, 126, 144, 154, 162
Parrish, J. 54, 55, 68
Partanen, J. 85
Pascual-Marqui, R. D. 201, 202
Pasqualetti, P. 161
Passadori, A. 181, 182
Pate, D. S. 203
Patriot, A. 205
Patterson, S. M. 249
Paul, R. H. 154
Paulsen, J. 203
Paulsen, J. S. 127, 129, 130, 131, 139
Paulson, G. W. 163, 207
Paulson, O. B. 144
Pearlson, G. D. 231
Pedersen, N. L. 91
Pelchat, G. 29, 173, 176
Pell, M. D. 200
Pellegrino, J. W. 116
Pelosi, L. 87
Penney, J. B., Jr. 196, 200
Pennington, B. F. 91
Perianez, J. A. 181, 182
Perlstein, W. M. 55, 175, 181, 182
Pessiglione, M. 207
Peters, A. 231
Peters, S. 205
Peterson, J. 153
Peterson, P. K. 62
Petrill, S. A. 89
Peyser, J. M. 154
Pfefferbaum, A. 86, 233
Pfurtscheller, G. 85
Pham, D. L. 230, 231
Phillips, J. G. 84, 202, 204
Piccinin, A. M. 223
Pickard, J. D. 55, 174
Pickering, S. J. 114
Picton, T. 21, 88
Picton, T. W. 173, 176, 180
Pier, M. P. 127, 134
Pillon, B. 195, 201, 205, 207
Pilowsky, L. S. 59
Pirozzolo, F. J. 201, 202, 211, 206
Pivik, J. 21
Platsidou, M. 115
Plomin, R. 91
Plotnik, M. 205
Plucker, J. 21, 22
Plude, D. 250

Pluijm, S. M. F. 235
Podd, J. 201
Podell, K. 41
Poewe, W. 204
Poirier, J. 200
Polansky, M. 175, 185
Polich, J. 86, 87, 88
Polliack, M. 21, 155, 156
Pollock, B. G. 55
Polman, C. H. 144, 154, 155, 156, 160
Ponsford, J. 21, 22
Ponsford, J. L. 173, 174, 175, 176, 177, 179, 183, 184, 185
Poon, L. W. 245
Porjesz, B. 87
Posner, M. I. 195, 208
Posner, M. J. 90
Posthuma, D. 81, 84, 85, 86, 87, 88, 89, 91, 92
Postle, B. R. 175
Powell, D. H. 41
Powell, J. W. 41
Prabhakaran, V. 36
Prasher, D. 202
Price, A. L. 205
Price, L. R. 1, 16
Price, T. S. 91
Prifitera, A. 14
Prigatano, G. P. 173
Propping, P. 85
Prosperini, P. 136, 141
Provenzale, J. M. 234, 235, 228, 229
Przuntek, H. 205, 208
Psychological Corporation 13, 16, 35, 40, 127, 128
Pulley, L. 248
Purdon, S. E. 142
Putnam, S. H. 33

Quinn, N. 200

Rabbitt, P. M. A. 35, 223
Rabinowicz, E. F. 143
Radwan, S. 16
Rae, C. 84
Rafal, R. D. 195, 208
Ragland, J. D. 137, 142
Rai, G. S. 87
Raine, A. 127, 136
Rammsayer, T. H. 199
Randolph, J. J. 66, 161, 162, 165
Ransmayr, G. 204
Ransohoff, R. M. 153
Rao, S. M. 21, 66, 153, 154, 155, 156, 164
Ratti, M. T. 134
Raven, J. 34, 64
Rawlings, R. 129, 130, 135
Raz, N. 228, 230, 232
Razani, J. 256
Rebec, G. V. 199
Rebok, G. W. 249

Reed, T. E. 271
Reeder, K. P. 29, 178
Reeves, D. L. 40
Reger, M. 256
Reingold, S. C. 153
Reinvang, I. 12, 36
Reitan, R. M. 39
Reiter, G. 129, 130, 139
Renault, B. 87
Resnick, S. M. 230, 231
Reuling, I. E. 144, 154, 155, 156, 160
Richard, M. T. 21
Richard-Clark, C. 85
Richardson, C. E. 87
Richardson, J. T. 127
Rickard, T. C. 103
Ricker, J. H. 13, 39, 54, 62, 63, 154, 156, 161
Rickler, C. 85
Ridderinkhof, K. P. 227
Ridgeway, V. 66
Riemann, R. 34, 89, 90
Rietveld, M. J. 91
Rijsdijk, F. V. 83, 89
Ringel, N. 127
Rinne, J. O. 195
Riolo, L. 249
Rios, M. 181, 182
Rippeth, J. D. 127
Risser, A. 185
Ritchot, K. F. M. 112
Ritter, W. 143
Rizzo, M. 257
Robaey, P. 87
Robbins, T. W. 144
Roberts, W. 86
Robertson, I. H. 66, 175, 181, 182
Robertson, L. C. 142
Robinson, D. 129, 130, 139
Robinson, F. P. 256
Rock, A. 35
Rockel, C. 111
Rodrigue, K. M. 230
Roenker, D. 43, 186
Roenker, D. L. 41, 42, 43, 248, 249, 250, 252, 254, 255, 257
Roesch, S. C. 222
Rogers, D. 195, 207
Rogers, T. D. 87
Rohling, M. L. 174
Roman, M. J. 203
Romero, J. J. 37
Ron, M. A. 66
Rose, S. A. 91
Roseman, J. M. 248
Rosenstein, E. D. 29, 30, 62, 63, 68
Rosenthal R. 57
Rosenthal, D. 269
Rosenthal, M. 174, 183, 184, 187
Rosnick, C. B. 249
Ross, D. 4

Rossi, A. 136, 141
Rosso, I. M. 135
Rosson, M. B. 247
Rostrup, E. 144
Rostrup, E. 232
Roth, C. 103, 104
Roth, D. L. 29, 178, 248
Roth, W. T. 86
Rouch, I. 246
Rovet, J. 86
Rowan, E. N. 207
Royall, D. R. 209
Rozewicz, L 66
Rubert, M. 248
Rubin, D. C. 233
Rudick, R. 153
Ruff, R. 65, 174, 175, 187
Rule, B. G. 60
Rumrill, P. D. 153
Rushton, J. P. 12
Rust, J. 87, 88
Ryan, J. J. 41
Rypma, B. 228, 229

Sabbe, B. G. 127, 134, 140
Sachdev, P. S. 235
Sackheim, H. A. 126
Sagar, H. J. 202, 206, 208
Sahakian, B. J. 55, 174
Sailer, M. 156
Saint-Cyr, J. A. 200, 206
Saklofske, D. H. 13, 14
Sakuma, M. 139
Salat, D. 12, 36, 231, 233
Salazar, A. M. 175
Saling, L. L. 84, 204
Salive, M. E. 248
Salmon, D. P. 65, 198
Salmond, C. H. 55, 174
Salort, E. 162, 165
Salthouse, T. A. 19, 29, 31, 32, 57, 58, 59, 65, 67, 70, 126, 137, 139, 141, 143, 176, 221, 223, 224, 225, 244, 245, 247, 248, 267, 268, 271
Saltz, P. 173
Sammer, G. 166
Samson, M. M. 235
Sanchez, L. E. 135
Sanchez, M. P. 161, 166
Sandell, J. H. 231
Sander, A. 185
Sander, A. M. 174, 187
Sanders, A. F. 34
Sanders, M. D. 67
Santangelo, S. L. 91
Sarazin, M. 195
Sarna, S. 174, 187
Saults, J. S. 115, 265
Sawamoto, N. 29, 204
Saxby, B. 199

Saxton, J. A. 60
Saykin, A. J. 161, 165
Scaravilli, F. 200
Schafer, E. W. P. 87
Schaie, K. W. 244, 249
Schallice, T. 180
Schapira, A. H. 200
Schatz, J. 111
Schechtman, E. 205
Scheltens, P. 200
Schenck, C. H. 62
Schene, A. H. 59
Schiess, M. C. 205
Schiffer, R. B. 66
Schiffter, T. 84, 204
Schlosberg, H. 33
Schmidhuber-Eiler, B. 204
Schmitter-Edgecombe, M. E. 57, 179, 181
Schneider, R. 154
Schoenfeld, M. A. 156
Schrausser, D. G. 271
Schretlen, D. 174, 183, 231
Schroeder, C. E. 144
Schuepbach, D. 129, 130, 139
Schultheis, M. T. 30, 43, 175, 186, 268
Schulz, D. 156, 161, 162
Schupbach, M. 207
Schuschu, K. R. 161, 165
Schwartz, M. 203
Scott, G. 174
Scott, J. N. 54, 69, 160, 164
Scott, L. C. 87
Seckl, J. R. 235
Seibert, C. 163
Seiden, J. 86
Seidman, L. J. 58, 127, 129, 130, 131
Seignourel, P. J. 55, 175, 181, 182
Seitz, J. 36
Seitz, R. J. 200
Sekikawa, A. 247
Sekuler, A. B. 42
Sekuler, R. 244, 249
Seligman, D. 2
Selnes, O. A. 29
Sereno, A. B. 205
Sethares, C. 231
Seward, J. 164
Shaddish, W. R. 131, 132
Shafiq-Antonacci, R. 245
Shahar, I. 205
Shannon, C. E. 211
Shapiro, A. M. 174, 183
Shapiro, K. L. 86
Sharman, T. 127
Sharpe, J. A. 67
Shawaryn, M. A. 30, 43
Shelley, A. M. 144
Shenkin, S. D. 234
Sherer, M. 174, 183, 184, 185, 187
Sherman, E. M. S. 18, 61, 209

Sherman, E. S. E. 30
Shibasaki, H. 29, 204
Shimony, J. S. 231, 233
Shipley, B. A. 84, 204
Shite, L. E. 234, 235
Shnier, R. 235
Shtasel, D. 135
Shucard, D. 87
Shucard, D. W. 54, 55, 68
Shucard, J. L. 54, 55, 68
Shum, D. H. 174, 179
Shum, D. H. K. 38
Shute, V. J. 116
Shuttleworth, E. C. 163
Sibbitt, W. L. 235
Siegel, L. S. 113
Siegert, R. J. 206
Sigmundsson, H. 89
Silipo, G. 143
Silva, S. 141
Simms, E. 85
Simonoff, E. 91
Simonotto, E. 36
Simpson, D. A. 174
Sims, R. 248
Singarayer, R. 84, 202
Singerman, J. D. 228
Sitskoorn, M. M. 59, 127
Sivan, A. B. 65
Slade, T. 87
Slagboom, P. E. 91
Sletvold, H. 162
Slewa-Younan, S. 173, 174
Sliwinski, M. 37, 58, 61
Sloane, M. 248, 249, 254
Small, B. J. 223, 249
Smid, H. G. 156
Smit, D. J. A. 87
Smith, A. 39, 66
Smith, D. M. 250, 252
Smith, E. 207
Smith, E. E. 158
Smith, E. G. 107
Smith, G. A. 84, 87, 89, 92, 108
Smith, J. A. L. 36
Smith, M. C. 203, 207
Smith, M. E. 87
Smith, M. J. 141
Smith, P. L. 34
Smits, C. H. 247
Snow, K. L. 107
Snyder, A. M., 68,
Snyder, P. J. 21, 68, 155, 164
Sofer, S. 256
Soininen, H. 85
Sokal, M. M. 3, 4, 5, 6
Somsen, R. J. M. 89
Song, J. 118
Soni, W. 129, 130
Sonn, U. 247

Soragna, D. 134
Sörbom, D. 81
Soreq, H. 200
Soucy, J. P. 207
Spanoudis, G. 115
Spearman, C. 7
Spellacy, F. 18, 30, 61
Speller, J. 140
Spencer, J. 175
Spencer, K. M. 86
Sperling, R. A. 165
Spieler, D. H. 221
Spikman, J. M. 175, 176, 179, 180, 181, 183, 184
Spinath, F. M. 34, 89, 90
Spokes, K. 129, 130, 135
Spreen, O. 209, 266
Squire, L. R. 66
St. Aubin-Faubert, P. 154, 155, 156, 164
Staff, R. T. 232
Stalp, L. D. 200
Stalvey, B. 248
Stalvey, G. T. 248
Stanford, L. D. 38
Staplin, L. K. 248
Starkstein, S. E. 201
Starr, J. M. 84, 204, 234, 235
Stassen, H. H. 85
Stathopoulou, S. 85
Stawski, R. S. 127
Steen, B. 247
Steen, G. 247
Steffener, J. 54, 62, 156
Steif, B. L. 126
Steinschneider, M. 144
Steketee, M. C. 141
Stelmack, R. M. 36, 87
Steriade, M. 84, 85
Stern, G. M. 207
Stern, M. B. 205
Sternberg, R. J. 7
Sternberg, S. 54, 90, 91
Stethem, L. L. 21, 29
Stevens, M. M. 111
Stewart, D. G. 144
Stewart, L. 207
Stewart-Williams, S. 201
Stone, W. F. 86
Stough, C. 8, 9, 11, 29, 35, 36, 66, 84
Strachan, M. W. J. 36
Stratta, P. 136, 141
Strauss, E. 18, 30, 61, 209, 244, 266
Strayer, D. L. 149, 250
Strich, S. J. 174
Strick, P. L. 196, 197
Stroop, J. R. 54, 59
Strous, R. D. 143
Struss, D. T. 200
Strypstein, E. 182

Stuss, D. T. 21, 29, 173, 176, 180, 184
Suhr, J. A. 249
Sullivan, E. V. 208, 233, 234
Sultzer, D. 231
Summerall, S. W. 41
Summerfelt, A. 127
Summers, P. E. 233
Sunohara, G. A. 86, 87
Surwillo, W. W. 87, 88
Sutton, S. 86
Svetina, C. 129, 130, 135
Swank, P. R. 118
Swearer, J. M. 87
Sweeney, J. A. 31, 106, 129, 130, 139
Swerdlow, N. R. 203
Swirsky-Sacchetti, T. 164
Sworowski, L. A. 154
Synowitz, H. 174, 175
Szafran, J. 244
Szendi, I. 55

Takahashi, T. 201
Talbot, S. A. 33
Tan, J. 84, 204
Tanaka, H. 201, 202
Tandon, R. 142
Tant, M. L. M. 185, 187
Tate, D. F. 233
Tate, R. L. 174, 176
Taylor, A. E. 206
Taylor, D. 156
Taylor, M. J. 86, 87
Taylor, S. F. 142
Teasdale, T. W. 174, 183
Teichner, W. H. 211
Teixeira-Ferreira, C. 205
Tellegen, A. 85
Temkin, N. 174
Tennstedt, S. L. 250, 252
Teravainen, H. 203
Thaker, G. 125, 127, 129, 130, 136, 142
Thomas, V. S. 246
Thompson, A. J. 66, 153
Thompson, B. 175
Thompson, D. S. 33
Thompson, E. 1, 21, 29, 40, 181, 269
Thompson, J. C. 66, 84
Thompson, L. A. 89
Tian, S. 201
Tidswell, P. 202
Tierney, M. J. 235
Tiersky, L. A. 29, 61
Tisserand, D. J. 230
Tissingh, G. 200
Tofts, P. S. 153
Tordoff, V. 113
Torrey, E. F. 85, 142
Toster, A. I. 200
Townsend, J. 231
Towse, J. N. 115

Tramontano, G. 21, 22, 29, 55, 61, 68, 176, 178, 180, 181, 185, 256, 269
Tranh, M. 232
Trapp, B. D. 153
Treland, J. E. 209
Treves, T. A. 200
Trimble, M. 207
Tsatsanis, K. 91
Tsourtos, G. 66
Tsuang, M. T. 129, 130, 131
Tuch, D. S. 233
Tugwell, P. 129
Tuholski, S. W. 115
Tulsky, D. 1, 13, 14, 15, 16, 21, 31, 37, 38, 40, 54, 68, 79, 91, 157, 158, 161, 163, 256, 269
Turkington, T. G. 228, 229
Tuulio-Henriksson, A. 61
Tyler, P. 245

Udupa, J. 164
Ueberall, M. A. 111
Uekermann, J. 205
Ueshima, H. 247
Ullsberger, P. 87
Ungerer, J. A. 111
Unverzagt, F. 153
Unverzagt, F. W. 252
Urban, T. A. 31, 106
U. S. Army 65

Vaccaro, M. 185
Vakils, E. 176
Valenzuela, M. J. 235
Valle-Inclan, F. 88
van Baal, G. C. M. 87, 91
van Beijsterveldt, C. D. 91
Van Beijsterveldt, C. E. 87
van Boxtel, M. P. 230
van den Berg, W. V. 175, 187
van den Bosch, R. J. 59
van der Kouwe, A. J. 233
Van der Linden, M. 37, 176, 182
van der Meer, J. W. 62
van der Meers, J. J. 89
van der Molen, M. W. 227
van der Naalt, J. 175, 176, 179, 180
van der Werf, S. P. 62
Van Erp, T. 61
van Gijn, J. 232
van Hoof, J. J. 134, 140
van Weerden, T. W. 175, 176, 179, 180
van Zomeren, A. H. 175, 176, 179, 180, 181, 182, 183, 184, 185, 186, 187
Vance, D. E. 42, 43, 244, 250, 254, 255, 256, 257
Vance, K. T. 205
Vanderploeg, R. D. 174, 175
Vanneste, S. 244
Vardy, Y. 205
Varney, N. R. 67

Vazquez, C. 66
Veijola, J. 246
Veltmeyer, M. D. 85
Vendrell, P. 154, 155, 161
Verhaar, H. J. J. 235
Verhaeghen, P. 57, 58, 127
Verin, M. 205
Verleger, R. 86
Vernon, P. A. 8, 9, 12, 29, 56, 79, 83, 89, 106, 202, 271
Vickers, D. 34
Vincente, K. J. 247
Vink, M. 59
Visser, P. J. 230
Vlaar, A. M. M. 37
Vladir, V. 57
Vlar, R. 269
Vogel, E. K. 86
Vogel, F. 85
Volavka, J. 127
Volkow, N. D. 235
Voros, J. G. 86, 87

Waber, D. 106
Wade, D. T. 37
Wadley, V. G. 42, 43, 248, 250, 252, 254, 255, 257
Wadley, V. W. 244
Wadsworth, S. J. 91
Wagner, E. K. 248
Wahlin, A. 234, 235
Wahlin, T. B. 234, 235
Wainwright, H. 174
Waldman, I. 91
Walhovd, K. B. 12, 36
Walker, J. A. 195, 208
Walker, W. 185
Wallace, C. J. 54, 69, 160, 164
Wallesch, C.-W. 174, 175
Walsh, B. 80
Walsh, D. 135
Walsh, K. W. 174
Wang, D. 201
Wang, G. J. 235
Wang, H. 201
Wang, J. 201
Wang, L. 201, 202
Wang, Y. 200
Ward, T. 66
Wardlaw, J. M. 234
Warfield, S. K. 165
Warr, P. 65
Warr, P. B. 244
Warren, H. C. 2
Wasylyshyn, C. 127
Waters, F. A. 84
Weber, D. L. 127
Weber, G. A. 83
Weber, T. A. 249
Webster, D. D. 206

Wechsler, D. 13, 14, 15, 16, 54, 60, 61, 68, 70, 90, 125, 127, 139, 157, 209, 222
Weder, B. 200
Weers, D. C. 235
Weese, S. E. 79
Wehman, P. 173
Wei, L. 164
Wei, X. 54, 69, 160, 164
Weiler, M. D. 106
Weinberger, D. R. 142
Weins, A. N. 29
Weinstock-Guttman, B. 165
Weintraub, S. 41
Weirich, M. 129, 130, 135
Weiss, L. 16
Weiss, L. G. 14
Welford, A. T. 33, 34
Wells, J. 248
Wells, L. 235
Welsch, R. 256
Welsh, M. C. 65
Wen, W. 235
Wenegrat, B. G. 86
Wesch, J. 29
Wesnes, K. 199
Westin, C. F. 144
Whalley, L. J. 232
White, D. A. 65, 66, 256
White, M. 35
White, M. F. 248
Whitehouse, P. J., 200,
Whiting, W. L. 234, 235, 228, 229
Whitla, D. 41
Whittington, C. J. 201
Whyte, J. 175, 181, 182, 185
Wichern, D. W. 209
Wickett, J. C. 12
Widlocher, D. J. 126
Wiederholt, W. C. 65
Wieneke, M. 139
Wiersma, D. 59
Wilk, C. 125, 127, 129, 130, 136, 137, 138, 142
Wilkins, J. W. 59
Williams, C. J. 85
Williams, D. M. 245
Williams, L. E. 231, 233
Williams, M. A. 38
Williams, S. C. 233
Williamson, A. 230
Willies, R. C. 247
Willis, A. 195
Willis, S. L. 249, 250
Wills, S. 20, 38
Willson, J. 35
Wilson, C. 111, 117
Wilson, R. S. 204, 223
Winbald, B. 246
Winogron, H. W. 117

Wiseman, R. 199
Wishart, H. A. 161, 165
Withaar, F. K. 185, 186, 187
Wolfe, N. 207
Wolfson, D. 39
Wolinsky, F. D. 252
Wollmann, T. 161, 166
Wolters, E. C. 200
Wolters, T. 166
Wong, D. 153
Wood, N. L. 115
Wood, P. K. 115
Woodard, J. L. 38
Woodcock, R. W. 15, 16, 17, 107, 108, 222
Wood-Dauphinee, S. 256
Woods, S. P. 127
Woodward, T. S. 205
Woodworth, R. S. 33
Wright, E. 252
Wright, G. M. 87
Wright, M. J. 84, 87, 89, 91, 92
Wrightson, P. 19, 177

Yakovlev, P. I. 111
Yamaguchi, S. 206
Yamakawa, M. 247
Yardley, S. L. 135
Yehene, E. 205
Yeo, R. A. 235
Yiend, J. 175
Yordanova, J. 85
Young, A. B. 196, 200
Young, J. P. 85
Young, R. K. 34
Youngstrom, E. A. 127, 134

Zachs, R. 250
Zajdel, D. 167
Zakay, D. 64
Zakzanis, K. K. 125, 132, 140, 142
Zaleta, A. K. 233
Zarahn, E. 228
Zaucha, K. 173
Zentall, S. S. 116
Zetusky, W. J. 206
Zhang, L. 118
Zhang, Y. 54, 69, 160, 164, 201
Zhu, J. 1, 14, 15, 16, 21, 40
Zimprich, D. 244
Zitman, F. G. 134, 140
Ziv, I. 200
Zivadinov, R. 165
Zmuda, M. D. 55
Zoccolotti, P. 181, 182
Zonderman, A. B. 230, 231
Zorrilla, L. E. 135
Zubin, J. 86
Zukin, S. R. 144

Subject index

AAA (American Automobile Association) 257
Abnormalities
  cognitive functioning 91
  lipid metabolism 145
  major fiber tracts 144
  neurological 174
  neurotransmitter 144
  non-specific, affecting frontotemporal poles 175
  response patterns 206
  stimulus processing 142
  temporal coupling between deliberation and execution processes 207
  white matter 232
Academic skills/achievement 116–117, 118
Accelerate 250
Acceleration-deceleration forces 174
Accuracy 34, 68, 156, 158
  2-back 159
  decision 32
  decreased 179
  equal performance between groups 69
  global skills contribute to 116
  improved 67
  initial encoding 141
  performance criterion for 178
  scanning 204
  time estimation 65
  trade-off between speed and 108
  word problem solving 116, 117
  working memory 57, 154, 270
  see also Speed-accuracy trade-off
ACE models 81–82
Acetylcholine activity 199, 200
Acquired cerebral dysfunction 1
Acquisition/recall 57–64, 161
ACTIVE (single-blind trial) 250, 254, 258
Acute hospitalization 136
Addition 116, 117
Additive structural model (Sternberg) 179
ADHD (attention-deficit/hyperactivity disorder) 86–87, 127, 134
  biomarkers in 79, 89

  heritability of 91
  identifying genes for 92
Adjunctive medication strategies 127
ADL (activities of daily living) 246
Adolescence 31
  cognitive development 55–56
  speed of processing 101–123
Adoption designs 80
Affective regulation 197
Afferent information 199
Age 34
  index of executive abilities as a function of 65–66
  PS and WM show improvement with 56
  typical correlation between PS and 103
Age Group X Task Condition interactions 227
Age-related change 229
  cognitive 234, 235
  number of transient connections in CNS 111
  processing speed 104, 109, 112–114, 116, 244
  reading skill 116
  structural integrity of white matter 233
  working memory 113
Age-related decline 29, 57, 58, 61
  cognitive functioning 244
  generalized slowing of abilities underlies 244
  perceptual-motor skill 230
  performance on mental imagery task 230
  resting neural activity 227
  signal-to-noise ratio of measured brain activation 228
Age-related issues
  articulation rate 113
  damage 233
  differences 227, 234
  diseases 86
  influences 224
  slowing 85, 109
  variance in cognitive performance 233

Subject index

Aging 31, 40, 91, 126, 139
   cognitive 34
   diminished PS demonstrated in 154
   information processing speed and 221–241
   model for clinical populations 243–263
   vulnerability of PS to 29, 30
   working memory decline during 57
Agnosia 195
Alcoholism 83
   chronic 127, 133
Algorithms 103, 108
ALL (acute lymphoblastic leukemia) 111
Alpha peak frequency 91, 92
Alpha waves 85
Alphabet Backwards test 38
Alphabet recitation 41
Alphabet-arithmetic tasks 249
Alzheimer's disease 36, 60, 84, 85, 86, 127, 195
   processing speed in 208–211
   slowed IPS in 196
Amantadine 156
Amateur athletes 41
American Journal of Psychiatry 128
AMIPB (Adult Memory and Information Processing Battery) 37
Amnesia, *see* PTA
Amos (statistical software) 81
Amplitude 86, 88
Amygdala 196
ANCOVA (analysis of covariance) 70
   information processing speed entered as covariate in 63
Anterior cingulate circuit 198
Anterior-to-posterior areas 87, 233
Antero-temporal lobes 174
Anthropometric testing 1
   death knoll of 7
   first public criticism of 6
   significant decline of 6
Anticipatory risk avoidance 186
Antiparkinsonian therapy 204
Antipsychotics 127
Anxiety 38
APA (American Psychological Association) 5–6
Apathy 200–201
Aphasia 195
Apomorphine 208
Appearance 55
Apprehension speed 84
Apraxia 195
Archives of General Psychiatry 128
Arithmetic 14, 17, 128, 129, 141, 160
   decoding and solving 117
   underlying operations 116
Arousal 34, 246
   emotional 198
Arthritis 245
Articulation rate 56, 113
Articulatory loop 113, 114

Asymptotic values 106, 108, 113
AT-SAT (Auditory Threshold Serial Addition Test) 57, 68, 69
   percent correct 63
Attention 18, 31, 37, 41, 164, 201, 234, 244
   complex 30, 38
   divided 42, 175, 185, 186
   family ratings of 185
   focusing 175, 203
   impaired 195
   information regarding 39
   poor 55
   post-TBI 181
   problems with 195
   selective 42, 211
   sustained 185
   switching 175, 245
   visual 206
   see also Executive attention
Attentional blink 86, 205
Attentional control 54
   executive 175
   interference of 55
Attentional resources 86
   deployment of 205
Attentional tasks 179
Atypical children/development 102, 111, 117–118, 119, 270
Auditory detection CPT 130
Auditory functioning 38
Auditory tasks 54, 180
   identification 249
Autism
   biomarkers in 79
   heritability of 91
   identifying genes for 92
Autonomy 43, 246, 248
Axonal damage 153
   see also Diffuse axonal injury
Axons 83, 91, 231, 233
   loss of membrane potential 163

Backward masking paradigm 143
Balance 249
Ballismus 198
Basal ganglia 196–199, 200, 202, 205, 220, 233, 234
Behavior genetics 80–82
Benzodiazepine use 246
Bereitschaftspotential 88
Beta rhythms 85
Bilateral parkinsonism 200
Biomarkers 79, 89, 92
Bipolar depression 126
Bipolar disorder 61
Bivariate correlations 63
Block Design 137
Blood flow 200, 227, 228
Bootstrap approach 222

Subject index 297

Bottlenecks 143, 144
Bottom-up approach 83
Bradykinesia 196, 199, 206–208, 209
   cognitive slowing correlated significantly with 204
Bradyphrenia 195, 196, 201, 202, 203, 204, 208
   absence/presence of 205
   psychomotor retardation and 207
   relationship between executive function and 206
Brain
   amount or composition of tissue 228
   cell development and integrity 145
   continued development 111
   electrical activity 11, 84
   lesions 163
   periventricular areas 153
   posterior fossa region 69, 164
   PS especially sensitive to insult to 270
   sensitive markers of dysfunction 127
   structural changes 207
   widespread pattern of significant activation 36
Brain atrophy 165
Brain imaging studies 200
Brain injuries/damage 14–15, 34, 154, 270, 271
   see also TBI
Brain size/volume 12, 92, 230–231
Brass instruments 3, 4, 5
Breathing cycle 34
Broad abilities 16
Brodmann area 228–229
Brown-Peterson task 156

Calculation 41
Calibration problems 3
Carbon monoxide poisoning 200
Cardiovascular disease 256
   risk factors 232
Carroll's three-stratum theory 16
Category fluency 59, 129, 134, 135
Category learning 205
Cattell-Horn Gf-Gc theory 16
Caudate 196, 230
   dopamine D2 receptor binding 235
   dopamine reduction in 200
   subcortical lesions in 199
Central processing 245
Cerebellum 165, 166, 230
Cerebral blood flow 200, 227
Cerebral metabolites 235
Cerebral plaque development 156
Cerebrospinal fluid 207
CES (central executive system) 54, 55, 156, 160
CFS (chronic fatigue syndrome) 20, 29, 62
   impaired PASAT performance 54
   neurological dysfunction stemming from 53
Character classification paradigm (Sternberg) 204
Charcot-Marie-Tooth disease 83
CHC (Cattell-Horn-Carroll) theory 15–16
Chess experts 103–104
Childhood
   cognitive development 55–56
   learning disabilities 86, 89
   speed of processing 101–123
Chinese characters 116
Cholinergic dysfunction 208
Cholinergic function/transmission 36
Cholinergic system 174
Chorea 198
Chronic illness 139, 143, 246
   inflammatory conditions 83
   outpatients 136
Chronoscopes 3–4
Chunking strategy 68
Cingulate gyrus 36
Circadian rhythms 246
Circuit breaking 3
Classification 2
Clinical groups 21
   additional longitudinal research needed in 23
   diverse 39
   mediator/moderator models in 70
Clinical psychology 22
Clinical tools 15, 37, 42, 43
   labeling of 30
   tendency to assess multiple cognitive domains simultaneously 31
Clinical trials 185
CNS (central nervous system) 31
   age-related changes in number of transient connections 111
   children with insult 111, 112
   medication affecting functioning 167
   processing measure 83
   properties that mediate or contribute to variations in speed at behavioral level 227
   widespread lesions in 153
Coding subtest (WISC-III) 17, 117, 128
Coeruleo-cortical noradrenergic projections 87
Cognitive abilities 17, 31–32, 91, 92, 161–162, 224, 247
   deficits in, primary contributor to 31
   higher-order 245
   hypothesized variable of 10
   important consideration when assessing 245
   primary 249
   search for genetic variation causing individual differences in 79
   targeted 250
Cognitive constructs 59, 125, 267–268
Cognitive development 55–56
Cognitive disability 173

Cognitive dysfunction 208
  parameters of disease process more precisely related to 166
  predicted 164
Cognitive dysmetria 144
Cognitive functioning 37
  abnormal 91
  age-related declines in 244
  aging effects on 246
  athletes with concussion 41
  complex 19
  correlations between dopamine D2 receptor binding and 234
  global 19
  higher 126, 266
  impact of subcortical white matter lesions on 198
  impaired 118
  interventions known to improve 256
  lesion burden and 165
  low/lower order 38, 126
  multiple 165
  performance on tasks of everyday life and 162
  poor hydration can impact 246
  PS and 29, 30, 42, 43
  recovery 183
  strongly dependent on genetic make-up 91
  domains of 14
  summary scores organized into more specific tests of 250
Cognitive growth 112
  delayed, in atypical children 118
Cognitive impairments,
  generalized 127
  type and severity of 23
Cognitive inhibition 39
Cognitive processes 112–113
  adolescents and adults with mental retardation 117
  higher-order/higher-level 9, 11, 36, 102, 269
  PASAT dependent on a number of 38
  perceptual 126
  rapid and efficient 199
  slowing of 86, 195
  speed, distinction between motor speed and 31
  time needed for children to execute 110
Cognitive sequelae 174
Cognitive slowing 86, 126, 140, 195, 209
  co-expression of motor and 207
  correlated significantly with bradykinesia 204
  difficulty shifting mental set because of 204
  disease-related 201
  impairments in 175
  nondemented and demented PD patients 203
  nonmotoric 202
  nonspecific 203

Cognitive tasks 87, 102, 109, 126, 143, 221, 227, 228, 229
  complex 19, 30, 176, 188
  demanding 177
  demanding, assessing processing speed in 177
  IQ and 87
  nonmotoric 212
  processing speed and its impact on 176
  simple 19
  speed of performance in 228
  time taken to complete/execute 22, 30–31, 266
  timed 204–205, 209
  see also ECTs
Cognitive tests 1, 164
  multiple-choice responses 246
  time utilized to respond in 32
Cohen's, d 131
Color 180
  naming 38, 54, 142
Columbia College 5, 7
Coma 173–174, 175
Comparison 143
  elementary 32
  letter 32, 33
  pattern 32, 33
Compensation strategies 246
Complementary after-images 244
Complex figure test 59
Complex processing speed 23
Computational processing 245
Computer systems 247, 249, 250, 254
  simulation models 235
  see also PCs
Concentration 37
  poor 55
Concentration training 184, 185
Concrete abilities 16
Concussion 41, 173
Confidence intervals 132, 134
  non-overlapping 140
Conflict condition matching task 201
Conflicts 6
Congruent response cuing 203
Constant interstimulus interval 54
Construct validity 41, 57, 59, 63, 69
  analyses 222
  future research should pay more careful attention to 70
Context updating/closure 86
Continuous performance test 61
Controlled medication studies 185
Contusions 174
Corpus callosum 164, 233
  splenium for younger adults 234
Correlational techniques/method 8, 81
Cortex
  glutamate distributed throughout 144
  motor 88

parietal 166, 196, 229, 230
premotor 88
primary visual 231
reducing output to 198
ventral occipitotemporal (extrastriate) 228
visual 85
see also Frontal cortex; Prefrontal cortex
Cortical afferent projections 87
Cortical disorders 195, 196
  see also SCDs
Cortical mantle sparing 154
Cortical-subcortical connections 199
Cortical-subcortical loops 197
Cortico-cortical networks 85
COWAT (Controlled Oral Word Association Test) 65
CPMS (chronic progressive multiple sclerosis) 153, 165
CPT (continuous performance test) 130
CPUs (central processing units) 110–111
Critical flicker fusion 244
Cross-Out subtest 15, 107, 108, 115
Cross-sectional studies 107
CRT (Choice Reaction Time) 10, 13, 19, 33, 54, 206, 209
Crystalized abilities 20
CS (Computation Span) tasks 64
Cultures 246
CVLT (California Verbal Learning Test) 59, 60, 129

Daily living 20
  functioning 21, 22, 23
  important contribution of PS to activities of 43
  vocational, independent 143
  see also Everyday life; IADL
Danish cohort 232
Data collection 2
Data entry task 248
Death
  most common cause in young people 173
  unexpected 180
Decision-making 179
  self-generated, nonroutine 206
Decision speed 16, 32
Decision time 10, 35
Degeneration 200
Delayed auditory feedback 204
Delayed match-to-sample task 141
Dementia 29, 61, 200, 201, 202, 203, 233, 256
  absence of 209
  cerebrovascular 60
  cortical 208
  diagnosis of 209
  generalized 209
  higher incidence of 207
  subcortical 154
Demographic factors 62

Demyelination
  callosal fiber tracts 164
  neural 155, 163
  periventricular 164
  slowed conduction speed as a result of 163
Dendritic branching 176
Depression 140, 204, 208, 245
  acute 134
  apathy can occur in absence of 201
  associations between PS and 162
  bipolar 126
  comorbidity between MS and 66
  impact on cognition in MS 162
  major 127, 200, 207
  primary 207
  unmedicated 127
  see also Geriatric depression
Developmental change 102–115
Diabetes 83, 256
Differential Ability Scales (Speed of Information Processing test) 15, 17
Diffuse axonal injury 175, 176, 183
  slowing in processing speed reflected in invariant presence of 176
Digit Span 14, 63, 70, 114, 115, 128, 129, 141
  backwards 156
  reverse 85
Digit Symbol-Coding subtest (WAIS-III) 13, 14, 20, 21, 22, 37, 39, 40, 54, 60, 61, 90–91
Digit vigilance 136
Direct vision 34
Discrimination 80, 83–84
  duration 199
  object 200
  perceptual 83
  sensory 7
  size 202
  spatial information 203
  see also Visual discrimination
Disease course 126, 165
Disease presence 58
Disease risk 143
Distraction 89
  inhibiting 175
  susceptibility to 185
DLPFC (dorsolateral prefrontal cortex) 197, 198, 200, 229, 230
Domain-specific factors 116, 117
Dopamine 144, 202, 234
  reduction in caudate and putamen 200
  selective slowing effect on cognitive speed 208
  striatal 199, 200
  subcortical, depletion 207
Dopaminergic activity 196, 199
  decline in transmission 235
  dysfunction 208
  treatment 207
Dorsal vagal nucleus 200
Drawing a line 39

Driving 43, 185–187, 256
  competency 248
  on-the-road performance 43
  performance 252
Driving Simulator 252, 254
DSST (WAIS Digit-Symbol Substitution Test) 125–151, 207, 245, 248
DTI (diffusion tensor imaging) 144, 166, 233–234, 271
Dual-task performance 175, 181, 182
Dual-task training 249
  variable priority 250
Dyad quantification method 68
Dysarthria 38, 39
DZ (dizygotic) twins 81–82, 84, 87, 89, 90
  MZ versus 9

ECTs (elementary cognitive tasks) 8, 10
Edinburgh High Risk Study group 135
Educational psychology 7
Education 36, 38, 245
  PS related to 29
EEG (electroencephalographic) recording 80, 84–88, 92, 271
EFPT (Executive Functional Performance Test) 162–163
Electromagnets 3
Electrophysiological recording/changes 79, 202
Ellis Island 127
Emotional behavior 197
Employment 187–188
  post-injury stability 186
Encoding
  initial, poor 62
  problems 59
  speed of 90
Endophenotypes 79, 92
England 7
English learning 116
Environmental influences/factors
  additive genetic 82
  shared/non-shared 80, 81, 82, 89
Episodic memory 71, 140, 141, 234
  age-related decreases in 58
  age-related variance in tests of 235
  deficits in 59, 61, 62, 63, 175
  development of disturbance 161
  greatly improved 62
  impairments in 175
  improved in TBI 62
  long-term 30, 42, 154
  processing speed may be related to 54
  relationship between age and 57
  verbal and nonverbal 61
Episodic memory decline
  depression-related 60
  MS-related 63
  schizophrenia 59

EQS (statistical software) 81
ERPs (event-related potentials) 32, 84, 180, 195, 201–202, 212, 227, 271
  electrophysiological 36
  P3 86–87
Errors 81, 117, 178, 205
  minor 255
  recognizing specific types of 205
  response 32
  standard 81
Etiology 199
  elusive 153
  undetermined 200
Event categorization 86
Everyday life 20
  functioning abilities/skills 42, 125, 136
  impact of PS deficit in MS on 162–163
  roles 143
  tasks 173, 243–263
Evoked-response potentials 11–12, 271
  delays in and loss of 163
  long-latency 201
Evolution 2
Excitatory nerve cells 85
Excitatory output 198
Executive abilities 54
  as a function of age 65–66
Executive attention 177, 181–182
  deficits 176
  difficulties in tasks assessing 176
  dysfunction 182
  impairments in 175
  relationship in TBI between processing speed and 181
  skills of 178
  slowness on measures of 182
Executive control functions 198
  higher-order 196
  impairments in 143
Executive deficits 135
Executive dysfunction 200, 201, 206
Executive functions 59, 64–66, 70, 128, 141, 143, 232, 234
  bradyphrenia and 206
  deficits in 162
  DLPFC circuits primarily associated with 198
  frontal-mediated 205
  impaired 199, 201, 209
  measure involving cognitive inhibition 39
  problems with 195
  role for dopamine in 207
Executive processes 34, 37, 142, 144
Experimental psychology 22
Expertise hypothesis 104
Exponential function 106, 108
Extrapyramidal signs 209
Eye-hand coordination 39

Eye movements 107
    saccadic 197, 205
    smooth pursuit 197

Factor analysis 14, 20, 38, 39, 177, 209, 231, 266
    confirmatory 35, 222
    exploratory 15, 222
    see also SCFA
Falsification and fabrication 7
Family environment 80, 81
Family Pictures 137
Fast speech response 42
Fatigue 34, 162, 200, 246
    nerve fiber 163
    see also CFS
Figural Visual Scanning and Discrimination 248
Finger Tapping task 32, 128, 209
    motor speed effects for 140
Fitness to drive 186, 187
FLAIR (fluid-attenuated inversion recovery) 165
Fluency measures, *see* Category fluency; Letter fluency; Verbal fluency
Fluid abilities 16
    declines in psychometric measures of 20
    significant negative correlation between WMH and 232
Fluid intelligence 11
    age-related differences in 231
    associated with IADL disability 247
    relationship between IT and 35
fMRI (functional magnetic resonance imaging) 36, 228
Forgetfulness 195
Fourier transformation 84
Fractional anisotropy 233, 234, 235
Fraternal twins, *see* DZ
Freedom from Distractability factor 14
Frequency domain 84-85
Frontal cortex 199
    defective interactions between striatum and 144
    inhibitory functions in 205
Frontal lobe 230, 231
    changes in functioning 233
    inferior 174
    lateral areas of 36
    lower metabolic activity in 232
Frontal-striatal loops 144
Frontoparietal subcortical networks 165
Frontotemporal dysfunction 176
FSCs (frontal-subcortical circuits) 197, 199, 205, 206, 220
Functional disability 136
Functional reach 249
Functional status
    important contribution of PS to 42
    improved 43

g (general concept of intelligence) 12
g-Stratum III 16
GABA (gamma aminobutyric acid) 199, 200
Gait 249
    disturbance/difficulty 198, 199, 206, 207
Galtonian thinking 9
Gaze restriction 198
GCS (Glasgow Coma Scale) 173-174, 175
Gender 34
    PS related to 29
General intelligence 7, 20, 35, 85
Generalizability 58
    limited 61
Gene-environment interactions 200
Genetics 79-100, 127, 135
Geographic regions 153
Geometric figures 39
Geriatric depression 59-60
Germany 2
Glasgow Coma Scale, *see* GCS
Global development hypothesis 56
Globus pallidus 196, 198
Glucose levels 36
Glucose metabolism 12
Glutamate 144, 199, 200
Go task 206
Goal-attainment 173
Goal-setting deficits 205
Goodness-of-fit statistic 82
Gray matter 111, 165
    volume declines as a function of increasing adult age 230
Grip Strength 209
Grooved Pegboard task 128, 129, 136, 209
    motor speed effects for 140
Guillain-Barré syndrome 83

Haemorrhages 174
HCs (healthy controls) 21, 154-162, 165, 166, 180, 202-207, 269
Head injury 62
    closed 111, 117, 118
    mild 117, 118
    moderate 118
    severe 38, 117, 118
    see also TBI
Health status 249
Healthy adults 56-57
    older 65
    PET studies of 234
    young 65, 186
Hedges' g 131
Hemiparkinsonism 200
Hemodynamic properties 228
Hereditary selection 2
heritability 79, 84, 89, 90, 91, 92, 135
    estimation in behavior genetics 80
    high 86
    index of processing speed can fail to show 92

302 Subject index

moderate to high 87
moderate 88
significant 88
Heterogeneity 132
    traumatic injury within a clinical sample 173–174
Heterozygous parkin mutations 200
Hick's law 211–212
Hierarchical regression 59, 60, 70, 230, 231, 235
Hierarchical task analysis 187
Hipp chronoscope 3–4
Hippocampus 230
HIV (human immunodeficiency virus) 257
    aging with 256
    related cognitive impairment 127
    symptomatic 29
Homogeneity statistics 132, 133
Hong Kong 116
Hopkins Verbal Learning Test 129
Hormones 235
    elevated thyroid stimulating 60
HRQoL (health-related quality of life) 162, 250–252
Huntington's disease 89, 127, 195, 198, 203, 234, 270
HVA (homovanillic acid) 207
Hybrid training procedure 250
Hydration 246
Hyperintensities 231–234
Hypertension 232
Hypoglycemia 36, 84
Hypokinetic syndromes 198
Hypophonia 199
Hypothesis-driven research 17

IADL (instrumental activities of daily living) 43, 246, 247, 249
    see also TIADL
Identical Pairs CPT 130
identical twins, see MZ
Illness-related disability 143
Image-based information 114
Immune system 91
ImPACT (Immediate Post-Concussion Assessment and Cognitive Testing) 41
Incongruent conditions 142, 180
    response cuing 203
Independent living 136
Individual differences 2, 6, 221–222, 227
    controlling for 58
    dopamine D2 receptor binding 235
    genetic variation causing 79
    large, P3 characterized by 86
    markers of differences in mental health 86
    neurobiological substrate of 229–230
    one of the great proponents of measurement of 4
    prolific period of research in 3
    scientific study of 5

Infants 107
Inflammatory processes 145
Information decay 143
Information processing efficiency 156
Inhibitory control 206
Inhibitory nerve cells 85
Initiation 205
Insecticide exposure 200
Instrumental deficits 195
Intellectual abilities 17, 22
    general 16, 20
    valuable information on assessment of 18
Intellectual assessment batteries 15
Intellectual deficits 135
Intellectual functioning 21, 53
    diminished processing speed may compromise 32
Intellectual status 209
Intelligence
    association between IT and 35, 36
    findings that shaped understanding of 30
    higher 64, 65, 83
    history of processing speed, and relationship to 1–28
    lower 64
    moderate relationship between ERP and 36
    "neural speed and efficiency" hypothesis of 79, 83
    orthogonal visual processes aspect of 35
    PNCV and 83
    PS related to 29
    studies relating processing speed to 89
Intelligence tests 3, 8, 80, 83, 135
    CHC influenced revisions 16
    faster IT related to higher scores 84
    processing speed from 90–91
    standardized 232
    testing and scoring structure 13
    variance in scores 89
Interference condition 142
Interhemispheric communication 164
Internal responses 32
International Health Exhibition (London 1884) 3, 101
Iodine-beta-CIT 207
Ipsilateral hemisphere 88
IQ (intelligence quotient) 11, 14, 62
    attempts to demonstrate association between RT and 29
    calculation of four dimensions of 90
    children with severe head injury 118
    Full Scale score 13
    genome scan for 79
    genomic regions influencing 91
    high 65
    IT correlated with 92
    P3 latency and 86
    psychometric 86, 91

Verbal 13, 35, 209
  see also PIQ; VIQ
ISIs (inter-stimulus intervals) 68, 158
  fixed 57
IT (inspection time) 7, 17, 19, 30, 33, 83, 222
  association between intelligence and 36
  biological study of 36
  central cholinergic pathways influence 36
  correlated with IQ 92
  debate as to whether individual differences are related to high-level cognitive strategies 36
  experimental research on 9
  generally defined 10–11
  limited 143
  nonmotoric 204
  paradigms conceptualized as research strategies 35
  rapid feature extraction indexed by 88
  relationship between fluid intelligence and 35
  significantly reduced 36
  slowed 204
  theory applied to intelligence 11
  typical procedure 34
  visual 84

Jackknife procedure 209
JLOT (Judgement of Line Orientation Test) 67
Johns Hopkins University 4
juxtacortical lesions in MS 165

Knowledge 20
Korsakoff's psychosis 84, 127
KTT (Keeping Track Task) 160, 164

Laboratories 3
  anthropometric 2, 5, 101
  psychological 2, 4
Laboratory paradigms 154
Language tasks 109–110
Large effect (Cohen) 133
Latency 32, 212
  LRP peak 84, 88, 92
  N1 88, 92, 201
  N2 201
  P2 88, 92
  P3 86, 87, 92, 201, 202, 206
  P300 36
LC (locus coeruleus) 87, 200
Learning abilities 161
Learning deficits 140
Learning disabilities 86
Lesion burden 163, 166
  cognitive functioning and 165
Lesion volume
  frontal 164, 165
  parietal 165
  total 68, 164, 165
Lesions 233
  cortical 165
  detecting in neuroanatomical areas associated with multiple cognitive functions 165
  diffuse 174
  hyperintense 199
  juxtacortical 165
  neuroradiologists' ratings of size 163
  predominantly focal 183
  right-side 256
  subcortical 198, 199
  white matter 198, 232
  widespread in CNS 153
Letter Cancellation 209
Letter comparison 32, 33
Letter cues 129
Letter fluency 136
Leukemia, see ALL
Levodopa treatment 202, 207, 208, 209
Lewy bodies 200
Limbic functions 198
Limbic regions 234
Limited time mechanism 32, 143, 176
Lipid metabolism 145
LISREL (statistical software) 81
List-learning 60, 128
  initial encoding trial of 181
  verbal tasks 219
LNS (WAIS Letter-Number Sequencing) task 126, 144, 157
Location 55
Locus coeruleus, see LC
Logarithms 106, 108, 211
Logical memory 60, 61, 128, 134
London 2, 3, 4, 101
Long-term memory 9, 18, 55, 57, 115
  access to highly overlearned material stored in 90
  activating representations within 175
  episodic 30, 42, 154
  function concurrently in patients with MS 63
  phonological information retrieval from 114
  stimulus and response stored in 103
Loss of consciousness 175, 181
LRP (lateralized readiness potential) 84, 88, 92
Lupus, see SLE

Magnetic resonance spectroscopy 235
Major depressive disorder 134
Mamillary bodies 230
Manganese toxicity 200
Manual movements 140
Masking 244
  backward 143
Mathematical deficits 38

304 *Subject index*

Maximum Likelihood 82
MCI (mild cognitive impairment) 256, 257
Mediational hypothesis 61, 62
Mediator/moderator models in clinical groups 70
Medication 208, 256, 258
  adjunctive 127
  affecting CNS functioning, impact of 167
  controlled studies 185
  dopamine 207
  effect of treatment on ERPs 202
  prescription 246
  reading labels 249
  side effects 257
  tolerance to 208
Medication exposure 139
  long-term 143
MEDLINE 128
Memory 7, 41, 201, 222, 224
  active 126
  associative 61
  auditory 16
  complex 176
  declarative 57, 128, 132
  deficits in 140, 162, 176
  disease-related decline 70
  everyday 247
  explicit 230, 232
  indices of 164
  nonverbal 61
  poorest performance 164
  recent 200
  scanning 102
  semantic 59, 85
  spatial 114
  specialized temporary storage systems 175
  story 135
  tests of 232
  training techniques 249, 250
  visual learning 195
  see also Episodic memory; Long-term memory; STM; Verbal memory; Visual memory; WM
Mental abilities 8, 12
Mental control 41
Mental retardation 111, 117, 118
Mental rotation 102, 204
Mental speed 8, 10, 91
  Cattell's multidimensional view of 18
  higher intelligence a result of 29
  measure of 40
Mental tests 5, 6
  relationship between speed and 7
Mental tracking 211
Mesial prefrontal region 200
Mesiofrontal pathology 200
Mesocortical system 234
Mesostriatal system 199
Meta-analysis 56, 106, 128–139, 140, 142, 155
  cognitive declines in HIV 256

Metabolic activity 232
Method of Limits procedure 158
Methylphenidate 185
MicroCog 41
Micrographia 199
Mind 5
Misunderstandings 8
Mobility impairments 248
Monitoring tasks 249
Mood 245
Morbidity 173
Morphometric measures 164, 165, 166
Motivation 198
Motor behavior 199
Motor disability 202
  frontal-striatal dopamine deficiency postulated to underlie 208
Motor functioning 31, 33, 40
  elementary 70
  procedure used to remove the effects of 60
Motor processes 3
Motor programming 198
motor skills 248
  acquisition of 195
Motor-speech factors 39
Motor speed 17, 34, 40, 41, 91, 128, 140
  distinction between cognitive processing speed and 31
  measures 135
  perceptual 109
Motor tasks 209
Movement initiation 199
Movement time 10, 208
Movements
  facial 199
  internally determined 202
  limb 199
  rapid voluntary 202
  uncontrolled 198
MRI (magnetic resonance imaging) 12, 68, 69, 163, 198
  advances in processing technologies 164
  methods known to be sensitive to cortical and juxtacortical lesions 165
  scanning parameters 166
  structural 232
  T2-weighted or proton density-weighted scans 232
  see also fMRI
MRPs (movement-related potentials) 202, 212
MS (multiple sclerosis) 20, 22, 29, 30, 57, 63–64, 68, 256
  genetic predisposition to 83
  impaired performance on PASAT 54
  neurological dysfunction stemming from 53
  primary cognitive deficits seen in various subtypes of 21
  processing speed in 31, 37, 42, 54, 91, 144, 153–172

TOL in 66
visual processing impaired among patients 67
MSA (multiple system atrophy) 195, 198
Multiple abilities 16
Multiple cerebral infarcts 200
Multiple cognitive domains 245
deficits across 234
simultaneous assessment of 31
Multiple speed constructs 222
Multivariates 82
Muscle control 245
Mutations of genes 200
Mx (statistical software) 81
Myelin sheaths 67, 79, 91
disintegration of 231
neuronal, destruction of 153
Myelinization 83
age-related increases in 111
changes in 144
loss of 176
MZ (monozygotic) twins 82, 84, 87, 89
DZ versus 9
extent to which they do not resemble each other 81
intrapair resemblance 85
reaction time 90
reared apart/reared together 80

N-back test 60, 158
Name identity 90
Name Writing 209
Naming 116
color 38, 54, 142
Narrow abilities 16
National Adult Reading Test 129
National Collaborative Perinatal Project 135
Naturalistic tasks 185
Neocortex 234
Nerve conduction velocity 79, 83, 195
decreased 271
too low a level 222
see also PNCV
Nerve fiber shearing 174, 180
Nervous breakdown 6
Neural architecture change 111
Neural conduction speed 163
Neural degenerative disorders 86
Neural efficiency 9, 11, 12, 35
Neural functioning 111
metabolic 227
Neural networks 92, 230
Neural speed 11, 86
Neural substrates 270–272
PS deficits in MS 163–166
Neural transmission 176
Neural wiring 79
Neuroanatomical areas 165
Neurobehavioral alterations 195
Neurobiological correlates of speed 227–236

Neurobiological substrates 234
Neurochemical change 174
Neurochemical substrates 207
Neurocognitive disorders 29
Neurodegeneration 85, 199
Neuroimaging 156
localized activation in 227–229
Neuroleptic usage 200
Neurological disorders/conditions 58
vulnerability of PS to 29
Neurological dysfunction 53
Neurological insult 29, 30, 38, 266
primary contributor to deficits in cognitive abilities 31
Neurological measures 68
Neuronal efficiency processing 35
Neurons 84
thalamic 85
Neuropathological diseases/features 83, 200
Neuropathology 174–175, 199
frontotemporal dysfunction 176
Neuropetides 200
Neurophysiology 36
indices 195
low-level measures 83
Neuropsychiatric conditions 127
Neuropsychological assessments 21
commonly used instrument 39
Neuropsychological changes 175
Neuropsychological constructs 53
Neuropsychological data 209
Neuropsychological deficit 174, 183
Neuropsychological dysfunction 91
Neuropsychological impairments 14
Neuropsychological measures 37, 68
select computerized 40
Neuropsychological performance decline 232
Neuropsychological recovery 184
Neuropsychological tasks 177
Neuropsychological tests 1, 38, 40, 155, 164, 187
choice of 166
insensitivity of 166
performance 180, 186
scores 207
simple and complex attention tasks 179
slowness on 181
standardized 154
timed 230
Neurotransmission
glutamate 144
synaptic 79
Neurotransmitters 199, 200, 234
catecholamine systems 144
general system abnormalities 144
Neurotropic viral tracing techniques 197
Neurovascular coupling 228
Neutral conditions 142
New York 5
Nicotinic acetylcholine receptors 144

306 Subject index

Nigrostriatal dopaminergic denervation 207
NMDA receptors 144
No-go trials 206
Non-English speaking immigrants 127
Nongenetic factors 200
Nonlanguage skills 109
Nonverbal information 55
Nuclei
  pigmented brainstem, progressive degeneration of 200
  subthalamic 196
  thalamic 196, 198
Nucleus accumbens 196
Number facility 17

Object matching 41
Occupational problems 20
Occupational therapists 162, 256
Oculomotor loops 197
Odd's Ratios 157
Oddball paradigms 86, 87, 88, 180, 201, 202
Oedema 174
Olivopontocerebellar atrophy 195
Operational load 160
Operationalization 53, 60, 61, 79, 80
Optic nerve 67, 231
Orbitofrontal loops/circuits
  lateral 197
  medial 198
Orthopaedically injured control group 177
Output-related processes 180
Oxidative stress 200
Oxygen metabolism 227

p-paradigm 84
Paper and pencil tests 32
Paradoxical kinesis 206
Parahippocampal gyrus 230
Parietal lead 87
Parkinson's disease 29, 84, 89, 127, 234, 270
  diminished PS demonstrated in 154
  frontal-subcortical determinants of processing speed in 195–220
Pars compacta 200
PASAT (Paced Auditory Serial Addition Test) 19–20, 21, 36, 37–38, 39, 42, 57, 61–62, 63, 66–67, 69, 70, 154–155, 156, 157, 164, 177, 178
  computerized derivatives of 68
  performance issues 54, 155, 160
  relationship between performance and gray matter volume 165
  visual analogue to 158
Path analysis 230
Path coefficients 317
Path diagrams 82
Pathogenesis 200
Pathognomonic motor symptoms 195

Pathways
  central cholinergic 36
  cortical-subcortical 200
  direct/indirect 198
  dopaminergic 200
  frontal-subcortical 196
  mesocortical 200
  mesolimbic 200, 234
  multisynaptic 198
  nigrostriatal 234
  reciprocal cerebello-cortical 165
  serotonergic 200
  striatothalamocortical 196
  white matter, well-defined 233
Pattern comparison 32, 33
PCs (personal computers)
  central processing unit circuitry 110–111
  test versions 42
Pearson correlations 164
Peer review 17
Pegboard tasks 117–118, 128, 129, 136, 140, 209, 248
Perceptual-motor tasks 109
Perceptual Organization Index 14, 16, 40
Perceptual problems 67
Perceptual speed 32, 84, 109, 234
  age-related variance in tests of 235
  frequently used experimental measures of 32
Peripheral nervous system 83
Peripheral processing 245
Peripheral vision 34
Personality 34
  difficult 6
PET (positron emission tomography) 12, 228, 229, 232, 234
Phenotypic variance 80, 81
Philadelphia 135
Philosophy 2
Phonological awareness 116
Phonological information retrieval 114
Phonological loop 39, 55, 156, 268
Physical disability 162, 165
Physical identity 90
Physical maturity 111–112
Physiological processes 246
  changes 174
  features 12
Picture arrangement subtests 135
PIQ (performance intelligence quotient) 13, 35
  deficits in 155
Planning 205
PNCV (peripheral nerve conduction velocity) 83, 92
Polypharmacy 246
Posner Letter Matching task 90, 248
Postural instability 198, 199, 206, 207
Potential confounds
  age 202
  cognitive status 202

depression 202
PASAT 66, 68
WM capacity 58
PPMS (primary progressive multiple sclerosis) 153, 154, 162
Precentral gyrus 166
Prefrontal cortex 158, 199, 231
　bilateral 165
　dorsolateral 197, 198, 200, 229, 230
Premorbid ability 128
　intellectual 134–135
Probands 135, 136
Problem solving 113, 116–117, 267
Process-of-elimination 246
PSI (WAIS-III Processing Speed Index) 13–14, 14–15 21, 22, 40, 70, 90, 127, 157
　lower in patients with MS 91
　persons with MS show significant impairment on 54
　score deficits 68
PSP (progressive supranuclear palsy) 195, 198
Psychiatric groups 140
Psychiatric illness/conditions 34, 58, 126, 133, 134
Psychoeducational impairments 14
Psychological Corporation 13, 16
Psychological Review 5
Psychometric ability constructs 225
Psychometric "g" 136
Psychometric intelligence 10, 20, 21, 22
　correlations between brain volume and 12
　differences in 29
　　IT been found to correlate strongly with 35
　　moderate but consistent negative correlation with 3
　　research on information processing foundations of 34
　　shorter IT results in higher scores on tests of 11
Psychometric perspective 221–227
Psychometric science 3
Psychometric tests 11, 36
Psychometric theory 15
Psychomotor ability 245
Psychomotor retardation 207
Psychomotor speed 65–66
　assessing 32
Psychophysical speed 32
Psychosocial deficits 173
Psychosocial impairment 183
Psychostimulant effects 199
PTA (post-traumatic amnesia) 173, 174, 181
　initial, length of 183
Purdue Pegboard Test 209, 248
Pursuit Rotor 209
Putamen 230
　dopamine D2 receptor binding 235
　dopamine reduction in 200

PVSAT (Paced Visual Serial Addition Test) 54, 67
　computerized derivatives of 68

Q statistics 132
Quality of life 22, 23
　compromised 246
　decreased 20, 248
　health-related 162, 250–252
　importance of PS with regard to 30, 42, 43
　persisting cognitive deficit reduces 173

Racism 10
Radiation therapy 111
Random sampling 133
"Rate" 8
Raven's Progressive Matrices 34, 35, 36
　Advance test 64
rCBF (regional cerebral blood flow) 200, 201, 228
Reading
　cognitive skills known to predict 116
　early, in alphabetic and non-alphabetic languages 116
　impaired 118
Reading comprehension 116, 117
Reading disability
　biomarkers in 79, 89
　heritability of 91
　identifying genes for 92
Reading labels 249, 254
Reasoning 113, 205, 222
　abstract 41, 164
　fluid 40
　tests of 232
　training techniques 249, 250
Recall 114
　deficits in 63
　free 61
　problems with 195
　story 41
　see also Acquisition/recall
Recall and recognition
　long delay 59
　poor 32
Recognition paradigm 89
Recovery 183–184
　acute phase of 179
　post-acute phase of 185
　rapid 173
　residual deficits in post-acute phase of 175
Red nucleus 196
Reductionist measures 9
Reflexive antisaccades 205
Regression analyses
　linear 65, 81, 160
　multiple 161
　stepwise 248
Regression coefficients 223, 225, 226

Subject index

Rehabilitation 173
Rehearsal 55, 113, 114
   covert 56
   faster speed of 79
Relative deviation scores 33
Relative risk findings 135
Reliability 245
Remediation strategies 184
Repeated task performance 103
Resemblance 85–86
   DZ twins 81
   phenotypic 81
   relatives 80
Response-selection phase 179
Response-switching 205
Reticular formation 196
Rey Auditory Verbal Learning Test 129
Rheumatoid arthritis 62
Rigidity 209
   cogwheel-type 199
   limb 198
Road Sign Test 254
Road traffic accidents 174
RRMS (relapsing remitting multiple sclerosis) 153–155 157, 158, 161, 162, 164, 165
RT (reaction time) 2–9, 16, 17, 30, 36, 69, 89–90, 114, 202–203, 228, 249
   assessment of 41
   attempts to demonstrate association between IQ and 29
   broadly defined 33
   change associated with practice 103
   children's 108
   complex 31, 40, 183, 254
   computerized measures 41
   correlation between FA and 234
   cued 204
   declines rapidly during childhood 102
   developmental change in 107
   lexical decision 229
   lower 34
   MS participants 155
   recognition experiments 33
   simple 31, 33, 40, 54, 101, 177, 206, 209
   slower/slowed 179, 201, 205
   task-switching 205
   tasks may accentuate age differences in processing speed 245
   visual/auditory tasks 54
   youth-adult 106
   see also CRT
RUFF Figural Fluency Test 65

Safety concerns 20
SCA (spinocerebellar ataxia) 195, 198
Scalp midline 87
Scanning tasks 203, 204
SCDs (subcortical disorders) 195–220
SCFA (single common factor analysis) 137
Schizoaffective disorder 128
Schizophrenia 58–59, 70, 84, 154, 270
   diminished PS demonstrated in 154
   processing speed and DSST in 125–151
   remitted 55
Schizophrenia Research 128
Science 5
Scientific thinking 2
Sclerotic plaques 153, 164
Scottish cohort 232
SDMT (Symbol-Digit Modalities Test) 20, 38, 39, 40, 66, 129, 135, 156, 163, 183, 209, 266, 269
   significant correlation between PS and RT composites and 41
Search and substitution operations 32
Sedative effects 208
Segregating genes 81
Selective reminding procedure 62
Selective response activation 88
Self-administered training 255
Self-Ordered Pointing Task 57
Sensorimotor abilities 3
   tests of 18
Sensorimotor processing 245
Sensory functioning 31, 41
   elementary 70
Sensory processes 3
   measurement of 6
   study and clinical assessment of 8
Sensory sensitivity 5
Sensory speed 245
Sensory tests 7
Sentence comprehension 205, 206
Sequencing 142
Serial 7s test 38
Serotonin 200
Set-shifting 181, 182, 201
Sex differences 9
Shearing injuries 175, 180
Short Term Memory Search Task (Sternberg) 248
Shuffling gait 199
Shy-Drager syndrome 195
Sigmoid function 229
Simple processing speed 18–19
Simultaneity mechanism 19, 32, 176–177, 268
Simultaneous processing task 207
SKILL studies 250
Slave subsystems 54–55, 156, 160
Slave systems 175, 268, 269
SLE (systemic lupus erythematosus) 68
   impaired PASAT performance 54
   neurological dysfunction stemming from 53
Slowing of thought 208
SMST (Sternberg Memory Scanning Test) 54, 69, 90, 91, 155–156, 160, 164
Span tasks
   complex 115
   digit 63, 70, 85
   spatial 114

Spatial processing 41
Spearman rank correlations 165
SPECT (single photon emission computed tomography) 201, 207, 208
Speech-based information 55
Speech impairment 38
Speech output 204
Speech rate change 114
Speed-accuracy trade-off 22, 67, 89, 177–178, 185, 205, 269, 270
Spillover effect 245
SPMS (secondary progressive multiple sclerosis) 153–155 157, 158, 161, 163, 165
Spontaneous recovery 184
Spot pattern test 7
Stability indices 108
Standard deviations 128, 134
    pooled 131
STE (subjective time estimation) 64–65
Stimuli 42, 114
    abnormalities in processing of 142
    auditory 32, 33, 222
    briefest target duration needed to achieve specified accuracy rate 34
    chunking 68
    complex 244
    correct discrimination between, time taken to make 80
    differences in RT between 34
    distractor 89
    duration of exposure to 7
    elementary 11
    encoding 179
    equiprobable 211
    evaluation processes 180
    exposure duration 34
    external 244
    identification and selection of 179
    inconsistent 203
    internal 244
    motivational aspects of 87
    obvious, accurate perceptual discrimination on 83
    relevant to the task at hand 86
    reorganization between rehearsals of 126
    simple RT measures require persistent attention to 37
    simple 244
    task that assesses ability to alternate between sets of 39
    time needed to fully evaluate and classify 86
    time taken to react to 10
    visuospatial 55
    see also Stimulus and response; Target stimuli; Visual stimuli
Stimulus and response 11, 69, 89, 177, 199, 202
    amount of time between 33
    cognitive delays in linking 203
    neuronal electrophysiological 201
    simple or complex 34
    stored in long-term memory 103
    structural equation models limit the influence of confounds 70
    tasks involving a variety/range of modalities 142, 144
    time it takes to press a button in 80
STM (short-term memory) 102, 164
    assessed with simple span tasks 115
    influence of processing speed on 115
    manipulation of information held in 39
    nonmotoric, speed of 204
    speed of access to 90
    time required to retrieve a single item from 90
    verbal span 56
Stooped posture 199
Storage and retrieval 62, 244
Story memory 60
Strategic planning 68
Stress 38
Striatal dopamine 199
    contralateral 200
Striatum 196, 198, 208
    defective interactions between frontal cortex and 144
    mediodorsal 199
    synaptic connection to internal globus pallidus 198
Stroke 195
Stroop Color-Word Test 38–39, 54, 59, 127, 128, 136, 141, 182, 183
    abnormalities in processing of stimuli 14
    interference condition 142, 180
Stroop reading task 183
Structural equation models 70, 81, 83, 137
    mathematically complete description of 82
Structural load 160
Substantia nigra 196, 200, 234
Subtraction 33, 38, 116, 117
Susceptibility genes 200
Symbol decoding 211
Symbol-number matching task 41
Symbol recognition tasks 33
Symbol Search subtest (WAIS-III) 14, 17, 21, 22, 40, 54, 90, 91, 127
Symbols 222
    target 14, 91
Sympathetic ganglia 200
Symptomatology 125, 126
    depressive 161, 162
Synaptic activity 84

Target stimuli 34, 89
    low probability 86
Task switching 205
TBI (traumatic brain injury), 20, 22, 29, 40, 61–62, 68, 127, 195, 256, 269
    impaired PASAT performance 54

most commonly reported and significant
    cognitive impairments in 21
  neurological dysfunction stemming from 53
  processing speed and 154, 173–194
TCST (Timed Card Sorting Task) 209–211
Temporal information processing 199
Temporoparietal association areas 200
Test of Everyday Attention 66
Test-retest reliability 128
Thalamo-cortical feedback loops 85
Thalamus
  subcortical lesions in 199
  tonic inhibitory influence on 198
Theory-driven assessments 16
Thyroid stimulating hormone, *see* TSH
TIADL (Timed Instrumental Activities of
    Daily Living) 250, 254, 255
Tics 198
Time 53, 143
Time-pressure demands 183–184
Time-pressure management 184–185
  training in 187
Timing sequences 199
TLV (total brain lesion volume) 68, 164
  semiautomated methods to quantify 165
TMT (Trail Making Test) 20, 37, 38, 59, 126,
    141, 182
  oral version 39
  Test-A 39, 209, 226, 248
  Test-B 39, 183, 209
  Trails A 128, 135, 141, 142
  Trails B 65, 66, 128, 134, 135, 141, 142, 245
  variables 136
  variants 225
TOL (Tower of London) 66
Topographic mapping 196
Tourette's syndrome 195, 198
Training tasks 249
Traits 80, 81, 82
  high heritability of 86
  shared 92
Trauma 173
  see also TBI
Tremor 209
  negative correlation between cognitive
    decline and 206
  predominant 207
  resting 199
TSH (thyroid stimulating hormone) 60
Twin studies 86, 91
  see also DZ; MZ
Two Choice Visual Reaction Time Task 248
Two-Goal Tapping 209

UAB (University of Alabama) Training 250
UFOV (Useful Field of Vision) test, 41–42,
    43, 264–265
  Useful Field of View 41, 186, 248, 252, 258
Unaffected relatives 135, 136
Unconsciousness 173

Undergraduate students 64
United States 116
Univariate models 82
University of Pennsylvania 5
Untimed tasks 9

Validity 245
  convergent 222, 226
  discriminant 53, 222, 226
  see also Construct validity
variables 17, 29, 128–129, 132, 137, 145, 208,
    209
  attention 136
  behavioral 221
  cognitive 10, 222, 232, 247
  confounding 36, 43
  decisions about the meaning of 222
  demographic 30, 167
  dependent 58, 69, 70, 221, 223
  DSST 136
  fluency 226
  independent 58
  indicator 226
  latent 70, 81
  matching time 140
  measured 82
  memory 59, 70
  mental 3
  multidimensional 23
  multiple indicator 223, 224
  neurobiological 227, 234–236
  neuropsychological 130, 131
  observed 223
  one-to-one correspondence between
    223
  physical disability 30
  reading time 226
  RT 34, 226
  search 14
  sociodemographic 176
  Stroop Neutral 226
  substitution 224
  target 226
  TMT 136, 226
  unmeasured 82
  verbal list-learning 133
  WCST 136, 141
  WM 140
  writing time 140
Vascular functioning 145
Vascular pathology 228
Vehicle crash risk 186
Ventral mesencephalon 234
Ventral tegmentum 200
Verbal abilities 18, 30, 42, 128
  intact 20
Verbal Comprehension Index 14, 16
Verbal fluency 39, 128, 136, 164, 201
  HVA levels, IP speed and 207
  problems with 195

Verbal information 62
　acquisition of 63
　processing 55
　unstructured 63
Verbal learning 161
　deficits in 162
　impaired in CFS 62
　indices of 164
　processing speed as a mediator of 59
Verbal memory 60, 143, 183
　deficits 135
　episodic 61
　impairments in 165
　selective deficit in performance 125
　short-term span 56
Verbal output 39
Verbal response 40
Verbal retrieval 59
Verbal spatial span 114–115
Verbal tasks 109
Verbalization 245
Videotapes 255
VIQ (verbal intelligence quotient) 13, 35, 155, 209
Viral encephalitis 199
Virtual reality technology 186
Visceral functions 198
Visual Attention Analyzer 42
Visual Awareness, Inc. 248, 249
Visual discrimination 7, 90
　duration of exposure to a stimulus necessary to make 10–11
Visual Elevator subtest 66
Visual expectancy paradigm 107
Visual functioning 33, 41
Visual identification tasks 249
Visual impairment 67
Visual information
　acquisition of 63
　processing speed 248
Visual Matching subtest 15, 107, 108, 115
　numeric component to 17
Visual Memory 16, 18, 60, 137
　executive 134
　processing speed as a mediator of 59
Visual-motor coordination 91
Visual-motor scanning speed 38
Visual nervous system 244
Visual perception 35, 67, 91
Visual processing 35, 40
　impaired, among MS patients 67
　relationship between IT and 35
Visual reaction time tasks 54
Visual Reproduction 128
Visual scanning 39, 142
Visual skills 116
Visual tasks 35
Visual-spatial skills/abilities 30, 40, 201
Visual-spatial tasks 109

Visual stimuli 32, 33, 54, 61, 204, 222
　distracting 42
Visuoconstruction 183
Visuospatial ability 195
　perception 67
Visuospatial processing 164
Visuospatial sketchpad 55, 114, 156, 268
Visuospatial skills 42, 247, 248
Vocabulary 13, 20, 128, 135, 137, 224, 226
Vocational outcomes study 142
Voxel-based morphometry 165
VT-SAT (Visual Threshold Serial Addition Test) 42, 57, 63, 68, 69, 158, 159, 161

WAIS (Wechsler Adult Intelligence Scale) 155, 222
　changes carried out in revisions of 13–14
　digit symbol task 61
　Full Scale IQ 127, 181
　PASAT scores significantly correlated with all subtests 20
　picture arrangement subtest 206
　PIQ of 35
　six-factor model for 16
　subtests for speed added to 16
　see also Digit Symbol-Coding subtest; DSST; LNS; PSI; WMI
WCST (Wisconsin Card Sorting Test) 39, 128, 136, 206
　Categories 134, 141
　Perseverative Errors 141
Wechsler tests 2, 135
　see also WAIS; WISC; WPPSI-III
White matter 153, 165
　integrity 144, 231–234
　observable shearing and disruption of 180
　parietal 111
　pathology 154
　subcortical 175, 198
　volume declines as a function of increasing adult age 230
　well-defined pathways 233
Whole-task training 250
Williams syndrome 84
Wilson's disease 195
WISC (Wechsler Intelligence Scale for Children) 13
　factor analytic studies 14
　Processing Speed Index 14, 15
　speed subtests added to 16
　see also Coding subtest; Symbol Search subtest
WM (working memory) 16, 18, 30, 33, 54–57, 58, 70, 116, 128, 129, 135, 154, 157, 160
　age-related changes and 113, 114
　bad performers 85
　Baddeley's model 268, 269, 270
　central executive of 175
　deficit 141, 156, 161, 181
　development of 31

executive control 36
frontal-temporal changes to 200
functions 40
higher intelligence and 64, 65
higher-order, mesolimbocortical dopamine influence on 199
holding constant 42
impaired performance on PASAT can result from deficits in 38
impairments in 65, 143, 175
increasing the difficulty level of a task 158
index of 164
lower 269–270
maintenance of larger amount of information in 79
mediation of episodic memory deficits in MS 63
minimal 39
multiple component model of 54
potential confound of 58
PS and 54, 60, 113–115, 156–161, 268–270
rehabilitation of 31
relative role versus PS in MS 157
slowed processing of information in 204
STM often considered a subcomponent of 115
systemic changes in 117
tests that target 37
theoretical formulations of 265
visual test 141
see also Executive attention; WM-PS
WMH (white matter hyperintensity) 232–233
WMI (WAIS-III Working Memory Index) 14, 40, 157, 181
non-deficient scores on 68
WM-PS (working memory-processing speed) model 268, 270
WMS (Wechsler Memory Scale)
Technical Manual 127
Word Lists 129
see also Logical memory subtest
Woodcock-Johnson Tests
Cognitive Abilities 15, 17, 222
Decision Speed 15
Diagnostic Supplement 16
Psycho-Educational Battery 107
Word decoding 116, 118
Word frequency 229
Word reading 54, 142
World War I army recruits 127
WPPSI-III (Wechsler Preschool and Primary Scale of Intelligence Third Edition) 16
WRAT Reading 128, 129

Z-scores 255